Law & Ethics
For Health Professions
SEVENTH EDITION

Karen Judson, BS

Carlene Harrison, EdD, CMA (AAMA)
Hodges University

LAW & ETHICS FOR HEALTH PROFESSIONS, SEVENTH EDITION

Published by McGraw-Hill Education, 2 Penn Plaza, New York, NY 10121. Copyright © 2016 by McGraw-Hill Education. All rights reserved. Printed in the United States of America. Previous editions © 2013, 2010, and 2006. No part of this publication may be reproduced or distributed in any form or by any means, or stored in a database or retrieval system, without the prior written consent of McGraw-Hill Education, including, but not limited to, in any network or other electronic storage or transmission, or broadcast for distance learning.

Some ancillaries, including electronic and print components, may not be available to customers outside the United States.

This book is printed on acid-free paper.
1 2 3 4 5 6 7 8 9 0 RMN/RMN 1 0 9 8 7 6 5

ISBN 978–0–07–351383–6
MHID 0–07–351383–0

Senior Vice President, Products & Markets: *Kurt L. Strand*
Vice President, General Manager, Products & Markets: *Marty Lange*
Vice President, Content Design & Delivery: *Kimberly Meriwether David*
Director: *Chad Grall*
Brand Manager: *William Mulford*
Director, Product Development: *Rose Koos*
Product Developer: *Yvonne Lloyd*
Senior Product Developer: *Michelle L. Flomenhoft*
Executive Marketing Manager: *Roxan Kinsey*
Digital Product Analyst: *Katherine Ward*
Director, Content Design & Delivery: *Linda Avenarius*
Program Manager: *Angela R. FitzPatrick*
Content Project Managers: *Vicki Krug/Sherry L. Kane*
Buyer: *Susan K. Culbertson*
Senior Designer: *Srdjan Savanovic*
Content Licensing Specialists: *Carrie Burger/Ann Marie Jannette*
Cover Image: *Metal button border: ©Ingram Publishing; Middle button: -VICTOR-, iStock Vectors/Getty images; Doctor with hand on child patient's forehead: ©Creatas/PunchStock; CD and caduceus: ©Thinkstock/ Jupiterimages; DNA: ©Andrey Prokhorov/Getty Images; X-rays on tablet: ©Hero Images/Corbis; Background (Electrocardiogram): ©Getty Images/Steve Allen*
Compositor: *Laserwords Private Limited*
Printer: *R. R. Donnelley*

All credits appearing on page or at the end of the book are considered to be an extension of the copyright page.

Library of Congress Cataloging-in-Publication Data

Judson, Karen, 1941- author.
    Law & ethics for the health professions/Karen Judson, Carlene Harrison.—
Seventh edition.
        p. ; cm.
    Law and ethics for the health professions
    Includes bibliographical references and indexes.
    ISBN 978-0-07-351383-6 (alk. paper)—ISBN 0-07-351383-0 (alk. paper)
    I. Harrison, Carlene, author. II. Title. III. Title: Law and ethics for the
health professions.
    [DNLM: 1. Legislation, Medical–United States.   2. Ethics, Medical—United
States. 3. Health Personnel—United States.   W 32.5 AA1]
    R725.5
    174.2—dc23
                                                                        2014018372

The Internet addresses listed in the text were accurate at the time of publication. The inclusion of a website does not indicate an endorsement by the authors or McGraw-Hill Education, and McGraw-Hill Education does not guarantee the accuracy of the information presented at these sites.

www.mhhe.com

Brief Contents

Contents

Chapter 6

Defenses to Liability Suits 150

Chapter 7

Medical Records and Informed Consent 175

Chapter 8

Privacy, Security, and Fraud 204

PART THREE PROFESSIONAL, TRANSITIONAL, AND SOCIETAL HEALTH CARE ISSUES 233

Chapter 9
Physicians' Public Duties and Responsibilities 234

Chapter 10
Workplace Legalities 265

Chapter 13
Health Care Trends and Forecasts 356

About the Authors

Karen Judson, BS

Karen Judson taught biology laboratories at Black Hills University in Spearfish, South Dakota; high school sciences in Idaho; and grades one and three in Washington state. She is also a former laboratory and X-ray technician and completed two years of nurse's training while completing a degree in biology.

Judson has worked as a science writer since 1983. She has written relationship, family, and psychology articles for a variety of magazines, including a series of high school classroom magazines, making a total of 500 articles published. Judson writes science and relationship books for teenagers (Enslow and Marshall Cavendish publishers). Her book for teens, *Sports & Money: It's a Sell Out,* made the New York City Public Library's list of best books for teens in 1995. Her book for teens, *Genetic Engineering,* was chosen by the National Science Teachers' Association as one of the best science books for children in 2001 and was featured on the NSTA Web site.

Carlene Harrison, EdD, CMA (AAMA)

Carlene Harrison is Dean of the School of Allied Health at Hodges University and is also Program Director for the Master of Health Services Administration and Graduate Certificate in Health Informatics. She has been a member of the faculty at Hodges University since 1992, but came on board full time in 2000, serving first as Chair of the Medical Assisting Program. As Dean of the School of Allied Health, she has overall responsibility for the following degree programs: Health Services Administration, Biomedical Sciences, Medical Assisting, Health Information Management, and Physical Therapist Assistant. Her doctorate is from Argosy University. Her dissertation research looked at improvement in critical thinking in adult learners.

Before becoming a full-time educator, Dr. Harrison worked for over 20 years in the health care field as an administrator. Employed mostly in the outpatient setting, she has worked in the for-profit, not-for-profit, and public health sectors.

Have feedback or questions for the authors? Use email address judsonlawethics@gmail.com to reach them!

Preface

Law and Ethics for Health Professions explains how to navigate the numerous legal and ethical issues that health care professionals face every day. Topics are based upon real-world scenarios and dilemmas from a variety of health care practitioners. Through the presentation of Learning Outcomes, Key Terms, From the Perspective of, Ethics Issues, Chapter Reviews, Case Studies, Internet Activities, Court Cases, and Videos, students learn about current legal and ethical problems and situations. In the seventh edition, Chapters 3 and 8 have been substantially revised to reflect changes in today's health care world. As students progress through the text, they will get the opportunity to use critical thinking skills to learn how to resolve real-life situations and theoretical scenarios and to decide how legal and ethical issues are relevant to the health care profession in which they will practice.

Law & Ethics is also available with McGraw-Hill Education's revolutionary adaptive learning technology, McGraw-Hill LearnSmart® and now SmartBook®! You can study smarter, spending your valuable time on topics you don't know and less time on the topics you have already mastered. Succeed with LearnSmart . . . Join the learning revolution and achieve the success you deserve today!

New to the Seventh Edition

A number of updates have been made in the seventh edition to enrich the user's experience with the product:

- Chapter 3, "Working in Health Care," has been extensively updated to reflect the changing configuration of health care management and the impact of telemedicine and social media on all facets of health care.

- Chapter 8, "Privacy, Security, and Fraud," moves beyond the details of the Health Insurance Portability and Accountability Act (HIPAA) to include the recently enacted Patient Protection and Affordable Care Act (usually abbreviated as ACA). The chapter also reveals the tremendous impact of health care fraud and abuse on health care costs.

- Chapter 13, "Health Care Trends and Forecasts," has been updated to evaluate the current status of health care in the United States and to inform students of today's trends in health care.

- All statistics and court cases have been updated, as well as content relevant to laws passed since the sixth edition.

- New case studies have been added. As in previous editions, the authors made an effort to include a variety of allied health professions in case studies and in other examples throughout the text.

- The interior design and layout have been refreshed to make it easier for students to navigate through the content.

- *McGraw-Hill Connect® Law & Ethics* has been updated to reflect updates in the chapters and feedback from customers. Additional Case Studies are included in Connect, as well as Video Case Scenarios, to allow students to apply important skills learned from the text. Both the Case Studies and the Video Cases include related questions with immediate feedback for the students.

- *Law & Ethics* is now available with the LearnSmart Advantage, a series of adaptive learning products fueled by both LearnSmart and SmartBook.

For a detailed transition guide between the sixth and seventh editions of *Law & Ethics,* visit the Instructor Resources in *Connect!*

To the Student

As you study to become a health care provider, you have undoubtedly realized that patients are more than the sum of their medical problems. In fact, they are people with loved ones, professions, worries, hobbies, and daily routines that are probably much like your own. However, because patients' lives and well-being are at stake as they seek and receive health care, in addition to seeing each patient as an individual, you must carefully consider the complex legal, moral, and ethical issues that will arise as you practice your profession. And you must learn to resolve such issues in an acceptable manner.

Law & Ethics provides an overview of the laws and ethics you should know to help you give competent, compassionate care to patients that is also within acceptable legal and ethical boundaries. The text can also serve as a guide to help you resolve the many legal and ethical questions you may reasonably expect to face as a student and, later, as a health care provider.

To derive maximum benefit from *Law & Ethics*:

- Review the Learning Outcomes and Key Terms at the beginning of each chapter for an overview of the material included in the chapter.

- Complete all Check Your Progress questions as they appear in the chapter and correct any incorrect answers.

- Review the legal cases to see how they apply to topics in the text, and try to determine why the court ruled as it did.

- Study the Ethics Issues at the end of each chapter, and answer the discussion questions.

- Complete the Review questions at the end of the chapter, correct any incorrect answers, and review the material again.

- Review the Case Studies and use your critical thinking skills to answer the questions.

- Complete the Internet Activities at the end of the chapter to become familiar with online resources and to see what additional information you can find about selected topics.

- Complete the *Connect* assignments from your instructor, including any LearnSmart or SmartBook modules assigned, as well as additional Case Studies and Video Case Scenarios.

- Study each chapter until you can answer correctly questions posed by the Learning Outcomes, Check Your Progress, and Review questions.

Law & Ethics Preparation in the Digital World: Supplementary Materials for the Instructor and Student

McGraw-Hill Education knows how much effort it takes for instructors to prepare for a new course. Through focus groups, symposia, reviews, and conversations with instructors like you, we have gathered information about what materials you need in order to facilitate successful courses. We are committed to providing you with high-quality, accurate instructor support. Knowing the importance of flexibility and digital learning, McGraw-Hill Education has created multiple assets to enhance the learning experience no matter what the class format: traditional, online, or hybrid. This product is designed to help instructors and students be successful, with digital solutions proven to drive student success.

connect®

A ONE-STOP SPOT TO PRESENT, DELIVER, AND ASSESS DIGITAL ASSETS AVAILABLE FROM MCGRAW-HILL: MCGRAW-HILL *CONNECT* LAW & ETHICS

McGraw-Hill *Connect*® **Law & Ethics** provides online presentation, assignment, and assessment solutions. It connects your students with the tools and resources they'll need to achieve success. With *Connect*, you can deliver assignments, quizzes, and tests online. A robust set of questions and activities, including all of the Check Your Progress and End-of-Chapter Questions, additional Case Studies, Video Case Scenarios, and interactives are presented and aligned with the textbook's learning outcomes. As an instructor, you can edit existing questions and author entirely new problems. *Connect* enables you to track individual student performance—by question, by assignment, or in relation to the class overall—with detailed grade reports. You can integrate grade reports easily with learning management systems (LMSs), such as Blackboard, Desire2Learn, and eCollege, plus much more. *Connect* **Law & Ethics** also provides students with 24/7 online access to an ebook. This media-rich version of the textbook is available through the McGraw-Hill *Connect* platform and allows seamless integration of text, media, and assessments. To learn more, visit **http://connect.mheducation.com.**

Connect Insight™ is the first and only analytics tool of its kind, which highlights a series of visual data displays—each framed by an intuitive question—to provide at-a-glance information regarding how your class is doing. As an instructor or administrator, you receive an instant, at-a-glance view of student performance matched with student activity. It puts real-time analytics in your hands so you can take action early and keep struggling students from falling behind. It also allows you to be empowered with a more valuable, transparent, and productive connection between you and your students. Available on demand wherever and whenever it's needed, Connect Insight travels from office to classroom!

A SINGLE SIGN-ON WITH CONNECT AND YOUR BLACKBOARD COURSE: MCGRAW-HILL EDUCATION AND BLACKBOARD

Blackboard, the Web-based course management system, has partnered with McGraw-Hill Education to better allow students and faculty to use online materials and activities to complement face-to-face teaching. Blackboard features exciting social learning and teaching tools that foster active learning opportunities for students. You'll transform your closed-door classroom into communities where students remain connected to their educational experience 24 hours a day. This partnership allows you and your students access to McGraw-Hill's *Connect* and *Create* right from within your Blackboard course—all with a single sign-on. Not only do you get single sign-on with *Connect* and *Create,* but you also get deep integration of McGraw-Hill Education content and content engines right in Blackboard. Whether you're choosing a book for your course or building *Connect* assignments, all the tools you need are right where you want them—inside Blackboard. Gradebooks are now seamless. When a student completes an integrated *Connect* assignment, the grade for that assignment automatically (and instantly) feeds into your Blackboard grade center.

McGraw-Hill Education and Blackboard can now offer you easy access to industry-leading technology and content, whether your campus hosts it or we do. Be sure to ask your local McGraw-Hill Education representative for details.

Still want a single sign-on solution using another learning management system? See how **McGraw-Hill Campus** (**http://mhcampus.mhhe.com/**) makes the grade by offering universal sign-on, automatic registration, gradebook synchronization and open access to a multitude of learning resources—all in one place. MH Campus supports Active Directory, Angel, Blackboard, Canvas, Desire2Learn, eCollege, IMS, LDAP, Moodle, Moodlerooms, Sakai, Shibboleth, WebCT, BrainHoney, Campus Cruiser, and Jenzibar eRacer. Additionally, MH Campus can be easily connected with other authentication authorities and LMSs.

CREATE A TEXTBOOK ORGANIZED THE WAY YOU TEACH: MCGRAW-HILL CREATE

With **McGraw-Hill** *Create,* you can easily rearrange chapters, combine material from other content sources, and quickly upload content you have written, such as your course syllabus or teaching notes. Find the content you need in *Create* by searching through thousands of leading McGraw-Hill Education textbooks. Arrange your book to fit your teaching style. *Create* even allows you to personalize your book's appearance by selecting the cover and adding your name, school, and course information. Order a *Create* book and you'll receive a complimentary print review copy in three to five business days or a complimentary electronic review copy (eComp) via e-mail in minutes. Go to **www.mcgrawhillcreate.com** today and register to experience how McGraw-Hill *Create* empowers you to teach *your* students *your* way.

RECORD AND DISTRIBUTE YOUR LECTURES FOR MULTIPLE VIEWING: MY LECTURES—TEGRITY

McGraw-Hill Tegrity records and distributes your class lecture with just a click of a button. Students can view it anytime and anywhere via computer, iPod, or mobile device. It indexes as it records your PowerPoint presentations and anything shown on your computer, so students can use keywords to find exactly what they want to study. Tegrity is available as an integrated feature of **McGraw-Hill *Connect* Law & Ethics** and as a stand-alone product.

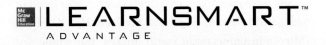

MCGRAW-HILL'S ADAPTIVE SUITE

New from McGraw-Hill Education, LearnSmart Advantage is a series of adaptive learning products fueled by LearnSmart. Since 2009, it has been the most widely used and intelligent adaptive learning resource proven to improve learning. Developed to deliver demonstrable results in boosting grades, increasing course retention, and strengthening memory recall, the LearnSmart Advantage series spans the entire learning process from course preparation to providing the first adaptive reading experience, and it's found only in SmartBook. Distinguishing what students know from what they don't, and honing in on concepts they are most likely to forget, each product in the series helps students study smarter and retain more knowledge. A smarter learning experience for students coupled with valuable reporting tools for instructors, and available in hundreds of course areas, LearnSmart Advantage is advancing learning like no other products in higher education today. **Go to www.LearnSmartAdvantage .com** for more information.

LEARNSMART®

LearnSmart is one of the most effective and successful adaptive learning resources available on the market today and is again available for *Law & Ethics*. More than 2 million students have answered more than 1.3 billion questions in LearnSmart since 2009, making it the most widely used and intelligent adaptive study tool. It has proven to strengthen memory recall, keep students in class, and boost grades. Students using LearnSmart are 13 percent more likely to pass their classes and 35 percent less likely to drop out. This revolutionary learning resource is available only from McGraw-Hill Education, so join the learning revolution, and start using LearnSmart today!

SMARTBOOK™

SmartBook is the first and only adaptive reading experience currently available. SmartBook personalizes content for each student in a continuously adapting reading experience. Reading is no longer a passive and linear experience, but an engaging and dynamic one where students are more likely to master and retain important concepts, thus coming to class better prepared. Valuable reports provide instructors with insight into how students are progressing through textbook content, and are useful for shaping in-class time and assessments. As a result of the adaptive reading experience found in SmartBook, students are more likely to retain knowledge, stay in class, and get better grades. This revolutionary technology is available only from McGraw-Hill Education for hundreds of course areas as part of the LearnSmart Advantage series.

Instructor Resources

You can rely on the following materials to help you and your students work through the material in this book. All of the resources in the following table are available in the Instructor Resources under the Library tab in *Connect*.

Need help? Contact McGraw-Hill Education's Customer Experience Group (CXG). Visit the CXG Web site at **www.mhhe.com/support**. Browse our FAQs (frequently asked questions) and product documentation and/or contact a CXG representative. CXG is available Sunday through Friday.

Want to learn more about this product? Attend one of our online webinars. To learn more about the webinars, please contact your McGraw-Hill sales representative. To find your McGraw-Hill representative, go to **www .mhhe.com and click "Find My Sales Rep."**

Supplement	Features
Instructor's Manual	Each chapter includes: • Learning Outcomes • Overview of PowerPoint Presentations • Teaching Points • Answer Keys for Check Your Progress and End-of-Chapter Questions
PowerPoint Presentations	• Key Concepts • References to Learning Outcomes
Electronic Test Bank	• EZ Test Online (computerized) • Word version • These questions are also available through Connect. • Questions are tagged with learning outcomes, level of difficulty, level of Bloom's taxonomy, feedback, topic, and the accrediting standards of ABHES and CAAHEP where appropriate.
Tools to Plan Course	• Transition Guide, by chapter, from *Law & Ethics*, 6e to 7e. • Correlations by learning outcomes to ABHES, CAAHEP, and more • Sample syllabi • Asset Map—a recap of the key instructor resources, as well as information on the content available through *Connect*

BEST-IN-CLASS DIGITAL SUPPORT

Based on feedback from our users, McGraw-Hill Education has developed Digital Success Programs that will provide you and your students with the help you need, when you need it.

• *Training for Instructors:* Get ready to drive classroom results with our Digital Success Team—which is ready to provide in-person, remote, or on-demand training as needed.

• *Peer Support and Training:* No one understands your needs like your peers. Get easy access to knowledgeable digital users by joining our Connect Community, or speak directly with one of our Digital Faculty Consultants, who are instructors using McGraw-Hill Education digital products.

• *Online Training Tools:* Get immediate anytime, anywhere access to modular tutorials on key features through our Connect Success Academy.

Get started today. Learn more about McGraw-Hill Education's Digital Success Programs by contacting your local sales representative or visiting **http://connect.customer.mheducation.com/start.**

Guided Tour

Chapter Openers

The **chapter opener** sets the stage for what will be learned in the chapter. **Key terms** are first introduced in the chapter opener so the student can see them all in one place; they are defined in the margins throughout the chapter for easy review, as well as in the glossary. **Learning Outcomes** are written to reflect the revised version of Bloom's Taxonomy, and to establish the key points the student should focus on in the chapter. In addition, major chapter heads are structured to reflect the Learning Outcomes and the Learning Outcomes are repeated next to these heads for easy reference. **From the Perspective of . . .** boxes illustrate real-life experiences related to the text. Each quotes health care providers as they encounter problems or situations relevant to the material about to be presented in the chapter.

1

Introduction to Law and Ethics

Key Terms

American Medical
  Association
  Principles
bioethicists
bioethics
code of ethics
common sense
compassion
courtesy
critical thinking
defendant
ethics
ethics committees
ethics guidelines
etiquette
fraud
health care
  practitioners
Hippocratic oath
law
liable
litigious
medical ethicists
moral values
plaintiff
precedent
protocol
summary judgment

LEARNING OUTCOMES

After studying this chapter, you should be able to:

LO 1.1 Explain why knowledge of law and ethics is important to health care practitioners.

LO 1.2 Distinguish among law, ethics, bioethics, etiquette, and protocol.

LO 1.3 Define *moral values* and explain how they relate to law, ethics, and etiquette.

LO 1.4 Discuss the characteristics and skills most likely to lead to a successful career in one of the health care professions.

FROM THE PERSPECTIVE OF. . .

BARBARA, AN EXPERIENCED CERTIFIED MEDICAL ASSISTANT (CMA) (AAMA) in a medical office with a walk-in clinic, instructs new employees in the reception area of the office to follow the medical office procedures whenever possible and prudent, but, above all, to use common sense in dealing with patients.

Barbara told Elaine, a new receptionist in the medical office, to politely ask walk-in patients why they needed to see a doctor. Elaine had been on the job for two weeks when an elderly man who was hard of hearing approached her, and she dutifully asked him the purpose for his visit. He was obviously too embarrassed to reply, but Elaine persisted, finally raising her voice. When the man shouted "I can't pee," all heads in the busy waiting room turned toward Elaine and the patient. A red-faced Elaine turned to arrange for the man to see a physician, but he quickly left the building. Barbara criticized Elaine's patient-handling technique, but the crux of the matter was that the patient left without seeing a doctor for his medical problem.

"Patients' needs always trump office routine," Barbara emphasizes. "If we somehow hurt or hinder a patient while doggedly sticking to a set routine, we may have risked legal liability, but more important, we haven't done our job."

From Barbara's perspective as the person responsible for training medical office personnel, Elaine failed to use common sense in communicating with a patient, and as a result, the man did not receive the medical treatment he needed.

From Elaine's perspective, she followed Barbara's instructions to the letter, and she failed to understand why Barbara had criticized her. She hadn't meant to embarrass the man, so was it her fault that he left without making an appointment?

From the patient's perspective as an elderly gentleman who seldom discussed personal matters, the young woman who was his first contact in the medical office embarrassed him, and he left rather than face further humiliation.

As you progress through *Law & Ethics for the Health Professions*, try to interpret the court cases, laws, case studies, and other examples or situations cited from the perspectives of everyone involved.

Why Study Law and Ethics?

There are two important reasons for you to study law and ethics:

- To help you function at the highest possible professional level, providing competent, compassionate health care to patients.
- To help you avoid legal entanglements that can threaten your ability to earn a living as a successful **health care practitioner.**

We live in a **litigious** society, where patients, relatives, and others are inclined to sue health care practitioners, health care facilities, manufacturers of medical equipment and products, and others when

LO 1.1
Explain why knowledge of law and ethics is important to health care practitioners.

health care practitioners
Those who are trained to administer medical or health care to patients.

litigious
Prone to engage in lawsuits.

Chapter 1 | Introduction to Law and Ethics   **3**

Court Cases

COURT CASE   911 Operators Sued

In 2006, just before 6 PM, a five-year-old boy called 911. He told the 911 operator that his "mom has passed out." When the operator asked to speak to the boy's mother, he said, "She's not gonna talk." The operator scolded the boy and logged the call as a child's prank. Three hours later the boy called 911 again. A different operator answered, and she also scolded the boy for playing a prank, but she did send a police officer to the boy's home. The officer discovered the boy's mother lying unresponsive on the floor and summoned emergency medical services. The EMS workers arrived 20 minutes later, and determined that the woman was dead, and had probably died within the past two hours.

The boy's older sister sued the two 911 operators on behalf of the dead woman's estate and on behalf of her son. The lawsuit alleged gross negligence causing a death and intentional infliction of emotional distress.

The 911 operators argued that they were entitled to government immunity, that they owed no duty to provide assistance to the woman who died, and that their failure to summon medical aid was not gross negligence.

A trial court and an appeals court found for the plaintiff, and the case was appealed to the Michigan Supreme Court, where in January 2012, the court denied further appeals.

Estate of Turner v. Nichols, 807 N.W.2d 164, 490 Mich. 988 (2012).

Several **court cases** are presented in every chapter. Each summarizes a lawsuit that illustrates points made in the text and are meant to encourage students to consider the subject's relevance to their health care specialty. The legal citations at the end of each case indicate where to find the complete text for that case. "Landmark" cases are those that established an ongoing precedent.

Check Your Progress Questions

These questions appear at various points in the chapters to allow students to test their comprehension of the material they just read. These questions can also be answered in *Connect*.

Check Your Progress

1. Name two important reasons for studying law and ethics.
2. Which state laws apply specifically to the practice of medicine?
3. What purpose do laws serve?
4. How is the enforcement of laws made possible?
5. What factors influence the formation of one's personal set of ethics and values?
6. Define the term *moral values*.
7. Explain how one's moral values affect one's sense of ethics.

Chapter Summary

Learning Outcome	Summary
LO 2.1 Describe and compare need and value development theories.	What classic need development theory is discussed in this chapter? • Abraham Maslow, in *Motivation and Personality* first published in 1954, identified a hierarchy of needs that motivates our actions: Deficiency or D-needs: 1. Need for basic life—food and shelter. 2. Need for a safe and secure environment. 3. Need to belong and to be loved. Being or B-needs: 4. Need for esteem, where status, responsibility, and recognition are important. 5. Need for self-actualization, for personal growth and fulfillment.

Ethics Issues   Making Ethical Decisions

Ethics ISSUE 1:

Joyce Weathers is a 62-year-old patient with emphysema. Mrs. Weathers is a grandmother who has smoked a pack of cigarettes a day for over 40 years. She enjoys smoking and does not want to quit. Her physician has become somewhat insistent that Mrs. Weathers quit. She tries, but each time she becomes nasty and irritable around her family. She lives with her daughter and two young grandchildren. The family members want her to quit, but it becomes very unpleasant at home when Mrs. Weathers tries to quit.

Discussion Questions

1. Using act-utilitarianism as a model, create a pain-avoided, pleasure-gained list to determine if Mrs. Weathers should continue smoking.

2. If your decision is that she should quit smoking, how can Mrs. Weathers's family help her?

Chapter 2 Review

Enhance your learning by completing these exercises and more at http://connect.mheducation.com!

Applying Knowledge

LO 2.1

1. What is another term for your personal concept of right and wrong?
   a. Utilitarianism

Case Studies

Use your critical thinking skills to answer the questions that follow each case study.

LO 2.3
Susan is a nursing student, arguing with her friend Linda, also a nursing student, over the benefits of getting a flu shot.

Internet Activities LO 2.3

Complete the activities and answer the questions that follow.

26. Locate the Web site for the organization representing the profession you plan to practice. Check the organization's code of ethics. Does the code conform to the seven principles of health care ethics? Explain your answer.

Resources

Edge, R., and J. Groves. *Ethics of Health Care: A Guide for Clinical Practice*. 3rd ed. New York: Thomson Delmar Learning, 2006.

Kohlberg, L. *The psychology of Moral Development: Essays on Moral Development*. Vol. 2. San Francisco: Harper and Row, 1984.

Kohlberg, L., and R. A. Ryncarz. "Beyond Justice Reasoning: Moral Development and Consideration of a Seventh Stage." In *Higher Stages of Human Development: Perspectives on Adult Growth*, ed. C. N. Alexander and E. J. Langer. New York: Oxford University Press, 1990.

End-of-Chapter Resources

The **Chapter Summary** is in a tabular, step-by-step format organized by Learning Outcome to help with review of the material. **Ethics Issues** are issues and related discussion questions based on interviews conducted with ethics counselors within the professional organizations for health care providers, as well as with bioethics experts. Each **Chapter Review** includes Applying Knowledge questions that reinforce the concepts the students have just learned. These questions can be answered in *Connect*. **Case Studies** are scenarios with exercises that allow students to practice their critical thinking skills to decide how to resolve the real-life situations and theoretical scenarios presented. **Internet Activities** include exercises designed to increase the students' knowledge of the chapter topics and help them gain more Internet research expertise. The **Resources** section presents a listing of additional references for the chapter.

Acknowledgments

Author Acknowledgments

Karen Judson

Thank you to the editorial team and production staff at McGraw-Hill, and all the reviewers and sources who contributed their time and expertise to making the seventh edition of Law & Ethics for Health Professions the best ever. Thank you, too, Carlene, for your hard work on this seventh edition.

Carlene Harrison

A big thank you to Karen Judson for getting me started on this marvelous adventure called writing.

To our reviewers, your contributions really make a difference. The editorial and production staff at McGraw-Hill did a great job. And last, to my husband Bill, your support and love keeps me going.

Reviewer Acknowledgments

Suggestions have been received from faculty and students throughout the country. This is vital feedback that is relied on for product development. Each person who has offered comments and suggestions has our thanks. The efforts of many people are needed to develop and improve a product. Among these people are the reviewers and consultants who point out areas of concern, cite areas of strength, and make recommendations for change. In this regard, the following instructors provided feedback that was enormously helpful in preparing the book and related products.

7e Reviewers

Multiple instructors reviewed the product while it was in development, providing valuable feedback that directly impacted the product. They include the following individuals:

Yvonne Alles, DHA
Davenport

Theresa Allyn, BS, MEd
Edmonds Community College

Doris Beran, MPH
Coconino Community College

Chantalle Blakesley-Boddie, BS, CMA (AAMA)
Lake Washington Institute of Technology

Marianne Bovee, CCMA, CET, CHI
Duluth Business University

Valerie Brock, MBA, RHIA, CDIP, CPC, CCP, CPAR
Tennessee State University

Joey L. Brown, MA/MS
Great Lakes Institute of Tech

Myra Brown, MBA, RHIA
East Carolina University

Patricia Brown Raphiel, MEd, MT/PBT (ASCP)
Southern University of Shreveport

Deborah Bryant, MS/ED.PSY, CMA (AAMA)
Chattahoochee Technical College

Cyndi Caviness, AAS, AHI, CMA (AAMA), CRT
Montgomery Community College

Christine Christensen, AAS, CCA, BAS
Williston State College

Marsha Eriks, BS, CST
Ivy Tech Community College

Kim Ford, AAS, MA
Catawba Valley Community College

Rebecca French, RN, BS, CRNI, MSN, ARNP-C, GNP-BC
Allen Community College (Iola, KS)

Brenda Garrett, MHA, CAM, CMOM, RMC
Danville Community College

Diane Gryglak, AA, BS, CMA (AAMA)
College of DuPage

Angela Hennessy, BS, MS
Corning Community College

Sandy Hunter, BS, MEd, PhD
Eastern Kentucky University

Robert Kieffer
Trocaire College

Karmon Kingsley, BS, CMA (AAMA)
Cleveland State Community College

Rhonda S. Lazette, BS, CMA (AAMA), CPC (AAPC)
Stautzenberger College

Kathy Locke, BA, CMA (AAMA), MS
Northwestern College

Sharon Luczu Thompkins
Gateway Community College

Erica Matteson, RHIA, BPS
Alfred State College

Mindy McDonald, BS, CMA (AAMA)
University of Northwest Ohio

Kelly Meyer, BS, MEd, CPhT, PhTR
Cisco College

Robert Micallef, MA
Madonna University

Pat Moody, MSN, RN
Athens Technical College (GA)

Brigitte Niedzwiecki, BSN, MSN, RN
Chippewa Valley Technical College

Cynthia S. Nivens
Forsyth Technical Community College

Ruth O'Brien, AAS, BA, CPFT, MHA, RRT, CPT, CPC-A
Miami-Jacobs Career College (OH)

Julie Pepper, CMA (AAMA)
Chippewa Valley Technical College

Berta Powers, AA, CCMA, CMA (AAMA)
De Anza College

Debra Pressley, BA, MBA
Blue Ridge Community College

Sue Pylant, CCS-P
Sanford-Brown College – San Antonio

Adrienne Reaves, EdD, RMA
Westwood College – DuPage

Starra Robinson-Herring, AAS, AHI, BA, BSHA, MS
Stanly Community College

Donna Rowan, MA, RMA
Community College of Baltimore County

Mary Ann Schaefer, RNC, BAABS, MBA, MJ
William Rainey Harper College

Jeanne Smoczyk, MS, RHIT
Chippewa Valley Technical College

Marlene Suvada, MHPE, RRT
National-Louis University

Charlene Thiessen
GateWay Community College

Lenette Thompson, CST
Piedmont Tech College

L. Joleen VanBibber, CDPMA, CFRDA
Davis Applied Technology College

Stacey Wanovich, MLT
Anoka Technical College

Gail Warchol
Mohawk Valley Community College

Claudia Williams, MS
Campbell University

Veronica Zurcher, BSAS, CMA (AAMA)
National College (Youngstown, OH)

Reviewers of Previous Editions

Cindy A. Abel, BS, CMA, PBT (ASCP)
Ivy Tech State College

Carol Adams-Turner
Lamar State College – Orange

Diane Alagna, RN, RMA Medical Assisting
Branford Hall Career Institute

Jeanne C. Ambrosio, BSN
Goodwin College

Thomas Ankeney, BA, RCP, RRT, CPFT, AE-C, NCPT
Maric College

Shkelzen Badivuku
Gibbs College

Julette Barta, CphT, BSIT
SJVC

Barbara C. Berger, BSN, RN, CMA, MS
Northwestern Connecticut Community College

Norma Bird, MEd, CMA (AAMA)
Idaho State University

Rebecca Bonefas, MA
Kaplan University

Rebecca Britt
Northwestern State University

Amelia Broussard, PhD, RN, MPH
Clayton College & State University

Joey L. Brown, MA/MS
Great Lakes Institute of Technology

Lou Brown
Wayne Community College

Martina Forte Brown, CCMA, CPT, CET
Brookstone College

Rita Bulington, RN, AS
Ivy Tech Community College

Lynn Callister, RN, PhD, FAAN
Brigham Young University

Cyndi Caviness, AAS, AHI, CMA (AAMA), CRT
Montgomery Community College

Linda Ciarleglio, BS
Stone Academy

Christine M. Cole, CCA
Williston State College

Rebecca Complin, BS, RDH, RDMS, RVT
American Career College

Dawn Felice Dannenbrink, MHA
High-Tech Institute

Barbara Desch
San Joaquin Valley College, Inc.

Deborah Eid
Carrington College

Christine Enz, CCS-P
Bryant & Stratton College

Dena A. Evans, BSN, MPH, RN, CMA
Richmond Community College

Cynthia Ferguson, AAS
Texas State Technical College

Terri Fleming
Ivy Tech Community College

Tammy B. Foles
Antonelli College

Kim Ford, AAS, MA
Catawba Valley Community College

Rebecca Anne French, RN, BS, CRNI, MSN, ARNP-C, GNP-BC
Allen Community College (Iola, KS)

Jill Frost
Tennessee Technology Center at Murfreesboro

Deborah Galanski-Maciak, MS, RHIT
Davenport University Online

Debbie Gilbert
Dalton State College

William D. Goren, JD, LLM
Northwestern Business College

James Goss, MHA, MICP
Loma Linda University

Gardiner M. Haight, BS Comm, JD
Bryant & Stratton College

Janet K. Henderson, CMA, AAT
North Georgia Technical College

Beulah A. Hofmann, RN, MSN
Ivy Tech Community College

Grant Iannelli, BS, DC
Kaplan University School of Health Sciences

Carol Lee Jarrell
Brown Mackie College

Wendyanne Jex, BA, MPA-HS
Kaplan University School of Health Sciences

Joyce S. Johnson, Department Head
Alamance Community College

Carrie Kaye, BA, MA
The Salter School

Katin Keirstead
Seacoast Career Schools

Karmon Kingsley, BS, CMA (AAMA)
Cleveland State Community College

Mary Koloski, CBCS, CHI
Florida Career College

Lynda M. Konecny
New York City College of Technology

Michelle Lovings, BA
Missouri College

Loreen MacNichol, CMRS, RMC, CCS-P
Andover College

Loreen W. MacNichol, BS
Kaplan University, Maine

Christine Malone, MHA
Everett Community College

Norma Mercado, MAHS, RHIA
Austin Community College

Robert Micallef, MA
Madonna University

Lane Miller, MBA/HCM
Medical Careers Institute

Lynne M. Muñoz, MEd
Everett Community College

Helen L. Myers
Hagerstown Community College

Kathleen Olewinski, MS, RHIA, NHA, FACHE
Bryant & Stratton College

Matthew R. Panzio, MD
Gibbs College

Cindy Pavel
Ivy Tech Community College

Sherry Pearsall, RN, MSN, CAS
Bryant & Stratton College

Michael W. Posey, PhD
Franklin University

Pamela B. Primrose, MLFSC, ABD, MT, ASCP
Ivy Tech Community College

Joan Renner, BSN, RNBC, Adjunct Faculty
Cecil Community College

Sharon M. Roberts, MBA, MS, PTA
Newbury College

Diane P. Roche, CMA, BSHCA, MSA
South Piedmont Community College

Kim Rock
Branford Hall Career Institute

Elizabeth Salazar, AS, BS
Centura College

Tammy L. Shick
Great Lakes Institute of Technology

James Steen, MBA, SS, RHIA
San Jacinto College North

Pat Stettler, CMT, FAAMT
Everett Community College

Rita Stoffel, BS, MT, MBA
Red Rocks Community

Tammy Summerson, BSN
Westwood College

Marlene Suvada, MHPE, RRT
National-Louis University

Nina Thierer, CMA, BS, CPC
Ivy Tech State College – Fort Wayne

Geraldine M. Todaro, MSTE, CMA, CLPlb
Stark State College of Technology

Tova R. Wiegand-Green
Ivy Tech State College

Constance Winter
Bossier Parish Community College

Mary M. Zulaybar, BS, CBCS
ASA Institute, Division of Health Disciplines

Technical Editing/Accuracy Panel

A panel of instructors completed a technical edit and review of the content in the book page proofs to verify its accuracy.

Lynnae Lockett, RMA, CMRS, RN
Bryant and Stratton College

Marta Lopez, MD, LM, CPM, RMA, BMO
Miami Dade College

Angela M. B. Oliva, BS, CMRS
Heald College and Boston Reed College

Luz P. Rios-Garcia, CMA (AAMA)
Branford Hall Career Institute

Wendy Schmerse, CMRS
Charter College

Digital Tool Development

Special thanks to the instructors who helped with the development of Connect, LearnSmart, and SmartBook. They include:

Chantalle Blakesley-Boddie, BS, CMA (AAMA)
Lake Washington Institute of Technology

William Travis Butler, RMA, MHA
ECPI University

Gloryvee Diaz, MA
Branford Hall Career Institute

Terri Gilbert, BSBA
ECPI University

Debra Glover, RN, BSN
Goodwin College

Susan Harrison-Grant, RN, MS, EdD
William Rainey Harper College

Judy Hurtt, MEd
East Central Community College

Rhonda S. Lazette, BS, CMA (AAMA), CPC (AAPC)
Stautzenberger College

Kelli Lewis, MSHI, RHIA
Valencia College

Lynnae Lockett, RMA, CMRS, RN
Bryant and Stratton College

Carrie Mack, AS, CMA (AAMA)
Branford Hall Career Institute

Angela M. B. Oliva, BS, CMRS
Heald College and Boston Reed College

Luz P. Rios-Garcia, CMA (AAMA)
Branford Hall Career Institute

Wendy Schmerse, CMRS
Charter College

Mia C. Small, MBA, AHI, RMA, CMRS
Bryant & Stratton College

Linda Sorensen, MPA, RHIA, CHPS
Davenport University

Alice L. Spencer, BS MT, MS, CQA (ASQ)
National College

Stacey Wanovich, MLT
Anoka Technical College

Art Witkowski, MEd,
Chemeketa Community College

The Foundations of Law and Ethics

1

Key Terms

Introduction to Law and Ethics

LEARNING OUTCOMES

After studying this chapter, you should be able to:

LO 1.1 Explain why knowledge of law and ethics is important to health care practitioners.

LO 1.2 Distinguish among law, ethics, bioethics, etiquette, and protocol.

LO 1.3 Define *moral values* and explain how they relate to law, ethics, and etiquette.

LO 1.4 Discuss the characteristics and skills most likely to lead to a successful career in one of the health care professions.

FROM THE PERSPECTIVE OF. . .

BARBARA, AN EXPERIENCED CERTIFIED MEDICAL ASSISTANT (CMA) (AAMA) in a medical office with a walk-in clinic, instructs new employees in the reception area of the office to follow the medical office procedures whenever possible and prudent, but, above all, to use common sense in dealing with patients.

Barbara told Elaine, a new receptionist in the medical office, to politely ask walk-in patients why they needed to see a doctor. Elaine had been on the job for two weeks when an elderly man who was hard of hearing approached her, and she dutifully asked him the purpose for his visit. He was obviously too embarrassed to reply, but Elaine persisted, finally raising her voice. When the man shouted "I can't pee," all heads in the busy waiting room turned toward Elaine and the patient. A red-faced Elaine turned to arrange for the man to see a physician, but he quickly left the building. Barbara criticized Elaine's patient-handling technique, but the crux of the matter was that the patient left without seeing a doctor for his medical problem.

"Patients' needs always trump office routine," Barbara emphasizes. "If we somehow hurt or hinder a patient while doggedly sticking to a set routine, we may have risked legal liability, but more important, we haven't done our job."

From Barbara's perspective as the person responsible for training medical office personnel, Elaine failed to use common sense in communicating with a patient, and as a result, the man did not receive the medical treatment he needed.

From Elaine's perspective, she followed Barbara's instructions to the letter, and she failed to understand why Barbara had criticized her. She hadn't meant to embarrass the man, so was it her fault that he left without making an appointment?

From the patient's perspective as an elderly gentleman who seldom discussed personal matters, the young woman who was his first contact in the medical office embarrassed him, and he left rather than face further humiliation.

As you progress through *Law & Ethics for the Health Professions*, try to interpret the court cases, laws, case studies, and other examples or situations cited from the perspectives of everyone involved.

Why Study Law and Ethics?

There are two important reasons for you to study law and ethics:

- To help you function at the highest possible professional level, providing competent, compassionate health care to patients.
- To help you avoid legal entanglements that can threaten your ability to earn a living as a successful **health care practitioner.**

We live in a **litigious** society, where patients, relatives, and others are inclined to sue health care practitioners, health care facilities, manufacturers of medical equipment and products, and others when

LO 1.1
Explain why knowledge of law and ethics is important to health care practitioners.

health care practitioners
Those who are trained to administer medical or health care to patients.

litigious
Prone to engage in lawsuits.

medical outcomes are not acceptable. This means that every person responsible for health care delivery is at risk of being involved in a health care–related lawsuit. It is important, therefore, for you to know the basics of law and ethics as they apply to health care, so you can recognize and avoid those situations that might not serve your patients well, or that might put you at risk of legal liability.

In addition to keeping you at your professional best and helping you avoid litigation, knowledge of law and ethics can also help you gain perspective in the following three areas:

1. *The rights, responsibilities, and concerns of health care consumers.* Health care practitioners not only need to be concerned about how law and ethics impact their respective professions, but they must also understand how legal and ethical issues affect the patients they treat. With the increased complexity of medicine has come the desire of consumers to know more about their options and rights and more about the responsibilities of health care providers. Today's health care consumers are likely to consider themselves partners with health care practitioners in the healing process and to question fees and treatment modes. They may ask such questions as, Do I need to see a specialist? If so, which specialist can best treat my condition? Will I be given complete information about my condition? How much will medical treatment cost? Will a physician treat me if I have no health insurance?

    In addition, as medical technology has advanced, patients have come to expect favorable outcomes from medical treatment, and when expectations are not met, lawsuits may result.

2. *The legal and ethical issues facing society, patients, and health care practitioners as the world changes.* Nearly every day the media report news events concerning individuals who face legal and ethical dilemmas over biological/medical issues. For example, a grief-stricken husband must give consent for an abortion in order to save the life of his critically ill and unconscious wife. Parents must argue in court their decision to terminate life-support measures for a daughter whose injured brain no longer functions. Patients with HIV/AIDS fight to retain their right to confidentiality.

    While the situations that make news headlines often involve larger social issues, legal and ethical questions are resolved daily, on a smaller scale, each time a patient visits his or her physician, dentist, physical therapist, or other health care practitioner. Questions that must often be resolved include these: Who can legally give consent if the patient cannot? Can patients be assured of confidentiality, especially since telecommunication has become a way of life? Can a physician or other health care practitioner refuse to treat a patient? Who may legally examine a patient's medical records?

    Rapid advances in medical technology have also influenced laws and ethics for health care practitioners. For example, recent court cases have debated these issues: Does the husband or the wife have ownership rights to a divorced couple's frozen embryos? Will a surrogate mother have legal visitation rights to the child she carried to term? Should modern technology be used to keep those patients alive who are diagnosed as brain-dead and have no hope of recovery? How should parenthood disputes be resolved for children resulting from reproductive technology?

3. *The impact of rising costs on the laws and ethics of health care delivery.* Rising costs, both of health care insurance and of medical treatment in general, lead to questions concerning access to health care services and allocation of medical treatment. For instance, should the uninsured or underinsured receive government help to pay for health insurance? And should everyone, regardless of age or lifestyle, have the same access to scarce medical commodities such as organs for transplantation or very expensive drugs?

COURT CASES ILLUSTRATE RISK OF LITIGATION

As you will see in the court cases used throughout this text, sometimes when a lawsuit is brought, the trial court or a higher court must first decide if the **plaintiff** has a legal reason to sue, or if the **defendant** is **liable.** When a court has ruled that there is a standing (reason) to sue and that a defendant can be held liable, the case may proceed to resolution. Often, once liability and a standing to sue have been established, the two sides agree on an out-of-court settlement. Depending on state law, an out-of-court settlement may not be published. For this reason, the final disposition of a case is not always available from published sources. The published cases that have decided liability, however, are still case law, and such cases have been used in this text to illustrate specific points.

In addition, sometimes it takes time after the initial trial for a case to be settled. For example, perhaps a patient dies after surgery in 2010, and the family files a wrongful death suit soon after. The case may go through several appeals and finally be settled in 2014.

It is also important to remember that while the final result of a case is important to the parties involved, from a legal standpoint the most

plaintiff
The person bringing charges in a lawsuit.

defendant
The person or party against whom criminal or civil charges are brought in a lawsuit.

liable
Legally responsible or obligated.

COURT CASES Patients Sue Hospitals

In 2013, lawsuits against hospitals that were moving through various courts included:

- A man entered a hospital emergency room suffering from severe headaches, dizziness, nausea and vomiting that were found to be connected to a fall the patient had just over two weeks earlier when he lost consciousness. A nurse gave the patient an enema, administered a sedative, and placed him on a bedpan. The patient fell asleep on the bedpan as the sedative took effect, and when he was discovered 4 ½ hours later, the man's lower extremites were swollen and painful. In his lawsuit, the man alleged that he developed deep vein thromboses in both legs.

- A woman visiting a hospital patient slipped on a spill caused by the other patient in the room and claimed she was injured. Hospital staff were notified, but allegedly failed to adequately clean up the spill.

- A woman who underwent a thyroid biopsy had to undergo the procedure again, when hospital staff lost the first specimen. The woman alleged insufficient staff training and supervision were responsible for her having to undergo a second biopsy.

- A hospital employee underwent minor surgery only to awaken and find that her anaesthesiologist and another person had drawn a moustache and tears on her face and snapped photos with their cell phones. Since the patient knew the plaintiffs, they said they thought she would be amused. The patient alleged a violation of her privacy, among other charges.

(All of the above cases were still in litigation as the 7th edition of *Law & Ethics for the Health Professions* was prepared for publication, but perhaps the underlying reasons for filing the lawsuits are already apparent to you.)

911 Operators Sued

In 2006, just before 6 PM, a five-year-old boy called 911. He told the 911 operator that his "mom has passed out." When the operator asked to speak to the boy's mother, he said, "She's not gonna talk." The operator scolded the boy and logged the call as a child's prank. Three hours later the boy called 911 again. A different operator answered, and she also scolded the boy for playing a prank, but she did send a police officer to the boy's home. The officer discovered the boy's mother lying unresponsive on the floor and summoned emergency medical services. The EMS workers arrived 20 minutes later, and determined that the woman was dead, and had probably died within the past two hours.

The boy's older sister sued the two 911 operators on behalf of the dead woman's estate and on behalf of her son. The lawsuit alleged gross negligence causing a death and intentional infliction of emotional distress.

The 911 operators argued that they were entitled to government immunity, that they owed no duty to provide assistance to the woman who died, and that their failure to summon medical aid was not gross negligence.

A trial court and an appeals court found for the plaintiff, and the case was appealed to the Michigan Supreme Court, where in January 2012, the court denied further appeals.

Estate of Turner v. Nichols, 807 N.W.2d 164, 490 Mich. 988 (2012).

---

important aspect of a court case is not the result, but whether the case represents good law and will be persuasive as other cases are decided.

Although the most recent cases published have been sought for illustration in this text, sometimes a dated case (1995, 1985, 1970, etc.) is used because it established important **precedent**.

Court cases appear throughout each chapter of the text to illustrate how the legal system has decided complaints brought by or against health care service providers and product manufacturers. Some of these cases involve **summary judgment**. Summary judgment is the legal term for a decision made by a court in a lawsuit in response to a motion that pleads there is no basis for a trial because there is no genuine issue of material fact. In other words, a motion for summary judgment states that one party is entitled to win as a matter of law. Summary judgment is available only in a civil action. (Chapter 4 distinguishes between criminal and civil actions.)

The following court cases illustrate that a wide variety of legal questions can arise for those engaged directly in providing health care services, whether in a hospital, in a medical office, or in an emergency situation. Health care equipment and product dealers and manufacturers can be held indirectly responsible for defective medical devices and products through charges of the following types:

- Breach of warranty.
- Statements made by the manufacturer about the device or product that are found to be untrue.
- Strict liability, for cases in which defective products threaten the personal safety of consumers.
- **Fraud** or intentional deceit. (Fraud is discussed in further detail in Chapter 4.)

The extent of liability for manufacturers of medical devices and products may be changing, however, since a 2008 U.S. Supreme Court decision held that makers of medical devices such as implantable defibrillators or breast implants are immune from liability for personal

precedent
Decisions made by judges in the various courts that become rule of law and apply to future cases, even though they were not enacted by a legislature; also known as case law.

summary judgment
A decision made by a court in a lawsuit in response to a motion that pleads there is no basis for a trial.

fraud
Dishonest or deceitful practices in depriving, or attempting to deprive, another of his or her rights.

Supreme Court Shields Medical Devices from Lawsuits

An angioplasty was performed on a patient, Charles Riegel, in New York. During the procedure, the catheter used to dilate the patient's coronary artery failed, causing serious complications. The patient sued the catheter's manufacturer, Medtronic, Inc., under New York state law, charging negligence in design, manufacture, and labeling of the device, which had received FDA approval in 1994. Medtronic argued that Riegel could not bring state law negligence claims because the company was preempted from liability under Section 360k(a) of the Medical Device Amendments (MDA) of the U.S. Food, Drug, and Cosmetic Act. State requirements are preempted under the MDA only to the extent that they are "different from, or in addition to" the requirements imposed by federal law. Thus, 360k(a) does not prevent a state from providing a damages remedy for claims premised on a violation of FDA regulations; the state duties in such a case "parallel," rather than add to, federal requirements (*Lohr,* 518 U.S., at 495, 116 S.Ct. 2240).

The *Riegel* case reached the U.S. Supreme Court, where the question to be decided was this: Does Section 360k(a) of the Medical Device Amendments to the Food, Drug, and Cosmetic Act preempt state law claims seeking damages for injuries caused by medical devices that received premarket approval from the Food and Drug Administration?

In February 2008, the U.S. Supreme Court held in this case that makers of medical devices are immune from liability for personal injuries as long as the FDA approved the device before it was marketed and it meets the FDA's specifications.

Appeals Court Case: *Riegel v. Medtronic, Inc.,* 451 F.3d 104 (2006); Supreme Court Case: *Riegel v. Medtronic, Inc.,* 552 U.S. 312, 128 S.Ct. 999, 2008.

injuries as long as the Food and Drug Administration (FDA) approved the device before it was marketed and it meets the FDA's specifications. (See the previous *Medtronic Inc.* case.)

Drugs and medical devices are regulated under separate federal laws, and an important issue in deciding drug injury cases is whether or not the drug manufacturer made false or misleading statements to win FDA approval. For example, the case *Warner-Lambert Co. v. Kent,* filed in 2006, involved a group of Michigan residents who claimed injury after taking Warner-Lambert's Rezulin diabetes drug. The case was brought under a Michigan tort reform law that said a drug company could be liable for product injury if it had misrepresented the product to win FDA approval. In this case, the question before the court was, Does a federal law prohibiting fraudulent communications to government agencies preempt a state law permitting plaintiffs to sue for faulty products that would not have reached the market absent the fraud?

A federal appeals court eventually heard the case and ruled that the Michigan "fraud on the FDA" law was preempted by a federal law that allowed the FDA itself to punish misrepresentations. This decision was appealed to the U.S. Supreme Court, and in a March 2008 decision, the Roberts Supreme Court affirmed the appeals court, thus leaving the previous state of the law unchanged and unclarified.

In this case, the people who sued the drug manufacturer were not allowed to collect damages. But when courts find that drugs are misrepresented so that developers can win FDA approval, drug manufacturers could be held legally responsible and forced to pay damages.

Examples of how drug manufacturers could be held legally responsible before any Supreme Court decision protecting them from liability were the many lawsuits filed against Merck & Company, a pharmaceutical firm that manufactured the drug Vioxx, once widely recommended for pain relief for arthritis sufferers. The drug was suspected of causing heart attacks and strokes in some patients, and from 1999,

Patient Sues over Drug Labeling Issue

In 2000, Diana Levine, a Vermont woman in her fifties, sought medical help for migraine headaches. As part of the treatment, the antinausea drug Phenergan, made by Wyeth, was injected in her arm. An artery was accidentally damaged during the injection, gangrene set in, and Levine's right arm was amputated. The amputation was devastating for Levine, a professional musician who had released 16 albums, and she filed a personal injury action against Wyeth in Vermont state court.

Levine asserted that Wyeth should have included a warning label describing the possible arterial injuries that could occur from negligent injection of the drug. Wyeth argued that because the warning label had been deemed acceptable by the FDA, a federal agency, any Vermont state regulations making the label insufficient were preempted by the federal approval. The Superior Court of Vermont found in favor of Levine and denied Wyeth's motion for

a new trial. Levine was awarded $7 million in damages for the amputation of her arm. The Supreme Court of Vermont affirmed this ruling on appeal, holding that the FDA requirements merely provide a floor, not a ceiling, for state regulation. Therefore, states are free to create more stringent labeling requirements than federal law provides.

The U.S. Supreme Court eventually heard the case and issued a decision in March 2009. Wyeth had argued that because the warning label had been accepted by the FDA, any Vermont state regulations making the label insufficient were preempted by the federal approval. The U.S. Supreme Court affirmed the Vermont Supreme Court, holding that federal law did not preempt Levine's state law claim that Wyeth's labeling of Phenergan failed to warn of the dangers of intravenous administration.

Wyeth v. Levine, 555 U.S. 555, 173 L.Ed.2d 51 (2009).

the year Vioxx went on the market, to 2007, Merck faced lawsuits from 47,000 plaintiffs, including patients, health providers, unions, and insurers. Many of the lawsuits alleged that Merck knew of the drug's potentially harmful side effects when the company placed the drug on the market.

In November 2007, Merck agreed to settle most of the lawsuits relating to Vioxx for a total of $4.85 billion. The settlement was open to plaintiffs who filed cases before November 8, 2007, who could provide medical proof of their heart attack or stroke, and who could prove they had used at least 30 Vioxx pills within 14 days prior to their illness. In March 2010, Merck and the Securities and Exchange Commission (SEC) announced that all payouts through the settlement process would be paid out by the end of June 2010.

Merck anticipated that some plaintiffs would opt out of the settlement, continuing to fight the company on a case-by-case basis. The company projected that remaining claims could cost the firm between $2 and $3 billion, and as of 2012, claims against Vioxx were still moving through the courts.

Federal preemption—a doctrine that can bar injured consumers from suing in state court when the products that hurt them had met federal standards—has become an important concern in product liability law. One such case, *Wyeth v. Levine,* decided by the U.S. Supreme Court in 2009, will become precedent for future cases involving drug manufacturers and consumers.

LO 1.2 and LO 1.3

Distinguish among law, ethics, bioethics, etiquette, and protocol.

Define *moral values* and explain how they relate to law, ethics, and etiquette.

Comparing Aspects of Law and Ethics

To understand the complexities of law and ethics, it is helpful to define and compare a few basic terms. Table 1-1 summarizes the terms described in the following sections.

Table 1-1 Comparing Aspects of Law and Ethics

	Law	Ethics	Moral Values
Definition	Set of governing rules	Principles, standards, guide to conduct	Beliefs formed through the influence of family, culture, and society
Main purpose	To protect the public	To elevate the standard of competence	To serve as a guide for personal ethical conduct
Standards	Minimal—promotes smooth functioning of society	Builds values and ideals	Serves as a basis for forming a personal code of ethics
Penalties of violation	Civil or criminal liability. Upon conviction: fine, imprisonment, revocation of license, or other penalty as determined by courts	Suspension or eviction from medical society membership, as decided by peers	Difficulty in getting along with others

	Bioethics	Etiquette	Protocol
Definition	Discipline relating to ethics concerning biological research, especially as applied to medicine	Courtesy and manners	Rules of etiquette applicable to one's place of employment
Main purpose	To allow scientific progress in a manner that benefits society in all possible ways	To enable one to get along with others	To enable one to get along with others engaged in the same profession
Standards	Leads to the highest standards possible in applying research to medical care	Leads to pleasant interaction	Promotes smooth functioning of workplace routines
Penalties of violation	Can include all those listed under "Law," "Ethics," and "Etiquette"; as current standards are applied and as new laws and ethical standards evolve to govern medical research and development, penalties may change	Ostracism from chosen groups	Disapproval from one's professional colleagues; possible loss of business

LAW

A **law** is defined as a rule of conduct or action prescribed or formally recognized as binding or enforced by a controlling authority. Governments enact laws to keep society running smoothly and to control behavior that could threaten public safety. Laws are considered the minimum standard necessary to keep society functioning.

Enforcement of laws is made possible by penalties for disobedience, which are decided by a court of law or are mandatory as written into the law. Penalties vary with the severity of the crime. Lawbreakers may be fined, imprisoned, or both. Sometimes lawbreakers are sentenced to probation. Other penalties appropriate to the crime may be handed down by the sentencing authority, as when offenders must perform a specified number of hours of volunteer community service or are ordered to repair public facilities they have damaged.

Many laws affect health care practitioners, including criminal and civil statutes as well as state medical practice acts. Medical practice acts apply specifically to the practice of medicine in a certain state. Licensed health care professionals convicted of violating criminal, civil, or medical practice laws may lose their licenses to practice. (Medical practice acts are discussed further in Chapter 3. Laws and the court system are discussed in more detail in Chapter 4.)

law
Rule of conduct or action prescribed or formally recognized as binding or enforced by a controlling authority.

ETHICS

ethics
Standards of behavior, developed as a result of one's concept of right and wrong.

moral values
One's personal concept of right and wrong, formed through the influence of the family, culture, and society.

An illegal act by a health care practitioner is always unethical, but an unethical act is not necessarily illegal. **Ethics** are concerned with standards of behavior and the concept of right and wrong, over and above that which is legal in a given situation. **Moral values**—formed through the influence of the family, culture, and society—serve as the basis for ethical conduct.

The United States is a culturally diverse country, with many residents who have grown up within vastly different ethnic environments. For example, a Chinese student in the United States brings to his or her studies a unique set of religious and social experiences and moral concepts that will differ from that of a German, Japanese, Korean, French, Italian, or even Canadian classmate. Therefore, moral values and ethical standards can differ for health care practitioners, as well as patients, in the same setting.

In the American cultural environment, however, acting morally toward another usually requires that you put yourself in that individual's place. For example, when you are a patient in a physician's office, how do you like to be treated? As a health care provider, can you give care to a person whose conduct or professed beliefs differ radically from your own? In an emergency, can you provide for the patient's welfare without reservation?

CODES OF ETHICS AND ETHICS GUIDELINES

code of ethics
A list of principles intended to govern behavior—here, the behavior of those entrusted with providing care to the sick.

ethics guidelines
Publications that detail a wide variety of ethical situations that professionals (in this case, health care practitioners) might face in their work and offer principles for dealing with the situations in an ethical manner.

While most individuals can rely on a well-developed personal value system, organizations for the health occupations also have formalized **codes of ethics** to govern behavior of members and to increase the level of competence and standards of care within the group. Included among these are the American Nurses Association Code for Nurses, American Medical Association Code of Medical Ethics, American Health Information Management Association Code of Ethics, American Society of Radiologic Technologists Code of Ethics, and the Code of Ethics of the American Association of Medical Assistants. Codes of ethics generally consist of a list of general principles, and are often available to laypersons as well as members of health care practitioner organizations.

Many professional organizations for health care practitioners also publish more detailed **ethics guidelines**, usually in book form, for

Check Your Progress

1. Name two important reasons for studying law and ethics.
2. Which state laws apply specifically to the practice of medicine?
3. What purpose do laws serve?
4. How is the enforcement of laws made possible?
5. What factors influence the formation of one's personal set of ethics and values?
6. Define the term *moral values*.
7. Explain how one's moral values affect one's sense of ethics.

members. Generally, ethics guideline publications detail a wide variety of ethical situations that health care practitioners might face in their work and offer principles for dealing with the situations in an ethical manner. They are routinely available to members of health care organizations, and are typically available to others for a fee.

One of the earliest medical codes of ethics, the code of Hammurabi, was written by the Babylonians around 2250 B.C.E. This document discussed the conduct expected of physicians at that time, including fees that could be charged.

Sometime around 400 B.C.E., a pledge for physicians known as the **Hippocratic oath** was published. The oath was probably not actually written by Hippocrates, the Greek physician known as the Father of Medicine. Authorship has been attributed to one or more of his students and to the Pythagoreans, but scholars indicate it was probably derived from Hippocrates's writings (see Figure 1-1).

Hippocratic oath
A pledge for physicians, influenced by the practices of the Greek physician Hippocrates.

FIGURE 1-1
Hippocratic Oath

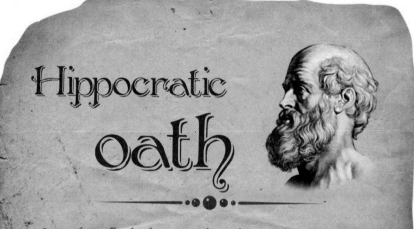

Hippocratic oath

I swear by Apollo, the physician, and Aesculapius, and Health, and Allheal, and all the gods and goddesses, that, according to my ability and judgment, I will keep this oath and stipulation, to reckon him who taught me this art equally dear to me as my parents, to share my substance with him and relieve his necessities if required; to regard his offspring as on the same footing with my own brothers, and to teach them this art if they should wish to learn it, without fee or stipulation, and that by precept, lecture, and every other mode of instruction, I will impart a knowledge of the art to my own sons and to those of my teachers, and to disciples bound by a stipulation and oath, according to the law of medicine, but to none other.

I will follow that method of treatment which, according to my ability and judgment, I consider for the benefit of my patients, and abstain from whatever is deleterious and mischievous. I will give no deadly medicine to anyone if asked, nor suggest any such counsel; furthermore, I will not give to a woman an instrument to produce abortion.

With purity and holiness I will pass my life and practice my art. I will not cut a person who is suffering with a stone, but will leave this to be done by practitioners of the work. Into whatever houses I enter I will go into them for the benefit of the sick and will abstain from every voluntary act of mischief and corruption; and further from the seduction of females or males, bond or free.

Whatever, in connection with my professional practice, or not in connection with it, I may see or hear in the lives of men which ought not to be spoken abroad, I will not divulge, as reckoning that all such should be kept secret.

While I continue to keep this oath unviolated, may it be granted to me to enjoy life and the practice of the art, respected by all men at all times, but should I trespass and violate this oath, may the reverse be my lot.

Percival's Medical Ethics, written by the English physician and philosopher Thomas Percival in 1803, superseded earlier codes to become the definitive guide for a physician's professional conduct. Earlier codes did not address concerns about experimental medicine, but according to Percival's code, physicians could try experimental treatments when all else failed, if such treatments served the public good.

When the American Medical Association met for the first time in Philadelphia in 1847, the group devised a code of ethics for members based on Percival's code. The resulting **American Medical Association Principles,** currently called the *American Medical Association Principles of Medical Ethics,* has been revised and updated periodically to keep pace with changing times (see Figure 1-2). The *American Medical Association Principles of Medical Ethics* briefly summarizes the position of the American Medical Association (AMA) on ethical treatment of patients, while the more extensive *Code of Medical Ethics: Current Opinions with Annotations* provides more detailed coverage.

When members of professional associations such as the AMA and the AAMA are accused of unethical conduct, they are subject to peer council review and may be censured by the organization

American Medical Association Principles
A code of ethics for members of the American Medical Association, written in 1847. (American Medical Association Web site: **www.ama-assn.org/ ama/pub/physicianresources/ medical-ethics/code-medical-ethics/ principles-medical-ethics.page.**)

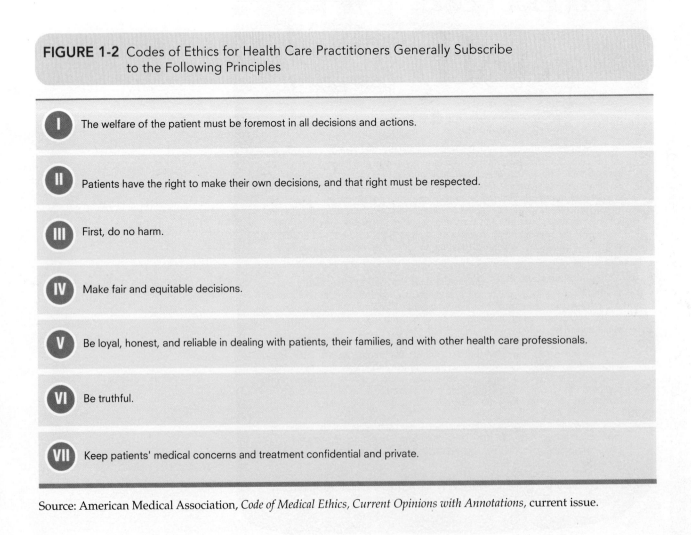

FIGURE 1-2 Codes of Ethics for Health Care Practitioners Generally Subscribe to the Following Principles

I   The welfare of the patient must be foremost in all decisions and actions.

II Patients have the right to make their own decisions, and that right must be respected.

III First, do no harm.

IV Make fair and equitable decisions.

V   Be loyal, honest, and reliable in dealing with patients, their families, and with other health care professionals.

VI Be truthful.

VII Keep patients' medical concerns and treatment confidential and private.

Source: American Medical Association, *Code of Medical Ethics, Current Opinions with Annotations,* current issue.

The Medical Assisting Code of Ethics of the AAMA sets forth principles of ethical and moral conduct as they relate to the medical profession and the particular practice of medical assisting.

Members of AAMA dedicated to the conscientious pursuit of their profession, and thus desiring to merit the high regard of the entire medical profession and the respect of the general public which they serve, do pledge themselves to strive always to:

A. Render service with full respect for the dignity of humanity.

B. Respect confidential information obtained through employment unless legally authorized or required by responsible performance of duty to divulge such information.

C. Uphold the honor and high principles of the profession and accept its disciplines.

D. Seek to continually improve the knowledge and skills of medical assistants for the benefit of patients and professional colleagues.

E. Participate in additional service activities aimed toward improving the health and well-being of the community.

The Medical Assisting Creed of the AAMA sets forth medical assisting statements of belief:

I I believe in the principles and purposes of the profession of medical assisting.

II I endeavor to be more effective.

III I aspire to render greater service.

IV I protect the confidence entrusted to me.

V I am dedicated to the care and well-being of all people.

VI I am loyal to my employer.

VII I am true to the ethics of my profession.

VIII I am strengthened by compassion, courage and faith.

Source: **http://www.aama-ntl.org/about/overview#.UzRbqIXLJBA.**

(see Figure 1-3). Although a professional group cannot revoke a member's license to practice, unethical members may be expelled from the group, suspended for a period of time, or ostracized by other members. Unethical behavior by a medical practitioner can result in loss of income and eventually the loss of a practice if, as a result of that behavior, patients choose another practitioner.

BIOETHICS

Bioethics is a discipline dealing with the ethical implications of biological research methods and results, especially in medicine.

bioethics
A discipline dealing with the ethical implications of biological research methods and results, especially in medicine.

As biological research has led to unprecedented progress in medicine, medical practitioners have had to grapple with issues such as these:

- What ethics should guide biomedical research? Do individuals own all rights to their body cells, or should scientists own cells they have altered? Is human experimentation essential, or even permissible, to advance biomedical research?

- What ethics should guide organ transplants? Although organs suitable for transplant are in short supply, is the search for organs dehumanizing? Should certain categories of people have lower priority than others for organ transplants?

- What ethics should guide fetal tissue research? Some say such research, especially stem cell research, is moral because it offers hope to disease victims, while others argue that it is immoral.

- Do reproductive technologies offer hope to the childless, or are they unethical? Are the multiple births that sometimes result from taking fertility drugs an acceptable aspect of reproductive technology, or are those multiple births too risky for women and their fetuses and even immoral in an allegedly overpopulated world?

- Should animals ever be used in research?

- How ethical is genetic research? Should the government regulate it? Will genetic testing benefit those at risk for genetic disease, or will it lead to discrimination? Should cloning of human organs for transplantation be permitted? Should cloning of human beings ever be permitted?

Society is attempting to address these questions, but because the issues are complicated, many questions may never be completely resolved.

THE ROLE OF ETHICS COMMITTEES

Health care practitioners may be able to resolve the majority of the ethical issues they face in the workplace from their own intuitive sense of moral values and ethics. Some ethical dilemmas, however, are not so much a question of right or wrong but more a question like, "Which of these alternatives will do the most good and the least harm?" In these more ambiguous situations, health care practitioners may want to ask the advice of a medical ethicist or members of an institutional ethics committee.

medical ethicist or bioethicist
Specialists who consult with physicians, researchers, and others to help them make difficult ethical decisions regarding patient care.

ethics committee
Committee made up of individuals who are involved in a patient's care, including health care practitioners, family members, clergy, and others, with the purpose of reviewing ethical issues in difficult cases.

Medical ethicists or **bioethicists** are specialists who consult with physicians, researchers, and others to help them make difficult decisions, such as whether to resuscitate brain-damaged premature infants or what ethics should govern privacy in genetic testing. Hospital or medical center **ethics committees** usually consist of physicians, nurses, social workers, clergy, a patient's family, members of the community, and other individuals involved with the patient's medical care. A medical ethicist may also sit on the ethics committee if such a specialist is available. When difficult decisions must be made, any one of the individuals involved in a patient's medical care can ask for a consultation with the ethics committee. Larger hospitals have standing ethics committees, while smaller facilities may form ethics committees as needed.

When a case is referred to the ethics committee, the members meet and review the case. The committee does not make binding decisions, but helps the physician, nurse, patient, patient's family, and others clarify the issue and understand the medical facts of the case and the alternatives available to resolve the situation. Ethics committees may also help with conflict resolution among parties involved with a case. They do not, however, function as institutional review boards or morals police looking for health care workers who have committed unethical acts.

See Chapter 2 for a more detailed discussion of the processes involved in making ethical decisions.

ETIQUETTE

While professional codes of ethics focus on the protection of the patient and his or her right to appropriate, competent, and humane treatment, **etiquette** refers to standards of behavior that are considered good manners. Every culture has its own ideas of common courtesy. Behavior considered good manners in one culture may be bad manners in another. For example, in some Middle Eastern countries, it is extremely discourteous for one male acquaintance to ask another, "How is your wife?" In Western culture, such a question is well received. Similarly, within nearly every profession, there are recognized practices considered to be good manners for members.

Most health care facilities have their own policies concerning professional etiquette that staff members are expected to follow. Policy manuals written especially for the facility can serve as permanent records and as guidelines for employees in these matters.

By the same token, health care practitioners are expected to know **protocol,** standard rules of etiquette applicable specifically to their place of employment. For example, when another physician telephones, does the receptionist put the call through without delay? What is the protocol in the diagnostic testing office when the technicians get behind because of a late patient or a repair to an X-ray machine?

Within the health care environment, all health care practitioners are, of course, expected to treat patients with the same respect and courtesy afforded others in the course of day-to-day living. Politeness and appropriate dress are mandatory.

etiquette
Standards of behavior considered to be good manners among members of a profession as they function as individuals in society.

protocol
A code prescribing correct behavior in a specific situation, such as a situation arising in a medical office.

Qualities of Successful Health Care Practitioners

Successful health care practitioners have a knowledge of techniques and principles that includes an understanding of legal and ethical issues. They must also acquire a working knowledge of and tolerance for human nature and individual characteristics, since daily contact with a wide variety of individuals with a host of problems and concerns is a significant part of the work. Courtesy, compassion, and common sense are often cited as the "three Cs" most vital to the professional success of health care practitioners.

LO 1.4

Discuss the characteristics and skills most likely to lead to a successful career in one of the health care professions.

COURTESY

courtesy
The practice of good manners.

The simplest definition of **courtesy** is the practice of good manners. Most of us know how to practice good manners, but sometimes circumstances make us forget. Maybe we're having a rotten day—we overslept and dressed in a hurry but were still late to work; the car didn't start so we had to walk, making us even more late; we were rebuked at work for coming in late . . . and on and on. Perhaps we're burned out, stressed out, or simply too busy to think. Regardless of a health care practitioner's personal situation, however, patients have the right to expect courtesy and respect, including self-introduction. ("Hi, I'm Maggie and I'll be taking care of you," is one nursing assistant's way of introducing herself to new patients in the nursing home where she works.)

Think back to experiences you have had with health care practitioners. Did the receptionist in a medical office greet you pleasantly, or did he or she make you feel as though you were an unwelcome intruder? (Remember Elaine in the chapter's opening scenario?) Did the laboratory technician or phlebotomist who drew your blood for testing put you at ease or make you more anxious than you already were? If you were hospitalized, did health care practitioners carefully explain procedures and treatments before performing them, or were you left wondering what was happening to you? Chances are that you know from your own experiences how important common courtesy can be to a patient.

COMPASSION

compassion
The identification with and understanding of another's situation, feelings, and motives.

Compassion is empathy—the identification with and understanding of another's situation, feelings, and motives. In other words, compassion is temporarily putting oneself in another's shoes. It should not be confused with sympathy, which is feeling sorry for another person's plight—typically a less deeply felt emotion than compassion. While "I know how you feel" is not usually the best phrase to utter to a patient (it too often earns the retort, "No, you don't"), compassion means that you are sincerely attempting to know how the patient feels.

COMMON SENSE

common sense
Sound practical judgment.

Common sense is simply sound practical judgment. It is somewhat difficult to define, because it can have different meanings for different people, but it generally means that you can see which solution or action makes good sense in a given situation. For example, if you were a nursing assistant and a gasping, panicked patient told you he was having trouble breathing, common sense would tell you to immediately seek help. You wouldn't simply enter the patient's complaint in his medical chart and wait for a physician or a nurse to see the notation. Likewise, if a patient spilled something on the floor, common sense would tell you to wipe it up (even if you were not a member of the housekeeping staff) before someone stepped in it and possibly slipped and fell. While it's not always immediately obvious that someone has common sense, it usually doesn't take long to recognize its absence in an individual.

Additional capabilities that are helpful to those who choose to work in the health care field include those that are listed in the following sections "People Skills" and "Technical Skills."

PEOPLE SKILLS

People skills are those traits and capabilities that allow you to get along well with others and to relate well to patients or clients in a health care setting. They include such attributes as the following:

- A relaxed attitude when meeting new people.
- An understanding of and empathy for others.
- Good communication skills, including writing, speaking, and listening.
- Patience in dealing with others and the ability to work as a member of a health care team.
- Tact
- The ability to impart information clearly and accurately.
- The ability to keep information confidential.
- The ability to leave private concerns at home.
- Trustworthiness and a sense of responsibility.

TECHNICAL SKILLS

Technical skills include those abilities you have acquired in your course of study, including but not limited to the following:

- Computer literacy
- Proficiency in English, science, and mathematics.
- A willingness to learn new skills and techniques.
- An aptitude for working with the hands.
- Ability to document well.
- Ability to think critically.

CRITICAL THINKING SKILLS

When faced with a problem, most of us worry a lot before we finally begin working through the problem effectively, which means using fewer emotions and more rational thinking skills. As a health care practitioner, you will be expected to approach a problem at work in a manner that lets you act as ethically, legally, and helpfully as possible. Sometimes solutions to problems must also be found as quickly as possible, but solutions must always be within the scope of your training, licensure, and capabilities. This problem-solving process is called **critical thinking**. Here is a five-step aid for approaching a problem using critical thinking:

1. **Identify and clarify the problem.** It's impossible to solve a problem unless you know the exact nature of the problem. For example, imagine that patients in a medical office have frequently complained that the wait to see physicians is too long, and several have protested

critical thinking
The ability to think analytically, using fewer emotions and more rationality.

loudly and angrily that their time "is valuable too." Rhea is the waiting room receptionist and the person who faces angry patients first, so she would like to solve this problem as quickly as possible. Rhea has recognized that a problem exists, of course, but her apologies to patients have been temporary fixes, and the situation continues.

2. **Gather information.** In the previous situation, Rhea begins to gather information. She first checks to see exactly why patients have been kept waiting, and considers the following questions: Are all the physicians simply oversleeping and beginning the day behind schedule? (Not likely, but an easy solution if this were the case would be to buy the physicians new alarm clocks.) Are the physicians often delayed in surgery or because of hospital rounds? Is the clinic understaffed? How long, on average, has each patient who has complained been left waiting beyond his or her appointment time?

3. **Evaluate the evidence.** Rhea evaluates the answers she has gathered to the earlier questions and determines that too many patients are, indeed, waiting too long beyond appointment times to see their physicians. The next step in the critical thinking process is to consider all possible ways to solve the problem.

4. **Consider alternatives and implications.** Rhea has determined that the evidence supports the fact that a problem exists and begins to formulate alternatives by asking herself these questions: Could the waiting room be better supplied with current reading material or perhaps television sets and a children's corner, so that patients both with and without children are less likely to complain about waiting? Is the waiting room cheery and comfortable, so waiting does not seem interminable? What solution would best serve the goals of physicians, other medical office personnel, and patients? Rhea must consider costs of, objections to, and all others' opinions of each alternative she considers.

5. **Choose and implement the best alternative.** Rhea selects an alternative and implements it. As a medical office receptionist, she cannot act alone, but she has brought the problem to the attention of those who can help, and her suggestions have been heard. As a result of Rhea's research, acceptable solutions to patients' complaints that they are forced to wait too long to see physicians might include the following:

    •   Patients are asked to remind receptionists when they have been waiting over 15 minutes so receptionists can check to see what is causing the delay.

    •   Additional personnel are hired to see patients.

    •   The waiting room is stocked with current news publications, television sets, and/or a child play center for patient comfort while waiting.

    Critical thinking is not easy, but, like any skill, it improves with practice.

DETERMINING IF A DECISION IS ETHICAL

While considering the legality of a certain act, health care practitioners must also consider ethical implications. According to many ethics

8. Tell how each of the following characteristics relates to law and ethics in the health care professions:

   The ability to be a good communicator and listener.

   The ability to keep information confidential.

   The ability to impart information clearly and accurately.

   The ability to think critically.

9. List and discuss each of the steps helpful to developing critical thinking skills.

10. Explain how you, as a health care practitioner, would use the critical thinking steps listed previously to reach a solution to the following problem: A patient from a different culture believes he has been cursed with a "liver demon" and will die unless the organ is surgically removed.

   _____

   _____

   _____

   _____

   _____

experts, the following questions can help you determine if an act you have decided on via critical thinking skills is ethical:

- If you perform this act, have you followed relevant laws, and kept within your employing company's policy?

- Will this act promote a win–win situation for as many of the involved individuals as possible?

- How would you feel if this act were to be publicized in the newspapers or other media?

- Would you want your family members to know?

- If you perform this act, can you look at yourself in a mirror?

The health care practitioner who demonstrates these qualities and skills, coupled with a working knowledge of law and ethics, is most likely to find success and job satisfaction in his or her chosen profession.

FIGURE 1-4 Assessing Your Strengths and Weaknesses Exercise:

Think carefully about each of the following statements; then put a check mark next to the statement that most accurately describes you. This is not a test, and there are no correct or incorrect answers; it is intended solely to help you evaluate those areas where you excel or need improvement.

☐ I like meeting new people and willingly place myself in situations where I can interact with someone new.

☐ I often make excuses in order to decline social invitations that would require me to meet and interact with new people.

☐ I can visit with anyone, and I enjoy listening to the opinions and experiences of others.

☐ I often have trouble initiating a conversation, and if forced to listen too long, my mind wanders or I find myself concentrating on my response, rather than on the conversation.

☐ If someone complains to me and I am in a position to help, I willingly explore solutions with the person who complains.

☐ I go out of my way to avoid people who chronically complain.

☐ I can tactfully tell a person the truth when necessary, without hurting feelings or fostering anger.

☐ I believe it's best to always tell others the truth, even if it risks making them angry or hurting their feelings.

☐ I know correct grammar, and always use it when writing reports or conversing with others.

☐ I can get my meaning across without always using good grammar.

☐ On the job I can listen to another person's complaints or criticism without becoming angry.

☐ Complaining about or criticizing my work always makes me angry.

☐ I can always keep private information about others to myself.

☐ One of my most endearing qualities is my inability to keep a secret.

☐ In stressful situations I keep my composure and think about the best way to proceed.

☐ I avoid stressful situations, because I tend to panic and would rather rely on someone else to tell me what to do.

☐ I am familiar with computers and enjoy learning new applications.

☐ I don't like using computers.

☐ I like science and math, and get good grades in those subjects.

☐ Science and math turn me off, and I avoid those courses whenever possible.

☐ Using my own words, both orally and in writing, I can explain technical or complicated material in a way others can easily understand.

☐ I don't like explaining complicated material to others, either orally or in writing.

Chapter Summary

Learning Outcome	Summary
LO 1.1 Explain why knowledge of law and ethics is important to health care practitioners.	**Why study law and ethics?** • Health care practitioners who function at the highest possible levels have a working knowledge of law and ethics. • Knowing the law relevant to your profession can help you avoid legal entanglements that threaten your ability to earn a living. Court cases illustrate how health care practitioners, health care facilities, and drug and medical device manufacturers can be held accountable in a court of law. • A knowledge of law and ethics will also help familiarize you with the following areas: • The rights, responsibilities, and concerns of health care consumers. • The legal and ethical issues facing society, patients, and health care practitioners as the world changes. • The impact of rising costs on the laws and ethics of health care delivery.
LO 1.2 & LO 1.3 Distinguish among law, ethics, bioethics, etiquette, and protocol; Define *moral values* and explain how they relate to law, ethics, and etiquette.	**What are the basic aspects of law and ethics, and how do they compare?** • Laws are considered the minimum standard necessary to keep society functioning. Many laws govern the health care professions, including criminal and civil statutes and medical practice acts. • Ethics are principles and standards that govern behavior. Most health care professions have a code of ethics members are expected to follow. • Bioethics is the discipline dealing with the ethical implications of biological research methods and results, especially in medicine. • Moral values define one's personal concept of right and wrong. • Etiquette refers to manners and courtesy. • Protocol is a code prescribing correct behavior in a specific situation, such as in a medical office.
LO 1.4 Discuss the characteristics and skills most likely to lead to a successful career in one of the health care professions.	**What characteristics and skills will most likely help a health care practitioner achieve success?** • People skills, such as listening to others and communicating well, are an asset to health care practitioners. • Technical skills, including a basic knowledge of computers, and a foundation in science and math are necessary to achieve an education in the health care sciences. • Critical thinking skills are required for you to correctly assess a situation and provide the proper response. Solving problems through critical thinking involves: 1. Identifying and clarifying the problem. 2. Gathering information. 3. Evaluating the evidence. 4. Considering alternatives and implications. 5. Choosing and implementing the best alternative. **What questions can help you decide if a decision is ethical?** 1. If you perform this act, have you followed relevant laws and kept within your employing company's policy? 2. Will this act promote a win–win situation for as many of the involved individuals as possible? 3. How would you feel if this act were to be publicized in the newspapers or other media? 4. Would you want your family members to know? 5. If you perform this act, can you look at yourself in a mirror?

Learning Outcomes for the Ethics Issues Feature at the End of Each Chapter

After studying the material in each chapter's Ethics Issues feature, you should be able to:

1. Discuss current ethical issues of concern to health care practitioners.

2. Compare ethical guidelines to the law as discussed in each chapter of the text.

3. Practice critical thinking skills as you consider medical, legal, and ethical issues for each situation presented.

4. Relate the ethical issues presented in the text to the health care profession you intend to practice.

Health care practitioners are bound by state and federal laws, but they are also bound by certain ethical standards—both personal standards and those set forth by professional codes of ethics and ethical guidelines, and by bioethicists. Many professional organizations for health care practitioners employ an ethics consultant who is available to speak with organization members who need help with an ethical dilemma. "We serve as a third party who can stand outside a situation and facilitate communication," says Dr. Carmen Paradis, an ethics consultant with the Cleveland Clinic's Department of Bioethics. At the Cleveland Clinic, ethics consultations are available to health care practitioners, patients, family members, and others involved with patient decisions.

Medical facility ethics committees can also serve as consultants. In larger health care facilities such committees usually deal with institutional matters, but in smaller communities where ethics consultants may not be available, members of an ethics committee may also function as ethics consultants.

Keep in mind as you read the Ethics Issues feature for each chapter that ethical guidelines are not law, but deal solely with ethical conduct for health care practitioners. Most guidelines published for professional health care practitioner organizations emphasize this difference. For example, as stated in *Guidelines for Ethical Conduct for the Physician Assistant Profession*, "Generally, the law delineates the minimum standard of acceptable behavior in our society. Acceptable ethical behavior is usually less clearly defined than law and often places greater demands on an individual. . . .

"Ethical guidelines for health care practitioners are not meant to be used in courts of law as legal standards to which practitioners will be held. Ethical guidelines are, rather, meant to guide health care practitioners and to encourage them to think about their individual actions in certain situations."

The ethical guidelines for various health care professions have several points in common, but first and foremost is that health care practitioners are obligated to provide the best care possible for every patient, and to protect the safety and welfare of every patient.

State and federal law may differ somewhat from an ethical principle. For example, a state's law may not require physicians to routinely inquire about physical, sexual, and psychological abuse as part of a patient's medical history, but the physician may feel an ethical duty to his or her patients to do so.

Furthermore, the fact that a health care practitioner who has been charged with illegal conduct is acquitted or exonerated does not necessarily mean that the health care practitioner acted ethically.

The term *ethical* as used here refers to matters involving the following:

1. Moral principles or practices.

2. Matters of social policy involving issues of morality in the practice of medicine.

The term *unethical* refers to professional conduct that fails to conform to these moral standards or policies.

The ethical issues raised are from the real-life experiences of a variety of health care practitioners and are recounted throughout the text to raise awareness of the ethical dilemmas many practitioners face daily, and to stimulate discussion.

Ethics ISSUE 1:

A physician assistant in a medical practice with several physicians contacts his professional association, the American Academy of Physician Assistants (AAPA), to report that one of his employing physicians often recommends chiropractic treatment for patients with persistent back pain issues that have resisted medical solutions. The PA knows it is legal to refer a patient for chiropractic treatments, but he adamantly opposes the practice, considering it "bogus medicine." The physician declines to discuss the matter.

Discussion Questions

1. In your opinion, how might the situation be resolved?

_____

_____

2. Is it ethical for the PA to continue working for the physician when their opinions differ so widely on this issue?

_____

_____

_____

Ethics ISSUE 2:

A registered nurse calls her professional organization's ethics consultant to ask for resources she can present to her employing medical clinic to support her intention to quit working with a physician she feels is providing sloppy and possibly dangerous care.

Discussion Questions

1. What is the most important principle for the nurse to consider here?

_____

_____

2. In your opinion, are there legal issues inherent in this situation, as well as ethical issues? Explain your answer.

_____

_____

_____

Ethics ISSUE 3:

A physician assistant (PA) has been helping treat a patient awaiting a heart transplant. The patient is depressed, and says he no longer wants to live. The PA is doubtful that the patient will cooperate in the demanding regimen required for posttransplantation patients.

Discussion Question

1. Is it ethical for the PA to say nothing to the patient's attending physician, or should he chart the patient's remarks and discuss the matter with the patient's physician?

_____

_____

Ethics ISSUE 4:

Family members of a certified medical assistant (CMA) (AAMA) employed by a medical clinic in a small community often ask the CMA for medical advice. Two of her family members have asked her to bring antibiotic samples home for them.

Discussion Question

1. In your opinion, would it be ethical for the CMA to give medical advice to her own family members? To bring drug samples home for them? Explain your answers.

_____

_____

Ethics ISSUE 5:

A radiology technician practicing in a small community is interested in dating a person he has seen as a patient.

Discussion Question

1. In your opinion, would it be ethical for the radiology technician to date one of his patients? Would it be ethical for him to date a coworker? Explain your answers.

_____

_____

Chapter 1 Review

Enhance your learning by completing these exercises and more at **http://connect.mheducation.com**!

Applying Knowledge

LO 1.1

1. List three areas where health care practitioners can gain insight through studying law and ethics.

_____

_____

_____

_____

2. Define *summary judgment*.

_____

_____

_____

_____

LO 1.2

3. Define *bioethics*.

_____

_____

_____

4. Define *law*.

_____

_____

5. Define *ethics*.

_____

_____

6. How is unethical behavior punished?

_____

_____

7. Define *etiquette*.

_____

_____

8. How are violations of etiquette handled?

_____

_____

9. What is the purpose of a professional code of ethics?

_____

_____

10. Name five bioethical issues of concern in today's society.

_____

_____

11. What duties might a medical ethicist perform?

_____

_____

12. Decisions made by judges in the various courts and used as a guide for future decisions are called what?

_____

_____

_____

_____

_____

13. Written codes of ethics for health care practitioners

   a. Evolved primarily to serve as moral guidelines for those who provided care to the sick

   b. Are legally binding

   c. Did not exist in ancient times

   d. None of these

14. What Greek physician is known as the Father of Medicine?

    a. Hippocrates

    b. Percival

    c. Hammurabi

    d. Socrates

15. Name the pledge for physicians that remains influential today.

    a. Code of Hammurabi

    b. Babylonian Ethics Code

    c. Hippocratic oath

    d. None of these

16. What ethics code superseded earlier codes to become the definitive guide for a physician's professional conduct?

    a. Code of Hammurabi

    b. Percival's Medical Ethics

    c. Hippocratic oath

    d. Babylonian Ethics Code

17. Unethical behavior is always

    a. Illegal

    b. Punishable by legal means

    c. Unacceptable

    d. None of these

18. Unlawful acts are always

    a. Unacceptable

    b. Unethical

    c. Punishable by legal means

    d. All of these

19. Violation of a professional organization's formalized code of ethics

    a. Always leads to prosecution in a court of law

    b. Is ignored if one's membership dues in the organization are paid

    c. Can lead to expulsion from the organization

    d. None of these

20. Law is

    a. The minimum standard necessary to keep society functioning smoothly

    b. Ignored if transgressions are ethical, rather than legal

    c. Seldom enforced by controlling authorities

    d. None of these

21. Conviction of a crime

    a. Cannot result in loss of license unless ethical violations also exist

    b. Is always punishable by imprisonment

    c. Always results in expulsion from a professional organization

    d. Can result in loss of license

22. Sellers and manufacturers can be held legally responsible for defective medical devices and products through what charges?

    a. Fraud

    b. Breach of warranty

    c. Misrepresentation of the product through untrue statements made by the manufacturer or seller

    d. All of these

23. The basis for ethical conduct includes

    a. One's morals

    b. One's culture

    c. One's family

    d. All of these

LO 1.2 & LO 1.3

24. What is bioethics concerned with?

    a. Health care law

    b. Etiquette in medical facilities

    c. The ethical implications of biological research methods and results

    d. None of these

LO 1.4

25. Critical thinking skills include

    a. Assessing the ethics of a situation

    b. First clearly defining a problem

    c. Determining the legal implications of a situation

    d. None of these

Case Studies

LO 1.2 & LO 1.3

Use your critical thinking skills to answer the questions that follow each case study. Indicate whether each situation is a question of law, ethics, protocol, or etiquette.

You are employed as an assistant in an ophthalmologist's office. Your neighbor asks you to find out for him how much another patient was charged for an eye examination at the eye clinic that employs you. Your neighbor also asks you how much the patient was charged for his prescription eyeglasses (the eye clinic also sells lenses and frames).

26. Can you answer either of your neighbor's questions? Explain your answer.

_____

_____

A physician employs you as a medical assistant. Another physician comes into the medical office where you work and asks to speak with your physician/employer.

27. Should you seat the physician in the waiting room, or show her to your employer's private office? Why?

_____

_____

You are employed as a licensed practical nurse (LPN) in a small town. (In California and Texas, the term for this profession is "licensed vocational nurse"—abbreviated as LVN.) A woman visits the clinic where you work, complaining of a rash on her body. She says she recently came in contact with a child who had the same symptoms, and she asks, "What did this child see the doctor for, and what was the diagnosis?" She explains that she needs to know, so that she can be immunized if necessary. You explain that you cannot give out this information, but another LPN overhears, pulls the child's chart, and gives the woman the information she requested.

28. Did both LPNs in this scenario act ethically and responsibly? Explain your answer.

_____

_____

LO 1.4

A physician admitted an elderly patient to the hospital, where she was treated for an irregular heartbeat and chest pain. The patient was competent to make her own decisions about a course of treatment, but her opinionated and outspoken daughter repeatedly second-guessed the physician's recommendations with medical information she had obtained from the Internet.

29. In your opinion, what responsibilities, if any, does a physician or other health care practitioner have toward difficult family members or other third parties who interfere with a patient's medical care?

_____

_____

30. What might the physician in this situation have said to her patient's daughter to help resolve the situation?

_____

_____

Internet Activities LO 1.1 and LO 1.2

Complete the activities and answer the questions that follow.

31. Use a search engine to conduct a search for Web sites on the Internet concerned with bioethics. Name two of those sites you think are reliable sources of information. Explain your choices. How does each site define the term *bioethics?*

_____

_____

32. Locate the Web site for the organization that represents the health care profession you intend to practice. Does the site provide guidance on ethics? If so, how? Does the site link to other sites concerning ethics? If so, list three ethics links; then explore these links.

_____

_____

33. Visit the Web site sponsored by the National Institutes of Health called Bioethics Resources (**http://bioethics.od.nih.gov/casestudies.html**). Click on the "Case Studies" link, and pick a case study and review it. Do you agree or disagree with the conclusions reached about the issue? Explain your answer.

_____

_____

Resources

Differences among law, ethics, and etiquette:

Answers.com Web site: **http://wiki.answers.com/Q/How_do_medical_ethics_differ_from_medical_etiquette.**

Critical thinking:

Sanchez, M. A. "Using Critical-Thinking Principles as a Guide to College-Level Instruction." *Teaching of Psychology* 22, no 1. (1995), pp. 72–74.

Telephone interview with Dr. Carmen Paradis, Dept. of Bioethics, Cleveland Clinic.

University of Dayton School of Law Web site: **http://academic.udayton.edu/legaled/CTSkills/CTskills01.htm.**

Other:

Barnett, Kyle. "Man Sues Hospital Who Allegedly Left Him on Bedpan for over Four Hours." *The Louisiana Record* (February 12, 2013). **http://louisianarecord.com/news/249019-man-sues-hospital-who-allegedly-left-him-on-bedpan-for-over-four-hours.**

Barnett, Kyle. "Ochsner Hospital Sued by Woman Who Slipped on Spill while Visiting Patient." *The Louisiana Record* (September 2, 2013). **http://louisianarecord.com/news/254481-ochsner-hospital-sued-by-woman-who-slipped-on-spill-while-visiting-patient.**

Barnett, Kyle. "Hospital Accused of Losing Woman's Biopsy Specimen, Necessitating a Second Biopsy." *The Louisiana Record* (September 13, 2013). **http://louisianarecord.com/news/254876-hospital-accused-of-losing-womans-biopsy-specimen-necessitating-a-second-biopsy.**

Terhune, Chad. "Surgery Photo Leads to Privacy Lawsuit against Torrance Memorial." *Los Angeles Times* (September 4, 2013). **http://articles.latimes.com/2013/sep/04.**

2

Key Terms

autonomy

beneficence

categorical imperative

confidentiality

deontological or duty-
    oriented theory

justice

needs-based
    motivation

nonmaleficence

principle of utility

role fidelity

teleological or
    consequence-
    oriented theory

utilitarianism

veracity

virtue ethics

Making Ethical Decisions

LEARNING OUTCOMES

After studying this chapter, you should be able to:

LO 2.1 Describe and compare need and value development theories.

LO 2.2 Identify the major principles of contemporary consequence-oriented, duty-oriented, and virtue ethics reasoning.

LO 2.3 Define the basic principles of health care ethics.

FROM THE PERSPECTIVE OF...

TOM AND BILL ARE RADIOLOGY TECHNICIANS at a 300-bed hospital in a large metropolitan area. Tom has been employed by the hospital for 10 years, and Bill is a recent graduate from radiology technician school and has been on the job for four months. Their supervisor, Anna, has been with the hospital for 20 years, moving up the ranks from radiology technician to manager of the department. Because they are short staffed, Anna has been helping the staff complete the required X-rays throughout the day.

One afternoon, Bill notices that Anna is late coming back from lunch. He doesn't give it a second thought because Anna is the boss and often has lunch meetings. However, while working with her that afternoon, Bill realizes that he smells alcohol on Anna's breath. He decides not to say anything. Several days later, Bill once again smells alcohol when around Anna.

Bill decides to talk with Tom about the problem. Tom confirms that he has noticed the problem also. Tom advises Bill not to say anything and offers three pieces of advice. First, Anna's behavior is not Bill's problem. Second, Anna is a supervisor, and it is difficult to understand the pressure she is under. For his final piece of advice, Tom reminds Bill that the last person hired is often the first person fired.

From Bill's perspective, he has seen a clear violation of hospital policy on the part of his supervisor.

From Tom's perspective, he has already decided he doesn't want to get involved in what could be a messy situation. The department is already short staffed, and if Anna were fired, that would mean he would have to work even harder until a new manager was found.

From Anna's perspective, she may not realize that she has a problem with alcohol. Even if she does realize that she has a problem, she may believe that the problem is not serious or she would never be fired because she has been with the hospital for so long.

Ethical decision making requires you to tap into your values, morals, and sense of fair play, so that you can be comfortable with the decisions you implement, and so that your decisions do not harm others. Study the following theories for further understanding of your own decision-making process.

Value Development Theories

LO 2.1

Describe and compare need and value development theories.

In Chapter 1, the differences between law, ethics, and etiquette were briefly discussed. Ethics was defined as standards of behavior, developed as a result of one's concept of right and wrong. One's personal concept of right and wrong, called moral values, is formed through the influence of the family, culture, and society. Because each individual experiences different family, cultural, and societal influences, like Tom and Bill in the opening scenario, individuals may see the same situation, yet determine different methods to handle the problem.

Psychologists, philosophers, and social scientists all study human behavior. Many subscribe to the idea that human behavior is a reflection of our attention to our needs or to our values. A classic work by Abraham Maslow, *Motivation and Personality,* first published in 1954, identified a hierarchy of needs that motivates our actions (see Figure 2-1). According to Maslow's theory, there are five stages of need that influence our behavior. We must satisfy each need in order, and the resulting progression is called a hierarchy. Maslow defined needs 1 to 3 as *deficiency,* or D-needs. Needs 4 and 5 are growth needs, also known as *being,* or B-needs.

1. The need for *basic life*—food and shelter.
2. The need for a *safe and secure environment.*
3. The need to *belong and to be loved.*
4. The need for *esteem,* where status, responsibility, and recognition are important.
5. The need for *self-actualization,* for personal growth and fulfillment.

Originally, Maslow believed that the needs followed a strict order, but in his later years he allowed for the possibility that some

FIGURE 2-1 Maslow's Hierarchy of Needs Pyramid

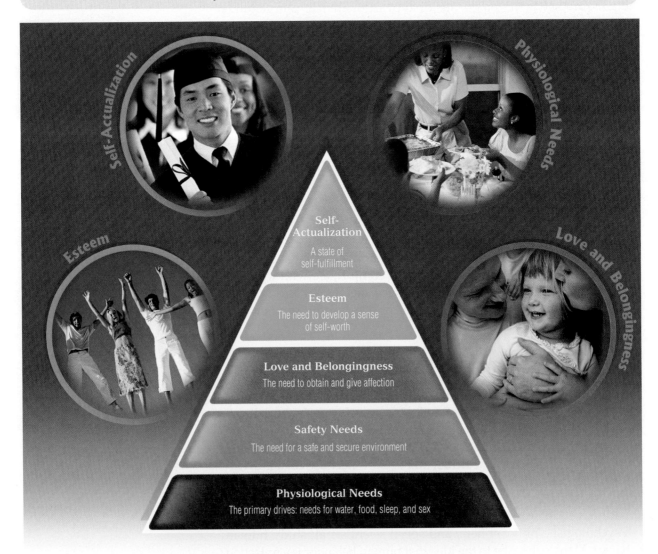

people may not require meeting all the D-needs before moving on to the B-needs.

Maslow's theory may help us understand what motivates people, but it does not always help us determine how we developed the values that guide us in ethical decision making.

Many psychologists believe that individuals move from **needs-based motivation** to a personal value system that develops from childhood. When we are born, we have no values. The value system we develop as we grow and mature is dependent on the cultural framework in which we live. If one grows up in an Asian culture, for example, honoring ancestors and tradition may emerge as prominent values; growing up in a Western culture, such as in the United States, may encourage one to place more value on materialism.

needs-based motivation
The theory that human behavior is based on specific human needs that must often be met in a specific order. Abraham Maslow is the best-known psychologist for this theory.

A variety of theories exist about how we develop values. Most focus on our stages of development from childhood to adulthood. One of the most famous researchers in this area is Jean Piaget (see Figure 2-2). By observing children at play, Piaget described four levels of moral development.

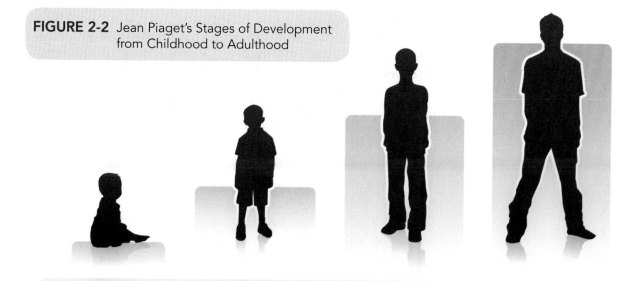

FIGURE 2-2 Jean Piaget's Stages of Development from Childhood to Adulthood

1. The first stage occurs from birth to age 2 and is called the *sensorimotor* stage, during which the child is totally self-centered. Children at this stage of development explore the world with their five senses, and cannot yet see from another's point of view.

2. As infants grow, they develop an awareness of things and people even if not in their direct sight, leading to the second stage, called the *preoperational* or egocentric stage, which extends from ages 2 to 7. During this time period, the child views the world from his or her own perspective. For example, when playing a game, the child is not particularly concerned with rules of play; the focus is on fun, not rules.

3. The third stage of Piaget's theory is called the *concrete operational* stage, extending from ages 7 to 12. In this stage, children tend to see things as either right or wrong, and to see adults as powerful and controlling.

4. Finally, during the *formal operational* stage, children develop abstract thought and begin to understand that there may be different degrees of wrongdoing. For example, children in earlier stages of development, when asked why telling a lie is wrong, may simply reply "because it's bad" whereas children in the formal operational stage can explain "because a lie isn't true." During this stage and through adulthood, intentions, such as lying (I intend to deceive you) and stealing (I intend to take that object) are central to decisions made.

Lawrence Kohlberg modified and expanded Piaget's work, laying the groundwork for modern studies on moral development. Consistent with Piaget, he proposed that children form ways of thinking through their experiences that include understandings of moral concepts such as justice, rights, equality, and human welfare. Kohlberg differed from Piaget in that he followed the development of moral judgment beyond the ages studied by Piaget, and he determined that the process of attaining moral maturity took longer and was more gradual than Piaget had proposed.

Kohlberg suggested that moral reasoning can best be understood as sequenced in six stages, grouped into three major levels:

1. Kohlberg's first major level is called *pre-conventional morality.* In the early stages of this level, children from ages 2 to 7 are egocentric, as in Piaget's first stage, and they accept the authority of others. In the second stage of pre-conventional morality, children begin to recognize that there may be more than just one view as to what is right or wrong. They begin to look at their own self-interest and begin to see advantages in the exchanging of favors.

2. The second level in Kohlberg's theory is called *conventional morality.* This level, with two stages, is when children ages 7 to 12 begin to conform to societal expectations as established by parents and social groups. The first stage in this level is sometimes referred to as "good boy/good girl" where children focus on following the expected social conventions and demonstrating good intentions. In the second stage, children become more aware of doing one's duty. The focus is on the rules and respect for authority.

3. *Post-conventional morality* (ages 12 and above) is the last level of Kohlberg's moral development theory. There are two stages to this level:

   a. The first stage of post-conventional morality focuses on the social contract and individual rights. A social contract is accepted when people freely enter into work for the benefit of all and for a pleasant society. During this stage, individuals explore how to balance individual rights and a fair society for all.

   b. The second stage of post-conventional morality is called universal principles. In this stage, the individual makes a personal commitment to such universal principles as social justice, equal rights, and respect for the dignity of all people and realizes that conventional norms and conventions are necessary to uphold society. If there is a conflict between these values and the social contract, the individual follows his or her basic principles. For example, some people want strict control of U.S. borders so that immigrants cannot cross into America illegally, and they want all illegal immigrants deported. Other individuals want people who cross into America illegally to have a fair route to citizenship.

Kohlberg's theory has recently been criticized, since much of his data were gathered from observing young males. As a result, he has revised his research methodology to account for possible gender bias.

A pharmacist/researcher has invented a drug that is very effective against a certain type of cancer. He determines that he will sell the drug for $3,000 a treatment. The drug is effective only if it is taken once every week. Harry's young wife is dying from this specific type of cancer. Harry sells everything he can and borrows money from anyone who will lend it to him, but cannot come up with enough money to pay for the drug. He approaches the pharmacist asking if the pharmacist will agree to payments or a lower fee. The pharmacist refuses, stating that he had worked very hard for many years to develop the drug and was entitled to profit from it. Harry decides to break into the pharmacy and steal the drug. (This dilemma was outlined in Kohlberg's writings and used as an example of how different levels of moral reasoning could be identified.)

1.–6. Using Kohlberg's levels of pre-conventional, conventional, and post-conventional moral reasoning, complete the following table by filling in the moral reasoning.

Level	In Favor of Stealing the Drug	Against Stealing the Drug
Pre-conventional—reward and punishment		
Conventional—please others and maintain a good society		
Post-conventional—moral principles broader than any society		

Value Choices Theories

Maslow, Piaget, and Kohlberg devised theories to help explain how we develop our values, but their theories do not tell us why moral individuals often come to different conclusions based on reasoning. Tom and Bill, the radiology technicians presented in the chapter's opening scenario, illustrate how two moral individuals can reach different solutions for a problem they both face.

As health care practitioners, we know how to perform the tasks required in doing our jobs. That is, we know the right way to take a patient's history, give an injection, take an X-ray, draw blood, or bill the insurance company for the services provided. We know what is right or wrong in performing each medical procedure. That part of the job is straightforward.

Our values, however—our concepts of right or wrong, good or evil as related to our behavior—can be subjective. Universal ethics—problems such as abortion, stem cell research, and euthanasia—are discussed in later chapters, but it is the everyday problems like Bill and Tom faced that are frustrating. They frustrate us because individuals often come to different conclusions, and thus actions, based on their personal beliefs. When faced with a difficult problem, some of us will draw conclusions based on formal religious beliefs or philosophies, while others will place more emphasis on weighing the outcomes of actions, and still others will rely heavily on past experience.

Because no professional code of ethics can address every situation found in health care, we may often find ourselves facing a problem that has no perfect and specific right or wrong solution. Moral people

LO 2.2

Identify the major principles of contemporary consequence-oriented, duty-oriented, and virtue ethics reasoning.

may agree to differ; therefore, it is important to determine a common framework for examining our value decisions.

At least three frameworks or theories exist in the literature that determine how value choices are made: teleological or consequence-oriented theory, deontological or duty-oriented theory, and virtue ethics.

TELEOLOGICAL OR CONSEQUENCE-ORIENTED THEORY

teleological or consequence-oriented theory
Decision-making theory that judges the rightness or wrongness based on the outcomes or predicted outcomes.

utilitarianism
A consequence-oriented theory that states that decisions should be made by determining what results will produce the best outcome for the most people.

Teleological or consequence-oriented theory judges the rightness of a decision based on the outcome or predicted outcome of the decision. **Utilitarianism** is the most well known of these theories. In *act-utilitarianism*, a person makes value decisions based on results that will produce the greatest balance of good over evil, everyone considered. In *rule-utilitarianism*, a person makes value decisions based on a rule, that if generally followed would produce the greatest balance of good over evil, everyone considered (Mappes and Degrazia, 2006). In Tom and Bill's problem at the beginning of the chapter, Tom is perhaps using act-utilitarianism to decide that nothing should be done as there has been no harm done and by reporting Anna, harm may occur. Bill, on the other hand, may be using rule-utilitarianism because he knows there is a rule against drinking alcohol during work hours and intoxicated employees are potential safety hazards.

Whether one uses act- or rule-utilitarianism, the process is the same. Once the person has described the problem and determined possible solutions, the solution will be based on which solution is best for all concerned. Often when describing utilitarianism, writers indicate that the solution that provides happiness or a net increase in pleasure over pain for those involved should be selected.

principle of utility
Used in utilitarianism; requires that the rule used in making a decision must bring about positive results when generalized to a wide variety of situations.

Supporters of the utilitarian theory have created a **principle of utility**. The principle of utility requires that the rule used to make the decision be a rule that brings about positive results when generalized to a wide variety of situations. There are, however, no absolute truths in utilitarianism.

DEONTOLOGICAL OR DUTY-ORIENTED THEORY

deontological or duty-oriented theory
Decision-making theory that states that the rightness or wrongness of the act depends on its intrinsic nature and not the outcome of the act.

categorical imperative
A rule that is considered universal law binding on everyone and requiring action.

Deontological or duty-oriented theory focuses on the essential rightness or wrongness of an act, not the consequences of the act. Immanuel Kant (1724–1804) is considered the father of duty-oriented theory. He defined the **categorical imperative** as the guiding principle for all decision making. This principle means that there are no exceptions (categorical) from the rule (imperative). The right action is one based on a determined principle, regardless of outcome. The rule may come from religious or other beliefs, but it is a rule not to be ignored under any circumstances. A priest who maintains the absolute confidentiality of confession even if he knows harm has come to or will come to another human being is an example of using duty-oriented decision making.

Kant argued that people may never be used as a means to an end. The Golden Rule ("do unto others as you would have them do unto you") is often cited in support of duty-oriented theory. Duty-oriented theories provide a foundation for rules of morality and for the idea of individual rights. However, critics of Kant find some of his ideas difficult to use in real life. For example, Kant argues that it is not permissible to lie or break a promise in an effort to save a third party from harm. These absolutes may create problems. For example, if a person promises to write a letter of recommendation for someone, but has to stretch the truth in order to write a favorable recommendation, does not writing the letter make the person immoral? A terminally ill patient asks a nurse questions about physician-assisted death and asks that the nurse not say anything to the family about his questions. When the family asks if the patient has asked about euthanasia, should the nurse tell the truth, even if the patient has asked that his questions be kept confidential?

VIRTUE ETHICS

Rather than focusing on decision making or reasoning to arrive at a right action, **virtue ethics** focuses on the traits, characteristics, and virtues that a moral person should have. Virtue ethicists believe that someone who has appropriate moral virtues such as practical wisdom (common sense), a sense of justice, and courage will make the right decision. Ethicists who support this idea began with Aristotle (384 B.C.E.), but Alasdair MacIntyre (1929–present) is the most well-known ethicist to write about virtue ethics. MacIntyre argued that our practice of medicine has traditions and standards of practice that apply to every health care practitioner—whether one is a technician, medical assistant, physician, nurse, coder, or other professional. He stated that if we examine our actions in our roles as health care practitioners, we will see that we often follow the dictates of an idealized role. We ask ourselves, What would a perfect medical assistant (or physician or nurse) do in this situation? In virtue ethics, the loyalty to the role we play helps us make our decision. We look to what has been done in the past, assuming that it represents the right answer.

Like the other theories, virtue ethics has its critics. First, the past may not provide the right answer. As an example, the role of nurses or

virtue ethics
Refers to the theory that people who have moral virtues will make the right decisions.

Check Your Progress

The following questions involve making a decision. Answer each question with a *yes* or a *no*. Identify whether you arrived at your answer by consequence-oriented, duty-oriented, or virtue ethics.

7. Would it be acceptable to "stretch the truth" on insurance papers so that patients could get the care needed that they could not afford under their current insurance policy?

8. Is it acceptable to date a patient? Does it make a difference if, for example, you are a medical assistant dating a physician?

9. A patient asks about a physician in the community. You think that particular physician is rude and doesn't care about his patients. Should you tell the patient who is asking about the physician what you think?

10. Would a surgical assistant with strong pro-life views be wrong in refusing to take part in a therapeutic abortion for a patient?

11. The radiology technician you work with has just done a chest X-ray on the wrong person. The patient was not hurt. Do you have to report the error to your manager?

12. A pharmacist believes that a prescription for a patient will do little to improve the patient's medical condition and may actually be contraindicated for the patient's problem. Does the pharmacist have a responsibility to talk with the physician?

FIGURE 2-3 Ethical Problem-Solving Steps

I Describe the problem. Identify the principles involved. Who will be affected by the decision? Who is ultimately in charge of making the decision?

II Collect the facts. Be sure to differentiate between fact and opinion. Are there any legal problems? Has the problem been solved before? What documentation exists?

III List the options—as many as possible.

IV Evaluate the potential options from step 3. Who benefits by the decision? Who does not benefit? What principles are maintained? What principles may need to be sacrificed? Are you going to use utilitarianism, duty-oriented theory, or virtue ethics?

V Make your decision and act.

VI After a certain amount of time, assess the results.

medical assistants even 10 years ago is different than their roles today. Previously, virtues for nurses included always following the physician's orders and never questioning authority. Today, such virtues for nurses have been replaced with playing patient advocacy and education roles. Additionally, there are new situations coming up every day in health care that have never been at issue before, such as the possibility of cloning human organs for transplant, and new medical imaging techniques that utilize the principles of particle physics, so there is no established tradition. Last, practitioners may find themselves with conflicting roles. For example, in the case at the beginning of the chapter, Bill wants to be a team player, but he also may need to report Anna for violation of hospital policy.

Making ethical decisions is not easy regardless of what model you choose to use. But whatever ethical framework is used, there are several steps that are common to them all. Figure 2-3 lists six steps to consider.

LO 2.3

Define the basic principles of health care ethics.

The Seven Principles of Health Care Ethics

Several codes of ethics were quoted in Chapter 1. Each code, such as the AAMA Code or the AMA Code, addresses a specific profession, but there are common elements in all health care professional ethics codes. The seven universal principles of health care ethics include the following:

1. AUTONOMY OR SELF-DETERMINATION

autonomy
The capacity to be one's own person and make one's own decisions without being manipulated by external forces.

The word *autonomy* comes from the Greek words *auto* (self) and *nomos* (governance). It is generally understood as the capacity to be one's own person, to make decisions based on one's own reasons and motives, not manipulated or dictated to by external forces. Autonomous decisions are characterized by:

- Competency—a person must be competent to make his or her own decision.

- The ability to act on the decision.

- Respect for the autonomy of others.

Chapter 7 discusses informed consent, which derives from the principle of autonomy, as applied to health care. Paternalism, substituting the medical provider's opinion of what is "best" for the patient for the patient's own determination of his or her best interests, often threatens the concept of autonomy in health care. Because patients may disagree with medical providers about what is best, and may not know or understand viable alternatives, informed consent is vital to preserving a health care consumer's autonomy.

Right-to-die cases, as discussed in Chapter 12, deal with a person's autonomy in making critical decisions.

The court case "Physician Charged in Assisted Suicide" is a landmark legal case that dealt with a patient's autonomy, as well as the issues of informed consent and the right to die.

2. BENEFICENCE

Although most dictionaries define **beneficence** as acts of charity and mercy, beneficence means more for the health care provider. Regardless of specialty, health care practitioners perform acts to help people stay healthy or recover from an illness. In fact, their first duty is to promote health for the patient above all other considerations. Modern medicine, however, has given rise to questions about the futility of care when discussing beneficence. For example, is it more beneficial

beneficence
Acts performed by a health care practitioner to help people stay healthy or recover from illness.

LANDMARK COURT CASE · Physician Charged in Assisted Suicide Case

In the late 1980s to early 1990s, Jack Kevorkian, a physician in Michigan, began helping terminally ill patients commit suicide. Janet Adkins, newly diagnosed with Alzheimer's disease, was Kevorkian's first public-assisted suicide in 1989. Kevorkian was charged with murder, but the Oakland County District Court dropped charges on December 13, 1990, after a two-day preliminary hearing. The court ruled that Kevorkian did not break any law by helping Adkins commit suicide because there was, at that time, no Michigan law outlawing suicide or the medical assistance of it.

Prominent issues in the case were:

- Whether Adkins was in fact giving informed consent.
- The fact that Kevorkian did not have an established professional relationship with Adkins.

- The fact that Adkins was not terminally ill (facing death within six months).

- The issue of whether or not a person actually possesses the right to die.

- The limits of autonomy.

People v. Dr. Kevorkian, No. 90-20157 52nd Dist. Ct. Mich. (1991); 534 N.W.2d. 172 (1995). Jack Kevorkian, nicknamed "Dr. Death," eventually claimed to have assisted with 130 suicides. In 1999, he was convicted of second-degree manslaughter, for which he served 8 years of a 10-to-25-year sentence. Kevorkian was released from prison in 2007, and allegedly remained unrepentant until his death on June 3, 2011.

for a patient in his nineties, who is hospitalized after suffering a series of debilitating strokes, to be maintained on a ventilator and drugs during his last days, or to be allowed to die in comfort?

3. NONMALEFICENCE

nonmaleficence
The duty to do no harm.

Nonmaleficence, as paraphrased from the Hippocratic oath, means the duty to "do no harm." Technology has made this a difficult principle to follow, since many modern-day drugs and treatments have the potential to heal, but also have serious side effects. A common example given when discussing nonmaleficence is the administration of morphine to reduce pain. Morphine is a powerful pain-killer, but it also suppresses respiration. When administering morphine, the provider's intent, of course, is to reduce pain, not to stop the patient's breathing. Accordingly, under the principle of double effect, secondary effects, such as reduced respiration or any other harmful outcome, must never be the intended result of medical treatment. The benefit to the patient must always outweigh the harm.

4. CONFIDENTIALITY

confidentiality
Keeping medical information strictly private.

The Health Insurance Portability and Accountability Act (HIPAA), discussed in detail in Chapter 8, mandates privacy and **confidentiality** of medical records, but health care practitioners who take care to maintain confidentiality at all times are equally as effective as laws. Health care practitioners mindful of protecting privacy and confidentiality, for example, do not conduct conversations about patients in the hospital hallway, in the medical office break room, or with an acquaintance. They also take care to protect computerized medical information, as detailed in Chapter 7, and when patients ask that information be kept from concerned relatives, such requests are honored.

Health care practitioners are in the most likely position to violate confidentiality rules, but others who have access to protected health care information, as defined under HIPAA, may also violate confidentiality, as in the case "Attorney Guilty of Unauthorized Disclosure."

5. JUSTICE

justice
Providing to an individual what is his or her due.

Justice, defined as what is due an individual, seems simple when applied to the U.S. health care system, but it is often complicated. Many would argue, for example, that everyone is entitled to health care, regardless of the ability to pay for the care. Others argue that the distribution of scarce resources and the expense of providing them do not allow us to provide all care for all patients. Still others argue that people must take responsibility for their actions before assuming they can have justice. For example, should a lifelong smoker who refuses to quit and develops emphysema and continues to smoke be entitled to all available health care regardless of cost? Should a motorcycle owner who refuses to wear a helmet while riding his or her motorcycle, or an automobile driver who refuses to wear a seat belt, be entitled to all available health care in the event of an accident, regardless of cost?

Attorney Guilty of Unauthorized Disclosure of Medical Information

In January 2003, a man began meeting with a psychiatrist. He confided to his doctor that he was having homicidal thoughts about his wife. The physician determined that his patient had bipolar disorder, and treated him for this condition for the next seven months.

A month into the man's psychiatric treatment, his wife filed for divorce. The man filed a counterclaim, in which he sought legal custody of the couple's minor child. While both the divorce case and the man's psychiatric treatment were ongoing, the man allegedly assaulted his wife at their home, and criminal charges were brought against him. Shortly thereafter, his wife sought and received a civil domestic-violence protection order. The order gave her temporary custody of the couple's child and suspended the man's contact and visitation rights until a full hearing could be held.

In preparation for the hearing, the wife's attorney issued subpoenas to the psychiatrist seeking the production in court of the man's medical records. The attorney mistakenly believed that the man had waived his privilege to his medical records by filing the counterclaim for custody in the divorce action. On the date of the hearing, the wife's attorney met with the prosecutor in the criminal case against the man, and she gave the prosecutor a copy of the man's medical records that she had received from his psychiatrist.

Before the hearing, the man and his wife reached a separation agreement, and the man's medical records were therefore never admitted into evidence in the divorce/protection-order case. Likewise, the man's medical records were not admitted in the criminal matter, and the man was ultimately acquitted.

The man brought an action against his ex-wife's attorney, his ex-wife, his psychiatrist, and his psychiatrist's employer, alleging improper disclosure of his medical records without his authorization. Charges against the defendants were dropped, but a court of appeals eventually held that the ex-wife's attorney "over-stepped her bounds as [the ex-wife's] attorney when she disseminated information regarding the man's psychiatric condition to the prosecution."

The court held that by giving the psychological records she obtained in the divorce case to the prosecutor in the criminal case against Hageman, attorney Belovich violated Hageman's rights to keep that information confidential. Allowing attorneys with such information obtained through discovery to treat the information as public would violate the policy of maintaining the confidentiality of individual medical records. The court therefore recognized that waiver of medical confidentiality for litigation purposes is limited to the specific case for which the records are sought, and that an attorney who violates this limited waiver by disclosing the records to a third party unconnected to the litigation may be held liable for these actions.

Hageman v. Southwest General Health Center, 119 Ohio St. 3rd, 185, 893 N.E.2d 153 (2008).

Compensatory justice, a concept that applies to medical malpractice lawsuits, refers to an individual's right to seek monetary compensation in the form of damages for a wrong done. Compensatory justice is discussed in more detail in Chapters 5 and 6. The act of seeking compensatory justice—of suing for damages for medical malpractice—has become an important part of health care today.

Ethics and laws often interconnect, as illustrated in Figure 2-4. A third element interconnecting with ethics and the law in health care is risk management—taking steps to minimize danger, hazard, and liability. Risk management is an important concept in the prevention of medical lawsuits, and is discussed further in Chapter 6.

6. ROLE FIDELITY

All health care practitioners have a specific scope of practice, for which they are licensed, certified, or registered, and from which the law says they may not deviate, as discussed in Chapters 3 and 5.

FIGURE 2-4
Conceptual Models of Law
and Ethics

Conceptual Model—Linear

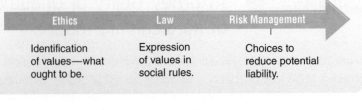

Ethics	Law	Risk Management
Identification of values—what ought to be.	Expression of values in social rules.	Choices to reduce potential liability.

Conceptual Model—Distinctions

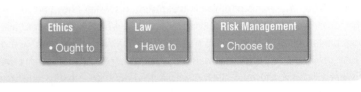

Ethics	Law	Risk Management
• Ought to	• Have to	• Choose to

Conceptual Model—Interconnectedness

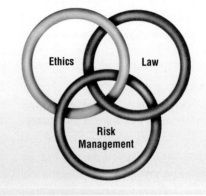

Ethics

Law

Risk Management

Source: "Understanding Relationships: Clinical Ethics, Law, and Risk Management," Lisa V. Brock, Assistant Attorney General/Senior Counsel Washington State, Anna Mastroianni, Professor, UW School of Law, March 27, 2014. **http://depts.washington.edu/bioethx/topics/law.html#models.**

role fidelity
Being faithful to the scope of the services for which you are licensed, certified, or registered.

In addition to the laws that affect scope of practice, it is a basic ethical principle that a practitioner must be true to (have **fidelity**) to his or her role. For example, a medical assistant should not diagnose a patient's condition, and a nursing assistant should not administer an intravenous drug to a patient, since such acts are not within the scope of practice for either profession.

7. VERACITY

veracity
Truth telling.

Veracity, or truth telling, has always had an ambiguous place in the health care practitioner's world. Because medical providers want to do what is best for the patient, they may not always tell the whole truth. For example, consider the use of placebos—biologically inert substances that will do no harm, but are sometimes given to patients under the guise of therapeutic treatment. Many studies have proven that if patients believe they are taking a drug that will help them, even if they are taking a placebo, their conditions may improve. In other cases, medical providers take a paternalistic view about truth telling, determining that what the patients don't know won't hurt them.

Health care ethics are drawn from the same pool of basic ethical principles that might be listed for any profession, but the nature of health care provides a unique focus. Primarily because a person's health is paramount to his or her living a successful and satisfying life, health care practitioners are routinely challenged to make sound decisions—concerning not only the appropriate medical care for each patient's condition but also the patient's future health and well-being, and sometimes the health and well-being of the patient's family. In our changing world, the use of technology, scarce resources, and the ever-increasing cost of health care all require that health care practitioners constantly strive to provide the best possible care for patients.

Check Your Progress

For each of the following actions, name a principle of health care ethics that was followed or violated, adding whether the principle was followed or violated.

13. A nurse tells a patient faced with the dilemma of deciding for or against debilitating surgery what he thinks is "best" for her.

14. A patient's medical malpractice lawsuit against a physician is dismissed in court because her HMO employer lost the patient's medical records.

15. A physician who knows one of his patients always wants to hear the truth tells him treatment for his cancer has not cured him of the disease, and he has less than a year to live.

16. An 85-year-old woman suffering from congestive heart failure is semiconscious and has been placed on a ventilator. Upon admission to the hospital, she filed a living will with the hospital, detailing her end-of-life requests, and signed a do-not-resuscitate (DNR) order. She is not expected to live beyond a matter of days, but her two daughters arrive from out of state and insist on overriding her DNR request. "Do everything to keep her alive," both daughters insist. The attending physician does not agree with the daughters, but cannot dissuade them and is obligated to comply.

17. A nurse's physician/employer asks her to dress the burn on a patient's hand after debriding the wound. The nurse knows correct procedure for dressing the burn, but she finds gloves uncomfortable and fails to wear them. The patient's burn later becomes infected.

18. A medical assistant believes her mother has a thyroid condition, so she steals samples of the appropriate medication from the clinic where she works and takes them home for her mother.

19. A medical coder who works for a group of physicians knows, through her access to patients' medical records, that Melanie, a single friend, is pregnant. When another friend asks her why Melanie is seeing a doctor, she refuses to admit even that Melanie is a patient of one of her physician/employers.

Chapter Summary

Learning Outcome	Summary

LO 2.1 Describe and compare need and value development theories.	**What classic need development theory is discussed in this chapter?**
	
	• Abraham Maslow, in *Motivation and Personality* first published in 1954, identified a hierarchy of needs that motivates our actions:
	
	Deficiency or D-needs:
	
	1. Need for basic life—food and shelter.
	2. Need for a safe and secure environment.
	3. Need to belong and to be loved.
	
	Being or B-needs:
	
	4. Need for esteem, where status, responsibility, and recognition are important.
	5. Need for self-actualization, for personal growth and fulfillment.
	
	What two value development theories are discussed in this chapter?
	
	• Jean Piaget's moral development stages:
	  • Sensorimotor stage, during which the child is totally self-centered—birth to age 2.
	  • Preoperational or egocentric stage, during which children view the world from their own perspective—ages 2 to 7.
	  • Concrete operational stage, when children see things as right or wrong and adults as all powerful—ages 7 to 12.
	  • Formal operational state, during which children practice more abstract thinking and learn there may be different degrees of wrongdoing—age 12, often extending into adulthood.
	
	• Lawrence Kohlberg's moral development stages:
	  • Pre-conventional morality—children ages 2 to 7 accept others' authority; at end of stage, recognize their own interests.
	  • Conventional morality—children ages 7 to 12 conform to others' expectations to win approval; at end of stage, focus on rules and respect for authority.
	  • Post-conventional morality (ages 12 and above).
	    a. Social contract and individual rights are balanced.
	    b. Universal principles—personal commitment to larger issues of society.

LO 2.2 Identify the major principles of contemporary consequence-oriented, duty-oriented, and virtue ethics reasoning.	**What is consequence-oriented ethics reasoning?**
	
	• Best known is utilitarianism—judge the rightness of a decision based on the outcome or predicted outcome.
	  • Act-utilitarianism—person makes value decisions based on results that will produce the greatest balance of good over evil.
	  • Rule-utilitarianism—person makes value decisions based on a rule that should produce greatest balance of good over evil.
	
	What is the principle of utility?
	
	• Requires that the rule used to make a decision bring about positive results when generalized to a wide variety of situations.
	
	What is duty-oriented ethics reasoning?
	
	• Focuses on the essential rightness or wrongness of an act, not the consequences of the act.
	• The right action is one based on a determined principle, regardless of outcome.
	
	What is virtue ethics reasoning?
	
	• People who have appropriate moral virtues will make the right decisions.

LO 2.3 Define the basic principles of health care ethics.

What ethical problem-solving steps are discussed in this chapter?

- Describe the problem and identify the principles involved.
- Collect the facts, differentiating between fact and opinion.
- List as many options as possible.
- Evaluate the potential options.
- Make your decision and act.
- After a certain amount of time, assess the results.

What are the basic principles of health care ethics?

- Autonomy or self-determination
- Beneficence
- Nonmaleficence
- Confidentiality
- Justice
- Role fidelity
- Veracity

Ethics Issues — Making Ethical Decisions

Ethics ISSUE 1:

Joyce Weathers is a 62-year-old patient with emphysema. Mrs. Weathers is a grandmother who has smoked a pack of cigarettes a day for over 40 years. She enjoys smoking and does not want to quit. Her physician has become somewhat insistent that Mrs. Weathers quit. She tries, but each time she becomes nasty and irritable around her family. She lives with her daughter and two young grandchildren. The family members want her to quit, but it becomes very unpleasant at home when Mrs. Weathers tries to quit.

Discussion Questions

1. Using act-utilitarianism as a model, create a pain-avoided, pleasure-gained list to determine if Mrs. Weathers should continue smoking.

2. If your decision is that she should quit smoking, how can Mrs. Weathers's family help her?

Ethics ISSUE 2:

An eight-year-old girl is suffering from a rare form of cancer and is in need of a bone marrow transplant. Despite searches for the past year, no donor match has been located. The parents decide to have another child, hoping that the younger child will be a blood marrow match for their eight-year-old. The baby will be born in the next three months.

Discussion Question

1. Compare consequence-oriented decision making and duty-oriented decision making in this case. In your opinion, which method of decision making will lead to the best decision for everyone concerned, or are the methods equal in that both will lead to the optimum decision?

Ethics ISSUE 3:

Martha is the administrative assistant to Valerie, the practice manager in a five-physician practice. Salaries of staff are confidential. Since payroll is handled by an outside company, only the practice manager has knowledge of who makes what salary. Valerie has gone to lunch and left her door open. Several people have been in and out of Valerie's office dropping off reports or other information. Martha goes in the office to place a report on Valerie's desk and notices that a budget worksheet, listing all staff salaries, is in clear view. It would be easy to take a quick look, especially since Martha believes she is paid less than other employees with fewer responsibilities. Martha backs out of the office and locks Valerie's door without looking at the sheet. She thinks to herself, If I should not know what everyone else is being paid, then no one else should either.

Curtis is one of the employees who had left information on Valerie's desk before Martha closed the door. He also sees the budget sheet, but does not stop to look at it. It did not occur to him to look at it, although it would have been great to know that he was being paid more than other employees. He puts his file down on Valerie's desk and thinks to himself, I will warn Valerie that she needs to be more careful about what she leaves on her desk for anyone to see.

Discussion Question

1. According to virtue ethics, who is more ethical—Martha, the one tempted to look but doesn't, or Curtis, who isn't even tempted to look? Defend your answer.

_____

_____

Chapter 2 Review

Enhance your learning by completing these exercises and more at
http://connect.mheducation.com!

Applying Knowledge

LO 2.1

1. What is another term for your personal concept of right and wrong?

   a. Utilitarianism

   b. Beneficence

   c. Moral values

   d. Role fidelity

2. Why did Tom and Bill in this chapter's opening scenario come to different decisions?

   a. Because of their age differences

   b. Because of differences in their societal, cultural, and family influences

   c. Because of their different relationships with their supervisor

   d. None of these

3. How is Abraham Maslow's theory of needs-based motivation best defined?

   a. It is a five-step progression that sees pleasure as the primary motivation for all human behavior.

   b. It is a progression called beneficence.

c. It is a theory that says human behavior is based on specific human needs that must often be met in a specific order.

d. It is a system of moral values.

4. Which of the following is *not* true of Jean Piaget's theory of value development?

a. Children in the sensorimotor stage of development see things as right or wrong.

b. During the sensorimotor stage of development, children explore the world with their five senses.

c. Children in the concrete operational stage of development see things as right or wrong.

d. Children begin to see different degrees of wrongdoing during the post-conventional stage.

5. How does Lawrence Kohlberg's theory of moral reasoning differ from Piaget's theory?

a. Kohlberg theorized that moral development occurs more gradually and takes longer than Piaget proposed.

b. Kohlberg studied adults instead of children.

c. Kohlberg studied both boys and girls, whereas Piaget did not.

d. Kohlberg does not break down moral development into stages, whereas Piaget did.

6. Which of the following is *not* true of Piaget's stages of value development?

a. During the sensorimotor stage of development, children use their five senses to explore the world.

b. The preoperational stage of development is characterized by abstract reasoning.

c. During the concrete operational stage of development, children see certain behaviors as right or wrong.

d. None of these

7. Which of the following is true of Lawrence Kohlberg's theory of the development of moral reasoning?

a. During the pre-conventional morality stage, children reject the authority of others.

b. A social contract is formed during the post-conventional morality stage.

c. Children become rebellious during the conventional morality stage.

d. None of these

LO 2.2

8. Teleological or consequence-oriented theories judge the rightness of a decision based on

a. The feelings of the person making the decision

b. The opinions of others who see the results of the decision

c. How many people agree that the decision was right

d. The outcome or predicted outcome of the decision

9. Which of the following best defines utilitarianism?

a. It is the same as pre-conventional morality.

b. It is a consequence-oriented theory that states that decisions should be made by determining what results will produce the best outcome for the most people.

c. It is a duty-oriented theory that says everyone has a duty to behave correctly.

d. It is a consequence-oriented theory that states that each individual should make decisions based on which outcome is best for him or her.

10. Which of the following best defines duty-oriented moral reasoning?

    a. Each individual's duty is to himself or herself first.

    b. Everyone should reject the authority of others and rely solely on self.

    c. It is a decision-making theory that states that the rightness or wrongness of the act depends on its intrinsic nature and not the outcome of the act.

    d. It is a form of post-conventional morality.

11. Immanuel Kant's categorical imperative states that

    a. Every rule has exceptions

    b. Only the outcome is important in decision making

    c. Feelings are not important in decision making

    d. The right action is one based on a determined principle, regardless of outcome

12. Virtue ethics focuses on

    a. The traits, characteristics, and virtues that a moral person should have

    b. The method one uses to make a moral decision

    c. Only the outcome of one's decisions

    d. The rule one uses in making a moral decision

13. Alasdair MacIntrye argues that

    a. All health care practitioners practice duty-oriented ethics reasoning

    b. Virtue ethics is the only theory that makes sense

    c. Individuals who have certain desirable qualities will make the right decisions

    d. None of these

LO 2.3

14.–20. List and define the seven basic principles of health care ethics.

_____

_____

_____

_____

_____

_____

_____

Case Studies

Use your critical thinking skills to answer the questions that follow each case study.

LO 2.3

Susan is a nursing student, arguing with her friend Linda, also a nursing student, over the benefits of getting a flu shot.

"I'm not getting a flu shot this year," Linda declares. "I paid $14 for one last year, and I still got sick. I had a horrible sinus infection that kept me out of school for days."

"I remember, but that wasn't the flu," Susan argues. "Since we see so many people in the clinic—especially older people with weakened immune systems—don't you think we, of all people, should be immunized against the flu?"

The argument continues at length, with Linda finally raising her voice and stomping off.

21. In your opinion, is the question of whether or not the nursing students should get a flu vaccine an ethical question? Explain your answer.

_____

_____

22. If you decide that this is an ethical question, which theory of moral reasoning best applies?

_____

_____

Ethan is an orderly in a skilled nursing care facility. He is charged with supervising patients in the dining room on a day when two of his coworkers have called in sick, leaving the facility shorthanded. On this day, several patients seem more irritable than usual, and Ethan is kept busy preventing outbursts and calming them. He also worries about patients prone to choking episodes, and finds himself feeling harried and stressed.

Wallace, an 80-year-old confined to a wheelchair, demands that Ethan help him back to his room. "It's a madhouse in here today," he shouts. Ethan knows he cannot leave his post, and panics when Wallace heads for the door.

Ethan runs ahead of Wallace, shuts the double doors to the dining room, and locks them.

23. Has Ethan acted ethically? Explain your answer.

_____

_____

24. What would you do in a similar situation? Use steps one through five for ethical decision making to reach a solution. Describe how each step was used.

_____

_____

25. Do you believe your solution is more ethical than Ethan's? Why or why not?

_____

_____

Internet Activities LO 2.3

Complete the activities and answer the questions that follow.

26. Locate the Web site for the organization representing the profession you plan to practice. Check the organization's code of ethics. Does the code conform to the seven principles of health care ethics? Explain your answer.

_____

_____

27. Visit the Web site for the National Center for Ethics in Health Care at **www.ethics.va.gov/resources/ethicsresources.asp.** Under the list of resource links, click on "Professionalism in Patient Care." What topics are listed under this link? How might these resources prove useful to you?

_____

_____

28. Visit Santa Clara University's Web site: **http://www.scu.edu/ethics/practicing/decision/.** Under "What is ethics?" list three things that, according to the site, ethics are _not_. Do you agree? Explain your answer. (If this URL is no longer available, do a Web search for "framework for thinking ethically." What was the number one result for this search, and how might you make use of the source?)

_____

_____

Resources

Edge, R., and J. Groves. _Ethics of Health Care: A Guide for Clinical Practice._ 3rd ed. New York: Thomson Delmar Learning, 2006.

Kohlberg, L. _The psychology of Moral Development: Essays on Moral Development._ Vol. 2. San Francisco: Harper and Row, 1984.

Kohlberg, L., and R. A. Ryncarz. "Beyond Justice Reasoning: Moral Development and Consideration of a Seventh Stage." In _Higher Stages of Human Development: Perspectives on Adult Growth,_ ed. C. N. Alexander and E. J. Langer. New York: Oxford University Press, 1990.

MacIntyre, Alasdair. _After Virtue._ Notre Dame: University of Indiana Press, 1984.

"Making Ethical Decisions," Arizona Character Education Foundation Web site: **www.azcharacteredfoundation.org/ethical.html.**

Mappes, T., and D. Degrazia. _Biomedical Ethics._ 6th ed. Boston: McGraw-Hill, 2006.

Power, F. C., A. Higgins, and L. Kohlberg. _Lawrence Kohlberg's Approach to Moral Education._ New York: Columbia University Press, 1989.

Working in Health Care

3

Key Terms

LEARNING OUTCOMES

After studying this chapter, you should be able to:

LO 3.1 Define *licensure, certification, registration,* and *accreditation.*

LO 3.2 Demonstrate an understanding of how physicians are licensed, how physicians are regulated, and the purpose of a medical board.

LO 3.3 Discuss the changing configuration of health care management.

LO 3.4 Distinguish among the different types of managed care health plans.

LO 3.5 Discuss the federal legislation that impacts health care plans.

LO 3.6 Discuss the impact of telemedicine and social media on the health care workplace.

To specialize, physicians must complete an additional two to six years of residency in the chosen specialty. When the residency is completed, specialists can then apply to the American Board of Medical Specialties (ABMS) to take an exam in their specialty. After passing this exam, physicians are board-certified in their area of specialization. For example, a specialist in oncology becomes a board-certified oncologist, and so on.

Doctor of Osteopathy (DO) Degree All 50 states also license physicians who have obtained a doctor of osteopathy (DO) degree from an accredited medical school, have successfully completed a licensing examination governed by the National Board of Osteopathic Medical Examiners, and have successfully completed the required internship and residency.

MDs and DOs spend 12 years or more training to become physicians. Both medical and osteopathic physicians prescribe drugs and practice surgery. The difference between the two is in their approach to medical treatment. Osteopathic doctors are trained to emphasize the musculoskeletal system of the body and the correction of joint and tissue problems. Medical doctors are trained in **allopathic** medicine, which means, literally, "different suffering" and emphasizes intervention in the form of drugs and/or surgery to alleviate symptoms.

Osteopathic and medical doctors can practice as generalists or primary care physicians—a designation that includes primary care specialties in family medicine/general practice, general internal medicine, and general pediatrics—or they can specialize in a specific type of medicine, such as obstetrics/gynecology, oncology, geriatrics, surgery, orthopedics, or a host of other specialties. Medical and osteopathic physicians may also further specialize in subspecialties, such as abnormalities of the hand within orthopedics, or diseases of the gastrointestinal system within internal medicine.

Recent U.S. government statistics show that in the United States, medical students are three times more likely to specialize than to remain generalists or primary care physicians. This has led to a ratio in the United States of 37.4 percent primary care physicians to 62.6 percent specialists. According to the American Medical Student Association (AMSA), reasons for the preference among medical students to specialize include these:

- Higher financial compensation for specialists (studies have found that a surgeon can earn up to seven times more than a primary care physician, per time spent with the patient).

- Decreased prestige for generalists.

- Medical training most often provided in tertiary care settings—those providing highly specialized services.

- Decreased exposure to generalist role models.

- Lack of attractiveness of general practices in, for example, rural and underserved areas because of relative isolation from technology and peer support.

A person educated in a foreign medical school who wants to practice in the United States must serve a residency and must take the Clinical Skills Assessment Exam (CSAE) before being licensed. The CSAE evaluates a candidate's ability to use the English language, to take medical histories, and to interact with patients and treat a case.

allopathic
Means "different suffering" and refers to the medical philosophy that dictates training physicians to intervene in the disease process, through the use of drugs and surgery.

THE PHYSICIAN'S LICENSE AND RESPONSIBILITIES

After physicians have finished their education and obtained licenses to practice medicine, their continued licensure falls under the jurisdiction of state medical boards (see Figure 3-1). Each state's medical board has the authority to grant or to revoke a physician's license. The federal government has no medical licensing authority except for the permit issued by the Drug Enforcement Administration (DEA) for any physician who dispenses, prescribes, or administers controlled substances, including narcotics and nonnarcotics (see Chapter 9).

When these conditions are satisfied and a license is granted, the physician who moves out of the licensing state may obtain a license in his or her new state of residence by:

- *Reciprocity*—the process by which a valid license from out of state is accepted as the basis for issuing a license in a second state if prior agreement to grant reciprocity has been reached between those states.

- *Endorsement*—the process by which a license may be awarded based on individual credentials judged to meet licensing requirements in the new state of residence.

FIGURE 3-1 Criteria for State Licensing of Physicians

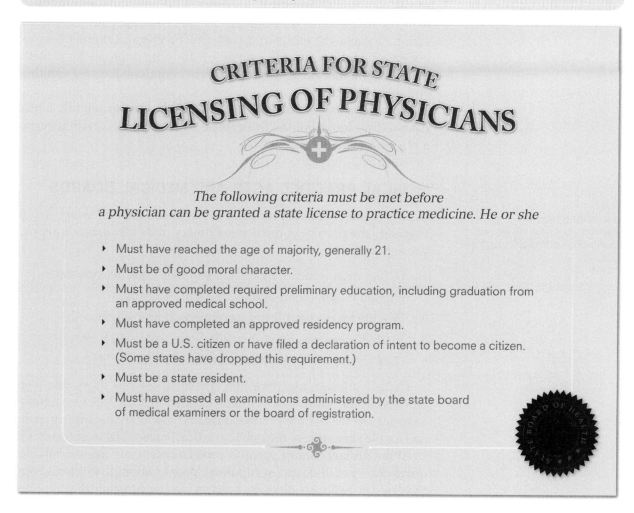

CRITERIA FOR STATE
LICENSING OF PHYSICIANS

*The following criteria must be met before
a physician can be granted a state license to practice medicine. He or she*

- Must have reached the age of majority, generally 21.
- Must be of good moral character.
- Must have completed required preliminary education, including graduation from an approved medical school.
- Must have completed an approved residency program.
- Must be a U.S. citizen or have filed a declaration of intent to become a citizen. (Some states have dropped this requirement.)
- Must be a state resident.
- Must have passed all examinations administered by the state board of medical examiners or the board of registration.

In some situations, physicians do not need a valid license to practice medicine in a specific state. These situations include the following:

- When responding to emergencies.
- While establishing state residency requirements in order to obtain a license.
- When employed by the U.S. armed forces, Public Health Service, Veterans Administration, or other federal facility.
- When engaged solely in research and not treating patients.

Physicians may be licensed in more than one state. Periodic license renewal is necessary; this usually requires simply paying a fee. However, many states require proof of continuing education units for license renewal; the average is 50 hours annually.

License Revocation or Suspension A physician's license can be revoked (canceled) or suspended (temporarily recalled) for conviction of a felony, unprofessional conduct, or personal or professional incapacity.

A felony is a crime that is punishable by death or a year or more in prison. Conviction of a felony is grounds for revocation or suspension of the license to practice medicine. Felonies include such crimes as murder, rape, larceny, manslaughter, robbery, arson, burglary, violations of narcotic laws, and tax evasion.

Unprofessional conduct is also cause for revoking or suspending a physician's license. Some states substitute the term *gross immorality* for *unprofessional conduct,* but offenses in either category are considered serious breaches of ethics and may also be illegal. Conduct deemed unprofessional includes falsifying records, using unprofessional methods to treat a disease, betrayal of patient confidentiality, fee splitting, and sexual misconduct.

Personal or professional incapacity may be due to senility, injury, illness, chronic alcoholism, drug abuse, or other conditions that impair a physician's ability to practice.

MEDICAL PRACTICE ACTS AND MEDICAL BOARDS

medical practice acts
State laws written for the express purpose of governing the practice of medicine.

In all 50 states, **medical practice acts** have been established by statute to govern the practice of medicine. Primary mandates of medical practice acts are to:

1. Define what is meant by "practice of medicine" in each state.
2. Explain requirements and methods for licensure.
3. Provide for the establishment of medical licensing boards.
4. Establish grounds for suspension or revocation of license.
5. Give conditions for license renewal.

Medical practice acts were first passed in colonial times, but were repealed in the 1800s, when citizens decided that the U.S. Constitution gave anyone the right to practice medicine. Quackery became rampant, and for the protection of the public, medical practice acts were reenacted.

Although laws are in place to protect consumers against medical quackery, even today unscrupulous people attempt to circumvent the law by hawking devices, potions, and treatments they say are "guaranteed" to cure any ailment or infirmity. Each state periodically revises its medical practice acts to keep them current with the times. Medical practice acts can be found in each state's code, which consists of laws for that state. Copies of state codes are available in most public libraries, in some university libraries, and on the Internet. (State codes as they apply to health care can be accessed electronically at official state Web sites under "medical practice acts.")

Each state's medical practice acts also mandate the establishment of **medical boards,** whose purpose is to protect the health, safety, and welfare of health care consumers through proper licensing and regulation of physicians and, in some jurisdictions, other health care practitioners. Board membership is composed of physicians and others who are, in most cases, appointed by the state's governor. Some boards act independently, exercising all licensing and disciplinary powers, while others are part of larger agencies such as departments of health. Funding for state medical boards comes from licensing and registration fees. Most boards include an executive officer, attorneys, and investigators. Some legal services may be provided by the state's office of the attorney general.

Through licensing, each state medical board ensures that all health care practitioners who work in areas for which licensing is required have adequate and appropriate education and training and that they follow high standards of professional conduct while caring for patients. Applicants for license must generally:

- Provide proof of education and training.
- Provide details about work history.
- Pass an examination designed to assess their knowledge and their ability to apply that knowledge and other concepts and principles important to ensure safe and effective patient care.
- Reveal information about past medical history (including alcohol and drug abuse), arrests, and convictions.

Each state's medical practice acts also define unprofessional conduct for medical professionals. Laws vary from state to state, but examples of unprofessional conduct include:

- Physical abuse of a patient.
- Inadequate record keeping.
- Failure to recognize or act on common symptoms.
- The prescription of drugs in excessive amounts or without legitimate reason.
- Impaired ability to practice due to addiction or physical or mental illness.
- Failure to meet continuing education requirements.
- The performance of duties beyond the scope of a license.
- Dishonesty
- Conviction of a felony.
- The delegation of the practice of medicine to an unlicensed individual.

Minor disagreements and poor customer service do not fall under the heading of misconduct.

medical boards
Bodies established by the authority of each state's medical practice acts for the purpose of protecting the health, safety, and welfare of health care consumers through proper licensing and regulation of physicians and other health care practitioners.

6. Define *medical practice acts.*

   _____

7. Where can you find the medical practice acts for your state?

   _____

8. What is the primary responsibility of state medical boards?

   _____

COURT CASE   ## Physician Disciplined by Board of Medical Examiners

A licensed pharmacist and a state pharmacy board investigator called a state's Board of Medical Examiners to express concern about a physician's prescription practices. The board investigated and found the physician had deviated from accepted standard of care by:

- Inadequately evaluating patients before prescribing antidepressants and failing to document reasons for prescriptions or following up on patients' use of the prescribed medications.

- Prescribing antibiotics for prolonged periods as treatment for urinary tract infections without determining that the infections had recurred or documenting the recurrence of the infections. The physician had also prescribed several antibiotics to a patient at once, allowing the patient to choose which antibiotic was the most effective.

- Prescribing narcotic and anxiolytic medications (drugs that relieve anxiety) to patients with nonterminal chronic pain without adequately pursuing and documenting use of available alternatives to narcotics and controlled medications.

Based on the above findings, the Board of Medical Examiners placed the physician on probation for two years and ordered him to take 60 hours of continuing education in the treatment of urinary tract infections, medical treatment of the elderly, management of chronic pain patients, and record keeping. He was also ordered to make prescription records available at all times for board inspection and was directed to stop making telephone refills for prescriptions of controlled medications.

Miller v. Board of Medical Examiners, 609 N.W.2d 478, 2000 Iowa Sup.

COURT CASE   ## State Board of Nursing Finds Nurse Incompetent

A state board of nursing found that a nurse violated the section of the state code that regulates nursing by repeatedly failing to conform to the minimum standards of practice with regard to the proper maintenance and documentation of controlled substances. Since the finding could have led to revocation of the nurse's license, the nurse filed a petition for judicial review. The district court affirmed the board's decision, and the nurse again appealed. The state court of appeals upheld both the district court and board decisions, clearing the way for temporary or permanent revocation of the nurse's license, or other penalty. (No final decision is available, since the opinion has not yet been published.)

Several times while on duty, the nurse failed to properly document and account for missing controlled substances. In one instance, she claimed containers of morphine and other drugs had fallen from her pocket while she was running down a stairwell. On other occasions, she claimed drug ampules had broken in her pocket, or she had misplaced syringes filled with controlled substances. Since her stories could not be corroborated, and she did not properly document losses or destruction of controlled drugs, the state court of appeals upheld the state board of nursing's finding that the nurse was incompetent in violating minimum standards of acceptable nursing practice.

Matthias v. Iowa Board of Nursing, 2-153/01-1019, 2002 Iowa App.

It is important to remember that while a variety of health care practitioners often work together as a team to provide medical care to patients, each individual is legally able to perform only those duties dictated by professional and statutory guidelines. Each health care practitioner is responsible for understanding the laws and rules pertaining to his or her job and for knowing requirements concerning renewal of licenses; recertification; and payment of fees for licensure, certification, and registration.

Fraud may, in some states, be considered unprofessional conduct, or it may be separately specified as grounds for revoking a physician's license. A physician is considered guilty of fraud if "intent to deceive" can be shown. Acts generally classified as fraud include:

- Falsifying medical diplomas, applications for licenses, licenses, or other credentials.
- Billing a governmental agency for services not rendered.
- Falsifying medical reports.
- Falsely advertising or misrepresenting to a patient "secret cures" or special powers to cure an ailment.

Check Your Progress

9. In the United States, physicians may be licensed to practice medicine as MDs or as DOs. Distinguish between the two.

_____

_____

_____

10. Name three types of unprofessional conduct for which a physician may lose his or her license.

_____

_____

_____

Fill in the blanks or answer the following questions in the spaces provided.

11. A physician is licensed by the _____ in which he or she wishes to practice.

12. The federal government's authority regarding medical licensing extends only to

_____ .

13. Give one example of fraud. _____ .

14. Name four situations in which physicians do not need a valid license to practice in a specific state.

_____

_____

_____

_____

Revocations and suspensions of license are never automatic. A physician is always entitled to a written description of charges against him or her and a hearing before the appropriate state agency. If a hearing is held, the physician also has the right to counsel, the right to present evidence in his or her defense, the right to confront and question witnesses, and any other rights granted by state law. Decisions are usually subject to appeal through the state's court system.

An honest mistake or a single incident of alleged incompetence or negligence is not usually sufficient grounds for license revocation.

Medical Practice Management Systems

LO 3.3

Discuss the changing configuration of health care management.

sole proprietorship
A form of medical practice management in which a physician practices alone, assuming all benefits and liabilities for the business.

Physicians have traditionally established medical management systems for the delivery of health care, but such systems have evolved over time, from the **sole proprietorships** most common before 1960, to various forms of staffing configurations and practice consolidations prevalent in today's health care marketplace. (A sole proprietorship consisted of a physician practicing alone, assuming all responsibility and liability for his services.)

Today's economic realities—for instance, the advent of managed care organizations, reduced Medicare reimbursements, and higher technology costs—are transforming the practice of modern medicine. Now fewer physicians practice alone. In fact, hospitals, private equity firms, and even health insurance companies are acquiring physician practices to the extent that according to a recent survey by Accenture, a global management consulting firm, just 39 percent of doctors nationwide are practicing independently, down from 57 percent in 2000.

group practice
A medical management system in which three or more licensed physicians share the collective income, expenses, facilities, equipment, records, and personnel for the business.

Consolidation arrangements may take the form of **group practices,** where three or more physicians engage full time in providing health care services. They share the collective income of the practice, as well as expenses, facilities, equipment, patient records, and personnel necessary for running the business. Physicians in group practice may be engaged in the same specialty, calling themselves, for example, Urology Associates, or they may provide care in two or three related specialties, such as obstetrics-gynecology and pediatrics. Alternatively, they may offer a variety of services, for example, obstetrics-gynecology, pediatrics, family practice, and internal medicine.

Some of the more familiar forms of group practice include:

associate practice
A medical management system in which two or more physicians share office space and employees but practice individually.

- **Associate Practice.** Two or more physicians decide to practice individually but agree to share office space and employees. This arrangement allows a sharing of expenses, but usually not a sharing of profits or liability.

partnership
A form of medical practice management system whereby two or more parties practice together under a written agreement specifying the rights, obligations, and responsibilities of each partner.

- **Partnership.** Two or more parties practice together under a written agreement specifying the rights, obligations, and responsibilities of each partner. Advantages of partnerships include sharing the workload and expenses, and pooling profits and assets. A major disadvantage is that each partner has equal liability for the acts, conduct, losses, and deficits of the partnership, unless specific provisions are made for these contingencies in the initial agreement.

professional corporation
A body formed and authorized by law to act as a single person.

- **Professional Corporation.** A body formed and authorized by law to act as a single person, although constituted by one or more persons and legally endowed with various rights and duties. State law governs corporations, so requirements for incorporation may vary. The corporation may own, mortgage, or sell property; manage its own business affairs; and sue or be sued. Physicians who form corporations are shareholders and employees of the organization. There are financial and tax advantages to forming a corporation, and fringe benefits to employees may be more generous than with a sole proprietorship or partnership. Forming a corporation also means that the incorporators and owners have limited liability in case lawsuits are filed.

In the past, hospitals were hubs within health care delivery systems serving specific areas. Physicians admitted patients to hub hospitals and were paid a fee for services rendered; hospitals were reimbursed separately for providing the facility, equipment, and personnel for servicing patients. Today, with the growing number of privately-owned ambulatory care centers, diagnostic facilities, surgical centers and specialty hospitals, the health care delivery system offers a complicated variety of services and staffing arrangements. For instance, with the advent of managed care organizations (MCOs), physicians are often salaried employees of hospitals, clinics, or other entities, which in turn are part of for-profit or not-for-profit corporate networks. (One example of such a not-for-profit arrangement is the Mayo Clinic Health Care and Research System, which employs salaried physicians and other health care practitioners in various locations within the United States.) In fact, large, for-profit health care service corporations, such as Hospital Corporation of America, the largest U.S. hospital chain as of 2014, are increasingly the norm for health care delivery.

Just as methods of health care delivery have morphed from sole physicians in private practice to the corporate model, managed care organizations have entered the health care marketplace as corporate entities that link health care financing, administration, and service delivery.

Types of Managed Care

Managed care organizations are corporations that pay for and deliver health care to subscribers for a set fee using a network of physicians and other health care providers. The network coordinates and refers patients to its health care providers and hospitals and monitors the amount and patterns of care delivered. The plans usually limit the services subscribers may receive under the plans. Managed care plans make agreed-upon payments to providers (hospitals or physicians) for providing health care services to health care subscribers. The payment from a managed care plan to providers may be one of several types, including contracted fee schedules, percentages of billed charges, capitation, and others. (*Capitation* is a set advance payment made to providers, based on the calculated cost of medical care of a specific population of subscribers.)

Before managed care plans, private health insurance policies were traditionally written as third-party indemnity health insurance. *Third party* means that the insurance company reimburses health care practitioners for medical care provided to policyholders. Indemnity is coverage of the

LO 3.4

Distinguish among the different types of managed care health plans.

managed care
A system in which financing, administration, and delivery of health care are combined to provide medical services to subscribers for a prepaid fee.

insured person against a potential loss of money from medical expenses for an illness or accident. Indemnity health insurance policies are fee-for-service and usually allow enrollees to see any doctor.

In an attempt to confront increasing health care costs—due in part to increasingly large awards in litigation, an aging population that requires more health care, the expensive technology used in modern-day medicine, and the impact of third-party payers for medical care—traditional fee-for-service health insurance companies now incorporate elements of managed care into their plans. (The impact of third-party payers is that there is little incentive to keep health care costs down when health care providers and recipients know that a third party—Medicare, Medicaid, other insurance—will pay.) Consequently, virtually all insured Americans have become familiar with such cost-containment/managed care measures as coinsurance, copayment fees, deductibles, formularies, and utilization review.

- *Coinsurance* refers to the amount of money insurance plan members must pay out of pocket, after the insurance plan pays its share. For example, a plan may agree to pay 80 percent of the cost for a surgical procedure, and the subscriber must pay the remaining 20 percent.

- *Copayment* fees are flat fees that insurance plan subscribers pay for certain medical services. For example, a subscriber might be required to make a $20 copayment for each visit to a physician office.

- *Deductible* amounts are specified by the insurance plan for each subscriber. For instance, the deductible for a single subscriber might be $500 a calendar year. In other words, the plan does not begin to pay benefits until the $500 deductible has been satisfied.

- *Formularies* are a plan's list of approved prescription medications for which it will reimburse subscribers.

- *Utilization review* is the method used by a health plan to measure the amount and appropriateness of health services used by its members.

HEALTH MAINTENANCE ORGANIZATIONS

Health maintenance organizations (HMOs) are one of several types of managed care organizations providing health care services to subscribers within the United States. HMOs and preferred provider organizations (PPOs) are the most common types of managed care plans. Under HMO plans, all health services are delivered and paid for through one organization. The three general types of HMOs are group model HMOs, staff model HMOs, and individual (or independent) practice associations (IPAs).

Group model HMOs contract with independent groups of physicians to provide coordinated care for large numbers of HMO patients for a fixed, per-member fee. They often provide medical care for members of several HMOs. Group model HMOs include prepaid group practices (PGPs). Physicians in PGPs are salaried employees of the HMO, usually practice in facilities provided by the HMO, and share in profits at the end of the year.

Staff model HMOs employ salaried physicians and other allied health professionals who provide care solely for members of one HMO. Subscribers to staff model HMOs can often see their doctors, get laboratory tests and X-rays, have prescriptions filled, and even order eyeglasses or contact lenses all in one location. Staff model HMOs also employ specialists or contract with outside specialists in some cases.

An **individual (or independent) practice association (IPA)** is an association of physicians, hospitals, and other health care providers that contracts with an HMO to provide medical services to subscribers. Health care practitioners who are members of an IPA may usually still see patients outside the contracting HMO. The providers who contract with an IPA practice in their own offices and receive a per-member payment, or capitation, from participating HMOs to provide a full range of health services for HMO members. These providers often care for members of several HMOs, which gives them a larger patient and income base than staff model HMOs.

individual (or independent) practice association (IPA)
A type of HMO that contracts with groups of physicians who practice in their own offices and receive a per-member payment (capitation) from participating HMOs to provide a full range of health services for members.

PREFERRED PROVIDER ORGANIZATIONS

Preferred provider organizations (PPOs), also called **preferred provider associations (PPAs),** are managed care plans that contract with a network of doctors, hospitals, and other health care providers who provide services for set fees. Subscribers may choose their primary health provider from an approved list and must pay higher out-of-pocket costs for care provided by health care practitioners outside the PPO group.

preferred provider organization (PPO)
A network of independent physicians, hospitals, and other health care providers who contract with an insurance carrier to provide medical care at a discount rate to patients who are part of the insurer's plan. Also called **preferred provider association (PPA).**

PHYSICIAN-HOSPITAL ORGANIZATIONS

Physician-hospital organizations (PHOs) are another type of managed care plan. PHOs are organizations that include physicians, hospitals, surgery centers, nursing homes, laboratories, and other medical service providers that contract with one or more HMOs, insurance plans, or directly with employers to provide health care services.

physician-hospital organization (PHO)
A health care plan in which physicians join with hospitals to provide a medical care delivery system and then contract for insurance with a commercial carrier or an HMO.

OTHER VARIATIONS IN MANAGED CARE PLANS

Managed care plans may also include the following identifying features:

- Gatekeeper or primary care plan. The insured must designate a **primary care physician (PCP).** Also known as a gatekeeper physician, the primary care physician directs all of a patient's medical care and generates any referrals to specialists or other health care practitioners.

primary care physician (PCP)
The physician responsible for directing all of a patient's medical care and determining whether the patient should be referred for specialty care.

- Point-of-service (POS) plan. Point-of-service plans allow plan members to seek health care from nonnetwork physicians, but the plan pays the highest benefits for care when given by the PCP or via a referral from the PCP. When care is provided without a referral, but still within the network, the plan pays benefits at a reduced level. Members also have out-of-network benefits, but at greatly reduced payment levels.

- Open access plan. Under open access plans, subscribers may see any in-network health care provider without a referral.

The National Committee for Quality Assurance (NCQA), the accrediting agency mentioned earlier, has introduced a new concept in primary care called the Patient-Centered Medical Home (PCMH). The organization offers accreditation to qualifying primary care practices implementing PCMH, and helps patients find those practices. The goal is to offer patients:

- Long-term partnerships between patients and clinicians, instead of patients being limited to sporadic, hurried visits.
- Physician-led teams that will coordinate care, especially for illness prevention and chronic conditions.
- An organization that will coordinate other clinicians' care and resources within the community, as needed.
- Enhanced access, which will include expanded hours and online communication.
- A share in decision making, ensuring informed choices and improved results.
- Improved quality of care without ever denying care.

An important added benefit, according to NCQA, is that insurers will pay for these services because they save more than they cost.

Managed care plans differ from one another in some respects, but all are designed to cut the cost of health care delivery. The impact of cost-cutting measures on the quality of health care remains a major point of contention. Advocates claim that managed care plans can deliver medical services more efficiently and at much less expense than traditional fee-for-service plans. Critics argue that necessary, quality medical services are often sacrificed for profit margins. The following questions are of special concern to patients enrolled in managed care plans:

- Will the most knowledgeable and experienced physician treat my medical conditions and those of my family?
- Is my physician too concerned with saving money?
- Must I fight to get routine procedures from my HMO?
- What if my HMO refuses to pay for a procedure I need?

In addition, physicians and other medical professionals, administrators of managed care plans, government officials, and HMO members are concerned with issues such as these:

- Do managed health care and competition actually drive down costs?
- Do regulations exist regarding patient rights in managed care plans?
- Do quality ratings for HMOs help consumers?
- Does managed health care provide higher-quality care than fee-for-service medicine?

Managed care is a fixture of modern medicine, but health care consumers and practitioners continue to debate its advantages and disadvantages, and may do so for many years to come.

15. Discuss two ways medical practice management systems have changed over time.

_____

_____

16. Define *managed care.*

_____

_____

17. What were two of the original objectives for establishing managed care?

_____

_____

18. Name and list distinguishing characteristics of three types of managed care plans.

_____

_____

19. Briefly define the concept *Patient-Centered Medical Home.*

_____

_____

Legislation Affecting Health Care Plans

PATIENT PROTECTION AND AFFORDABLE CARE ACT (PPACA)

When Barack Obama was elected President of the United States in 2008, he vowed to initiate comprehensive changes in the American health care system. After months of heated debate, H.R. 3590, the **Patient Protection and Affordable Care Act** (usually abbreviated **ACA**) was signed into law on March 23, 2010. Additional changes to the health care system were enacted by the **Health Care Education and Reconciliation Act,** signed into law on March 30, 2010. The two acts mandated major changes in the American health care system, which included the following (see Table 3-1) at the time they were passed:

LO 3.5
Discuss the federal legislation that impacts health care plans.

Patient Protection and Affordable Care Act (PPACA)
A federal law enacted in 2010 to expand health insurance coverage and otherwise regulate the health insurance industry.

Health Care Education and Reconciliation Act (HCERA)
Also enacted in 2010, a federal law that added to regulations imposed on the insurance industry by PPACA.

Table 3-1 PPACA Provisions Effective in 2010

Issue	Effect
Temporary high-risk insurance pool	Creates a national pool to provide health coverage for individuals with preexisting conditions who have been uninsured for six months.
Preexisting conditions	Prevents insurance companies from denying coverage to children with preexisting medical conditions.

(continued)

Table 3-1 (continued)

Issue	Effect
Adult children	Insurance companies must cover dependent children up to age 26.
Coverage limits	Insurance plans cannot place lifetime limits on coverage and cannot rescind coverage except for fraud.
Tanning salons	A 10 percent tax is imposed on indoor tanning services.
Preventive care	Insurance plans must cover preventive services such as vaccinations for children and cancer screening for women.
Medicare recipients	Some Medicare patients receive a $250 rebate to help cover the cost of medications.
*Tax credit for business	Small businesses with 25 or fewer employees can receive tax credits for the 2010 tax year to help pay for offering employees health insurance.

*In 2013, compliance for small businesses was pushed ahead to January 1, 2015.

Changes implemented in 2011 concerned annual fees imposed on pharmaceutical manufacturers, tax changes on health care savings accounts, closing the Medicare "doughnut hole" for seniors who experience a gap in drug coverage, paying bonuses through Medicare fees to primary care doctors and general surgeons practicing in underserved areas, funding community health centers for low-income people, and requiring insurance companies to pay rebates to enrollees if they spent less than 80–85 percent of premium dollars on health care as opposed to administrative costs.

In 2012 and 2013, the annual fees on drug makers were to increase, limits were placed on contributions to health care savings accounts, the threshold for out-of-pocket medical expenses on income tax forms increased, and the Medicare tax rate increased.

Table 3-2 PPACA Provisions Effective 2014 through 2018

Year	Issue	Effect
2014	Health insurance exchanges	State-run health care exchanges for uninsured individuals and small businesses created.
	Individual mandate	Everyone must have health insurance or pay a fine. Companies with 50 or more employees will pay a fine if any of their full-time workers qualified for federal subsidies.
	Medicaid expansion	Income eligibility increased for those under 65.
	Federal subsidies	Federal subsidies will help lower income people buy insurance.
	Annual insurance company fees	Annual fees imposed on health insurance companies.
2015–2016	Individual mandate	Penalties for not carrying insurance are increased each year.
	Annual insurance company fees	Annual fees imposed on health insurance companies increase.
2017–2018	Annual fee on drug manufacturing	Annual fee on pharmaceutical manufacturers is increased each year.
	Annual insurance company fees	Annual fees imposed on health insurance companies are increased each year.
	Excise tax on high-cost insurance plans	A 40 percent excise tax is imposed on the more expensive health care plans.

As a provision of the ACA, health care insurers were encouraged to unite with health care providers to form **accountable care organizations (ACOs).** The accountable care model emphasized preventive care, health care team coordination, electronic health records, treatment based on proof, and day or night access. Those ACOs that met quality standards might also reward doctors and hospitals for controlling costs and improving patient outcomes by allowing them to keep a portion of what they save.

The Affordable Care Act called for establishing ACOs for certain groups of patients, such as those receiving Medicare, the chronically ill, those with high hospital usage, and those with mild health risks such as asthma or high blood pressure. However, at the beginning of 2014, ACOs had been established just for patients on Medicare.

The extent of the effect of the 2010 legislation on health care plans in the United States remains to be seen as provisions are rewritten, postponed, or otherwise enacted over time.

Earlier legislation that has impacted health care insurers, providers, and consumers in the United States includes the following health care legislation.

HEALTH INSURANCE PORTABILITY AND ACCOUNTABILITY ACT

The **Health Insurance Portability and Accountability Act (HIPAA) of 1996** was an ambitious attempt by Congress to reform the American health care system. The HIPAA helps workers keep continuous health insurance coverage for themselves and their dependents when they change jobs, but its many provisions go far beyond this mandate. The primary objectives of the law were to:

1. Improve the efficiency and effectiveness of the health care industry by:
   - Accelerating billing processes and reducing paperwork.
   - Reducing health care billing fraud.
   - Facilitating tracking of health information.
   - Improving accuracy and reliability of shared data.
   - Increasing access to computer networks within health care facilities.

2. Help employees keep their health insurance coverage when transferring to another job.

3. Protect confidential medical information that identifies patients from unauthorized disclosure or use.

HIPAA also created the Healthcare Integrity and Protection Data Bank (HIPDB), but a provision of the 2010 Patient Protection and Affordable Care Act merged the HIPDB with the National Practitioner Data Bank. HIPDB is a national health care fraud and abuse data collection program for the reporting and disclosure of certain adverse actions taken against health care providers, suppliers, or practitioners. Data from the combined HIPDB and the NPDB are available to federal and state government agencies and to health plans, but are not available to the general public.

Accountable care organization (ACO)
A health care payment and delivery model that could reward doctors and hospitals for controlling costs and improving patient outcomes by allowing them to keep a portion of what they save if standards of quality are met.

Health Insurance Portability and Accountability Act (HIPAA) of 1996
A federal statute that helps workers keep continuous health insurance coverage for themselves and their dependents when they change jobs, protects confidential medical information from unauthorized disclosure or use, and helps curb the rising cost of fraud and abuse.

HEALTH CARE QUALITY IMPROVEMENT ACT

In creating the Health Care Quality Improvement Act (HCQIA) of 1986, Congress found that "the increasing occurrence of medical malpractice and the need to improve the quality of medical care have become nationwide problems that warrant greater efforts than those that can be undertaken by any individual state." Accordingly, the act requires that professional peer review action be taken in some cases. It also limits the damages for professional review and protects from liability those who provide information to professional review bodies.

One of the most important provisions of the HCQIA was the establishment of the National Practitioner Data Bank (NPDB). Use of the NPDB was intended to improve the quality of medical care nationwide by encouraging effective professional peer review of physicians and dentists. Information that must be reported to the NPDB includes medical malpractice payments, adverse licensure actions, adverse clinical privilege actions, and adverse professional society membership actions. The NPDB is a resource to assist state licensing boards, hospitals, and other health care entities in investigating the qualifications of physicians, dentists, and other health care practitioners.

National Practitioner Data Bank queries are mandatory for physicians when they apply for privileges at a hospital, and every two years for physicians already on the medical staff who wish to maintain their privileges. They are voluntary for hospitals conducting professional review, other health care entities with formal peer review programs, state licensing boards at any time, those who wish to self-query, and plaintiffs' attorneys under certain circumstances. The NPDB may not disclose information to a medical malpractice insurer, defense attorney, or member of the general public.

LO 3.6

Discuss the impact of telemedicine and social media on the health care workplace.

telemedicine
Remote consultation by patients with physicians or other health professionals via telephone, closed-circuit television, or the Internet.

Telemedicine

Telemedicine refers to remote consultation with physicians or other health care professionals via telephone (both landline and smartphone), closed-circuit television, fax machine, or the Internet. When telemedicine was first used, it generally involved transmission of X-rays, sonograms, or other medical data between two distant points. In some cases, usually through closed-circuit television, a physician could examine a patient in a distant location, thus allowing patients in rural areas more complete access to medical care. Today, transmitted medical data includes video, audio, and written or computerized patient data. In fact, increasing use of the Internet has made telemedicine an important component of the health care system, and one that health care practitioners should be prepared to use.

According to the American Telemedicine Association (ATA), telemedicine provides the following services:

- *Primary care and specialist referral services.* Primary care physicians can ask specialists to review a patient's medical history, laboratory and X-ray results, medications, and other data for help in making a diagnosis or in other aspects of the patient's care.

- *Remote patient monitoring.* Through remote transmission, medical data for homebound patients can be sent to home health agencies or remote diagnostic testing facilities for interpretation. Data can be specific to one condition, such as blood glucose levels, or it can cover a broader area of concern. These services often supplement home health care visits.

- *Consumer medical and health information.* Through use of the Internet and/or wireless devices, consumers can find specific information about medical conditions, locate support and discussion groups, learn about prescribed medications, and so on. This aspect of telemedicine includes the use of **patient portals** for patients with computers or smartphones to schedule appointments with physicians, review lab results, ask for medication refills, see educational materials, and otherwise communicate with health care providers.

- *Medical education.* Physicians and other health care professionals can enroll in online courses where relevant, attend professional seminars remotely, hear specialists speak, and otherwise participate in continuing education.

patient portal
A secure online Web site that gives patients 24-hour availability to health care providers.

Another aspect of telecommunication that the Health Research Institute says is actually "changing the nature of health-related interactions" is social media. The term social media includes social networking sites, such as Facebook, LinkedIn, and Twitter, as well as media sharing sites, blogs, microblogs, subject-specific discussion sites, and wikis, which are Web sites that allow collaborative editing of content and structure.

HRI's 2012 report, "Social Media 'Likes' Healthcare: From Marketing to Social Business," lists four characteristics of social media networks that are especially adaptable to health-related interactions:

1. User-generated content
2. Community
3. Rapid distribution
4. Open two-way dialogue

Consider the following documented incidents of health-related social media use:

- A diabetic patient tweets about her long wait in a hospital emergency room. Someone on the hospital staff sees her tweet and responds, even sending a person to talk to her.

- A high school student with a rare cancer posts her diagnosis on her Facebook page and a nurse sees the post and refers the student to a nearby specialist.

- Diabetic patients with problems controlling blood sugar and energy levels post journals, and even strangers respond with recipes and helpful tips about diet and exercise.

- A patient with multiple sclerosis posts a YouTube video showing how a new drug has helped him with movement issues, and 5,000 watchers post questions and comments.

- One large insurance company partnered with a social media company to offer Life Game, an online social game to help players with personal wellness goals.

The Health Research Institute survey found that 42% of respondents had used social media to access health-related consumer reviews;

Kubasek, Nancy, et al. *Dynamic Business Law.* New York: McGraw-Hill/Irwin, 2009.

Liuzzo, Anthony L. *Essentials of Business Law.* New York: McGraw-Hill, 2010.

Mappes, Thomas A., and David DeGrazea. *Biomedical Ethics.* New York: McGraw-Hill, 2005, chap. 3.

Moini, Jahangir. *Medical Assisting Review.* New York: McGraw-Hill, 2008, chap. 8.

"Social Media 'Likes' Healthcare: From Marketing to Social Business," *Health Research Institute,* April 2012.

Telephone interview November 5, 2007, with Dr. Carmen Paradis, Dept. of Bioethics, Cleveland Clinic. She provided a copy of the Cleveland Clinic Health System's "Code of Ethical Business and Professional Behavior," quoted in Ethics Issue 1.

Law, the Courts, and Contracts

4

Key Terms

administrative law
breach of contract
case law
civil law
common law
constitutional law
contract
criminal law
defendant
executive order
felony
jurisdiction
law of agency
legal precedents
minor
misdemeanor
negligence
plaintiff
procedural law
prosecution
respondeat superior
Statute of Frauds
statutory law
substantive law
tort
tortfeasor
void

LEARNING OUTCOMES

After studying this chapter, you should be able to:

LO 4.1 Discuss the basis of and primary sources of law.

LO 4.2 Discuss the classifications of law.

LO 4.3 Define the concept of torts and discuss how the tort of negligence affects health care.

LO 4.4 List and discuss the four essential elements of a contract and differentiate between expressed contracts and implied contracts.

LO 4.5 Discuss the contractual rights and responsibilities of both physicians and patients.

LO 4.6 Relate how the law of agency and the doctrine of *respondeat superior* apply to health care contracts.

FROM THE PERSPECTIVE OF. . .

"SOMETIMES PATIENTS DON'T UNDERSTAND that what they are asking us to do is insurance fraud," says Christine, a patient billing specialist who works for a hospital in the Pacific Northwest. When Babs, a hospital patient, was treated for breast cancer, her physician obtained her informed consent to use a new treatment that he had helped develop. A drug was injected into her breast that targeted for destruction just the small malignant tumor; no healthy tissue was destroyed. Babs's medical insurance company refused to pay for the procedure, claiming it was "experimental." The procedure was new, but Babs's physician had used it many times with success. "Can't you just say I had a traditional lumpectomy," Babs asked Christine, "so my insurance company will pay for it?"

"We had to explain to Babs that this would constitute insurance fraud, and we couldn't do it," Christine explains.

From Babs's perspective, she wanted her insurance company to help pay for the expensive procedure.

From Christine's perspective, lying about the procedure performed was not only illegal but also unethical.

LO 4.1

Discuss the basis of and primary sources of law.

The Basis of and Primary Sources of Law

THE FEDERAL GOVERNMENT

Federal laws governing the administration of health care and all other national matters derive from powers and responsibilities delegated to the three branches of government by the U.S. Constitution. As you probably recall from basic government classes, the three branches of government are legislative, executive, and judicial. Here is a quick review of the three branches' composition and responsibilities.

The two houses of Congress—the Senate and the House of Representatives—make up the *legislative branch.* Each member of Congress is elected by the people of his or her state. The House of Representatives, with membership based on state populations, has 435 seats, while the Senate, with two members from each state, has 100 seats. Members of the House of Representatives are elected for two-year terms, and senators are elected for six-year terms. The primary duty of Congress is to write, debate, and pass bills, which are then passed on to the president for approval.

Other powers of Congress include:

- Making laws controlling trade between states and between the United States and other countries.
- Making laws about taxes and borrowing money.
- Approving the printing of money.
- Declaring war on other countries.

Functions specific to the House of Representatives include the following. Members of the House can:

- Introduce legislation that compels people to pay taxes.
- Decide if a government official should be put on trial before the Senate if he or she commits a crime against the country. (Such a trial is called *impeachment*.)

Functions specific to the Senate include the following. Senators can:

- Approve and disapprove any treaties the president makes.
- Approve or disapprove any people the president recommends for jobs, such as cabinet officers, Supreme Court justices, and ambassadors.
- Hold an impeachment trial for a government official who commits a crime against the country.

The president of the United States is the chief executive of the *executive branch* of government, which is responsible for administering the law. Through his or her ability to issue **executive orders**, the president has limited legislative powers. Executive orders become law without the prior approval of Congress. They are usually issued for one of three purposes: to create administrative agencies or change the practices of an existing agency, to enforce laws passed by Congress, or to make treaties with foreign powers.

executive order
A rule or regulation issued by the president of the United States that becomes law without the prior approval of Congress.

The U.S. Supreme Court heads the *judicial branch* of government, which also includes federal judges and courts in every state. The judicial branch interprets the law and oversees the enforcement of laws.

The division of powers and responsibilities among three branches of government ensures that a system of checks and balances will keep any one branch from assuming too much power (see Figure 4-1).

STATE GOVERNMENTS

State governments also have three branches: *legislative, executive,* and *judicial.* The number of state legislators a state may elect is based on the number of political districts in each state, since citizens elect legislators from the various districts. Therefore, the numbers of members of state legislatures are not the same as the number of members in the U.S. Congress.

State legislative branches also consist of two chambers: the Senate and the House of Representatives. In some states, the House of Representatives is called the Assembly or General Assembly. Terms served may be the same as in the federal government—six years for senators and two years for representatives or assembly members—or they may differ.

The governor is the head of the state's executive branch. Each state has its own constitution, but state constitutions cannot conflict with the U.S. Constitution. Those responsibilities not delegated by the federal constitution are left to the states (see Table 4-1).

There are four types of law, distinguished according to their origin:

1. **Constitutional law** is based on a formal document that defines broad governmental powers. Federal constitutional law is based

constitutional law
Law that derives from federal and state constitutions.

office may be an accessory to insurance fraud if he or she takes no action, even though he or she knows that some health care practitioners are billing for services not rendered.

CIVIL LAW

civil law
Law that involves wrongful acts against persons.

Criminal law involves crimes against the state; **civil law** does not involve crimes but instead involves wrongful acts against persons. Under civil law, a person can sue another person, a business, or the government. Civil disputes often arise over issues of contract violation, slander, libel, trespassing, product liability, or automobile accidents. Many civil suits involve family matters such as divorce, child support, and child custody. Court judgments in civil cases often require the payment of a sum of money to the injured party.

Check Your Progress

Fill in the blanks or answer the following questions in the spaces provided.

7. The written law that says murder is a crime is an example of _____ law.

8. The law that says a law enforcement officer must read a prisoner his or her rights is an example of which type of law?

9. One who contributes to or aids in the commission of a crime. _____

10. The laws that determine the rules for one person's suing of another are broadly classified as

_____ law.

11. _____ law involves crimes against the state.

12. _____ law involves wrongful acts against persons.

13. Which two types of law are most likely to affect health care providers?

14. Under criminal law, practicing medicine without a license is classified as a(n)

_____ .

15. Which type of law does not involve crimes, but may involve one person suing another?

16. Court judgments in lawsuits against health care practitioners most often include what as a penalty?

LO 4.3

Define the concept of torts and discuss how the tort of negligence affects health care.

tort
A civil wrong committed against a person or property, excluding breach of contract.

Tort Liability

Civil law includes a general category of law known as torts. A **tort** is broadly defined as a civil wrong committed against a person or property, excluding breach of contract. The act, committed without just cause, may have caused physical injury, resulted in damage to someone's property, or deprived someone of his or her personal liberty and freedom. Torts may be intentional (willful) or unintentional (accidental).

INTENTIONAL TORTS

Some torts involve intentional misconduct. When one person intentionally harms another, the law allows the injured party to seek a remedy in a civil suit. The injured party can be financially compensated for any harm done by the **tortfeasor** (person guilty of committing a tort). If the conduct is judged to be malicious, punitive damages may also be awarded. Examples of intentional torts include the following:

tortfeasor
The person guilty of committing a tort.

Assault. The open threat of bodily harm to another, or acting in such a way as to put another in the "reasonable apprehension of bodily harm."

Battery. An action that causes bodily harm to another. It is broadly defined as any bodily contact made without permission. Battery may or may not result from the threat of assault. In health care delivery, battery may be charged for any unauthorized touching of a patient, including such actions as suturing a wound, administering an injection, or performing a physical examination.

Defamation of Character. Involves damaging a person's reputation by making public statements that are both false and malicious. Defamation can take the form of libel or slander. Libel is expressing in published print, writing, pictures, or signed statements content that injure the reputation of another. Libel also includes reading statements aloud or broadcasting for the public to hear. Slander is speaking defamatory or damaging words intended to prejudice others against an individual in a manner that jeopardizes his or her reputation or means of livelihood.

False Imprisonment. The intentional, unlawful restraint or confinement of one person by another. The offense is treated as a crime in some states. Refusing to dismiss a patient from a health care facility on his or her request, or preventing an employee or patient from leaving the facility might be seen as false imprisonment.

Fraud. Deceitful practices in depriving or attempting to deprive another of his or her rights. Health care practitioners might be accused of fraud for promising patients "miracle cures" or for accepting fees from patients for using mystical or spiritual powers to heal.

Invasion of Privacy. An intrusion into a person's seclusion or private affairs, public disclosure of private facts about a person, false publicity about a person, or use of a person's name or likeness without permission. Improper use of or breaching the confidentiality of medical records may be seen as invasion of privacy.

Intentional torts may also be crimes. Therefore, some civil wrongs may also be prosecuted as criminal acts in separate court actions. See Table 4-2 for a summary of intentional torts.

UNINTENTIONAL TORTS

The more common torts within the health care delivery system are those committed unintentionally. Unintentional torts are acts that are not intended to cause harm but are committed unreasonably or

Table 4-2 Intentional Torts

Tort	Description
Assault	Threatening to strike or harm with a weapon or physical movement, resulting in fear
Battery	Unlawful, unprivileged touching of another person
Trespass	Wrongful injury to or interference with the property of another
Nuisance	Anything that interferes with the enjoyment of life or property
Interference with contractual relations	Intentionally causing one person not to enter into or to break a contract with another
Deceit	False statement or deceptive practice done with intent to injure another
Conversion	Unauthorized taking or borrowing of personal property of another for the use of the taker
False imprisonment (false arrest)	Unlawful restraint of a person, whether in prison or otherwise
Defamation	Wrongful act of injuring another's reputation by making false statements
Invasion of privacy	Interference with a person's right to be left alone
Misuse of legal procedure	Bringing legal action with malice and without probable cause
Infliction of emotional distress	Intentionally or recklessly causing emotional or mental suffering to another
Fraud	Dishonest or deceitful practices in depriving, or attempting to deprive, another of his or her rights

negligence

An unintentional tort alleged when one may have performed or failed to perform an act that a reasonable person would or would not have done in similar circumstances.

with a disregard for the consequences. In legal terms, this constitutes **negligence**.

Negligence is charged when a health care practitioner fails to exercise ordinary care, and a patient is injured. The accused may have performed an act or failed to perform an act that a reasonable person, in similar circumstances, would or would not have performed. "Didn't intend to do it" or "should have known better" best describe a negligent act. Under principles of negligence, civil liability exists only in cases in which the act is judicially determined to be wrongful. A health care practitioner, for example, is not necessarily liable for a poor-quality outcome in delivering health care. He or she becomes liable only when his or her conduct is determined to be malpractice, the negligent delivery of professional services.

Negligence and defenses to liability suits are discussed in detail in Chapter 5.

Negligence is often alleged in lawsuits against health care practitioners, as in the case, "Chiropractor's Outrageous Conduct Results in Trial." As illustrated in the court case on page 93, hospitals are not immune to charges of negligence.

Most times we think of medical negligence cases as those brought against doctors or medical personnel individually, but a hospital or other institution is held to the same standard of care as a doctor or a physician. So when evaluating a case for institutional negligence, the standard is, What would/should a reasonably careful hospital do under similar circumstances?

There are two different ways a hospital can face liability under medical malpractice. A hospital can be held liable for the medical negligence conducted by its agents or employees, or it can be liable for

COURT CASE   Chiropractor's Outrageous Conduct Results in Trial

A chiropractor had two patients who became his employees. The two patients/employees sued the chiropractor for outrageous conduct and invasion of privacy, based on the fact that each plaintiff had a sexual relationship with the chiropractor, and when the two plaintiffs told the chiropractor they wanted to end their sexual relationships with him, he threatened to stop their medical treatment and to fire them. He also exposed himself to the two plaintiffs in his office, and allegedly otherwise harassed them sexually.

A trial court found for the two plaintiffs, and the chiropractor appealed. The appellate court concluded that the trial court did not err in determining that "reasonable people could find the chiropractor's conduct so outrageous in character, and so extreme in degree, as to go beyond all possible bounds of decency and be regarded as atrocious and utterly intolerable." The judgment of the trial court was affirmed.

The jury awarded Pearson $237,685 in compensatory damages on her chiropractic negligence claim, $100,000 in compensatory and punitive damages on her claim for outrageous conduct, and $200,000 in compensatory and punitive damages on her claim for invasion of privacy. The jury awarded Fahy $229,400 in compensatory damages on her chiropractic negligence claim and $100,000 in compensatory and punitive damages on her claim for outrageous conduct. The trial court entered judgment accordingly.

Note: Whether or not the chiropractor lost his license to practice was not decided by this court but was a matter for his state licensing board to decide.

Pearson and Fahy v. Kancilla, 70 P.3d 594 (Colo. App. 2003).

COURT CASE   Physician Sued for Negligence

A physician sterilized a female patient who had sought such a procedure to avoid having more children. The woman later became pregnant and delivered a healthy child. She sued her physician, alleging that the doctor's performance of a sterilization procedure had been negligent and seeking damages for the future expenses of raising a child. The physician filed a motion for preliminary determination. A trial court denied the motion, permitting the plaintiff to seek damages for raising the child. The physician appealed.

The appellate court held that the parents were not "injured" by delivering a healthy child, and, therefore, could not receive an award for damages. The court reversed the trial court's order denying the physician's motion for preliminary determination and remanded the case for "further proceedings consistent with this opinion."

Chaffee v. Seslar, 786 N.E.2d 705; 2003 Ind.

COURT CASE   Chicago Hospital's Negligence Clarified by Illinois Appellate Court

In 2008, the Illinois Appellate Court affirmed a Cook County jury's $2.7 million verdict for institutional negligence against Loyola Medical Center in a Chicago transplant error case.

The issue in *Longnecker* was whether Loyola University Medical Center was negligent when it transplanted the decedent with a severely hypertrophic replacement heart. The harvested heart was severely diseased and was considered for transplantation only because the harvesting doctors did not examine it. Despite the diseased state of the new heart, the decedent's heart surgeon went ahead with the transplant. The decedent died without ever waking up from the surgery.

Longnecker v. Loyola University Medical Center, 2008 WL 2550686 (1st Dist., June 25).

its own institutional negligence. According to legal experts, a hospital owes its patients a duty to exercise a reasonable degree of care when dealing with an apparent risk.

Various types of evidence are useful in establishing a hospital's standard of care, including expert testimony, existing federal and state laws, hospital bylaws, custom and community practice, and accreditation standards. And while expert testimony is typically required in medical malpractice cases, sometimes institutional negligence can be established without expert testimony.

THE COURT SYSTEM

The type of court that tries a case depends on the state law or federal law that was allegedly violated. The federal court system, with some exceptions, hears cases involving federal matters. State court systems are independent of one another, and each system has its own rules and regulations. Generally, state courts decide cases involving matters occurring within their own state borders.

Federal Courts **Jurisdiction** is the power of a court to hear and decide a case before it. In most common law systems, jurisdiction is conceptually divided between jurisdiction over the subject matter of a case and jurisdiction over the person of the litigants. Examples of cases over which federal courts have jurisdiction include federal crimes, federal antitrust law, bankruptcy, patents, copyrights, trademarks, suits against the United States, and areas of admiralty law (pertaining to the sea).

State Courts Each state has its own court system, but the general structure is the same in all states. The bottom tier consists of local courts. The next highest tier is trial courts, followed by appellate courts, and then the state supreme court. As with the federal court system, there are also special state courts with jurisdiction in certain kinds of cases.

Figure 4-3 shows the various federal and state court systems in the United States.

Players in the Court Scene When criminal and civil cases go to court, a complaining party—the **plaintiff**—must show that he or she was wronged or injured. The government—the **prosecution**—is the plaintiff in criminal cases. A private individual is the plaintiff in civil cases. The **defendant**, who is charged with an offense, must dispute the complaint.

Officers of the court are responsible for carrying out courtroom duties:

- *Judges* are elected or appointed to preside over the court and in most states must be licensed attorneys. They rule on points of law about trial procedure, presentation of evidence, and all laws that apply to the case. If there is no jury, the judge determines the facts in the case. Judges hand down sentences after a verdict is rendered.

- *Attorneys* represent plaintiffs and defendants, presenting evidence so that the jury or the judge can reach a verdict.

- *Court clerks* keep court records and seals, enter court orders and judgments into the record, and keep the papers of the court.

jurisdiction
The power of a court to hear and decide a case before it.

plaintiff
The person bringing charges in a lawsuit.

prosecution
The government as plaintiff in a criminal case.

defendant
The person or party against whom charges are brought in a criminal or civil lawsuit.

- *Bailiffs* keep order in the courtroom and may remove disruptive persons from the court at the judge's request.
- *Court reporters* make a running account of all court proceedings, using a stenotype machine that types shorthand symbols onto a tape.
- *Juries* are most often selected from lists of registered voters. Six or 12 jurors are chosen to hear the evidence presented in court and render a verdict.

FIGURE 4-3 Court Systems in the United States

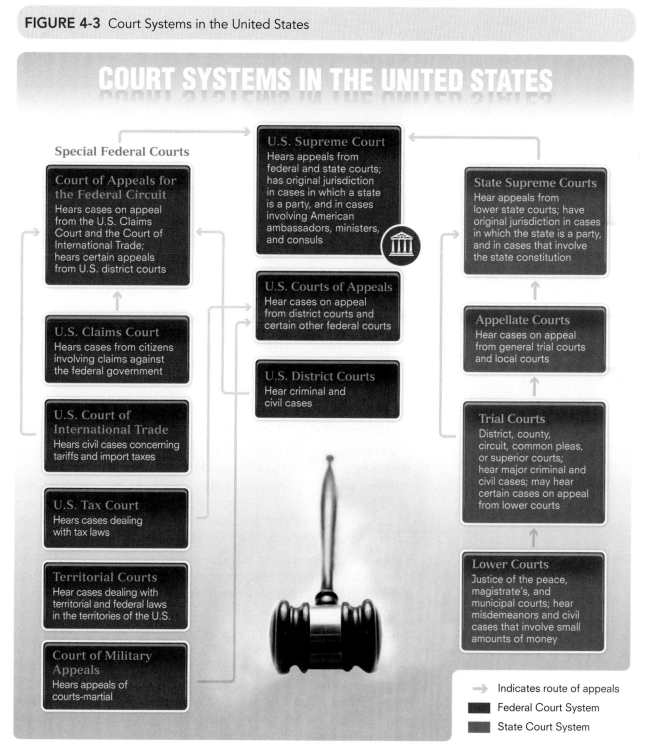

COURT SYSTEMS IN THE UNITED STATES

Special Federal Courts

Court of Appeals for the Federal Circuit
Hears cases on appeal from the U.S. Claims Court and the Court of International Trade; hears certain appeals from U.S. district courts

U.S. Claims Court
Hears cases from citizens involving claims against the federal government

U.S. Court of International Trade
Hears civil cases concerning tariffs and import taxes

U.S. Tax Court
Hears cases dealing with tax laws

Territorial Courts
Hear cases dealing with territorial and federal laws in the territories of the U.S.

Court of Military Appeals
Hears appeals of courts-martial

U.S. Supreme Court
Hears appeals from federal and state courts; has original jurisdiction in cases in which a state is a party, and in cases involving American ambassadors, ministers, and consuls

U.S. Courts of Appeals
Hear cases on appeal from district courts and certain other federal courts

U.S. District Courts
Hear criminal and civil cases

State Supreme Courts
Hear appeals from lower state courts; have original jurisdiction in cases in which the state is a party, and in cases that involve the state constitution

Appellate Courts
Hear cases on appeal from general trial courts and local courts

Trial Courts
District, county, circuit, common pleas, or superior courts; hear major criminal and civil cases; may hear certain cases on appeal from lower courts

Lower Courts
Justice of the peace, magistrate's, and municipal courts; hear misdemeanors and civil cases that involve small amounts of money

→ Indicates route of appeals
■ Federal Court System
■ State Court System

Fill in the blanks to accurately complete the following statements.

17. The highest tier of federal courts consists of _____.

18. A lawsuit brought by a patient against a health care practitioner would be heard first in a(n)

_____ court.

19. Torts are wrongs committed against _____.

20. The two broad types of torts include _____ and

_____.

21. The type of tort most likely to concern health care practitioners is

_____.

LO 4.4

List and discuss the four essential elements of a contract and differentiate between expressed contracts and implied contracts.

contract
A voluntary agreement between two parties in which specific promises are made for a consideration.

void
Without legal force or effect.

breach of contract
Failure of either party to comply with the terms of a legally valid contract.

Contracts

A **contract** is a voluntary agreement between two parties in which specific promises are made for a consideration. The elements of a contract are important to health care practitioners because health care delivery takes place under various types of contracts. To be legally binding, four elements must be present in a contract.

1. *Agreement.* One party makes an offer, and another party accepts it. Certain conditions pertain to the offer:

   - It can relate to the present or the future.
   - It must be communicated.
   - It must be made in good faith and not under duress or as a joke.
   - It must be clear enough to be understood by both parties.
   - It must define what both parties will do if the offer is accepted.

   For example, a physician offers his or her services to the public by obtaining a license to practice medicine and opening for business. Patients accept the physician's offer by scheduling appointments, submitting to physical examinations, and allowing the physician to prescribe or perform medical treatment. The contract is complete when the physician's fee is paid.

2. *Consideration.* Something of value is bargained for as part of the agreement. In the previous example, the physician's consideration is providing his or her services; the patient's consideration is payment of the physician's fee.

3. *Legal Subject Matter.* Contracts are not valid and enforceable in court unless they are for legal services or purposes. For example, a contract entered into by a patient to pay for services of a physician in private practice would be **void** (not legally enforceable) if the physician were not duly licensed to practice medicine. **Breach of contract** may be charged if either party fails to comply with the terms of a legally valid contract.

Breach of Contract Also Charged in Medical Negligence Lawsuit

A nurse treated an inmate at the county jail with an injection of 200 mg of Prolixin decanoate that resulted in the inmate's permanent impotence. He filed an action against the nurse, the hospital, and the health care organization for negligence and breach of contract. A jury found for the plaintiff and awarded him damages in the amount of $450,500. The defendants appealed the decision and the award. An appeals court upheld the trial court's decision and award, except for $100,000 awarded as part of the breach-of-contract claim. The appeals court held that since the plaintiff was not part of the contract between the nurse and her employer, he was not entitled to damages on that claim.

Dempsey v. Pease, Mercy Health Services, St. Joseph Mercy Hospital (Court of Appeals of Michigan, 2001).

4. *Contractual capacity.* Parties who enter into the agreement must be capable of fully understanding all of its terms and conditions. A mentally incompetent person cannot enter into a legal contract. For example, persons declared legally insane, persons in a drug-altered mental state, and in some cases, persons under extreme duress are considered incapable of entering into a contract. Exceptions may be made for situations in which a contract is necessary to sustain life.

If either of the concerned parties is incompetent at the time a contract is made, the agreement may be voidable, that is, able to be set aside or to be validated at a later date. Say, for example, a patient enters into a contract while under the effects of a medication that can interfere with judgment. After the effects of the medication have worn off, the patient may say, "No, I don't want the contract enforced" or "Yes, I want the contract enforced."

Of special concern to health care providers is the physician–patient contract as applied to minors. Because of the risk of being accused of battery or assault, health care practitioners cannot treat a minor without the consent of a responsible parent or legal guardian, except in cases where minors suffer a life-threatening emergency, or have been legally determined to be mature. A **minor** is defined as anyone under the age of majority, which is 18 in most states, and 21 in some jurisdictions. See Chapter 11 for a more extensive discussion of minors and the administration of medical services.

Sometimes breach of contract becomes an additional issue in medical negligence lawsuits, as in the above case, "Breach of Contract Also Charged in Medical Negligence Lawsuit."

minor
Anyone under the age of majority: 18 years in most states, 21 years in some jurisdictions.

Types of Contracts

The two main types of contracts are expressed contracts and implied contracts. Expressed contracts are explicitly stated in written or spoken words. Implied contracts are unspoken. Their terms result from actions of the involved parties.

EXPRESSED CONTRACTS

An expressed contract may be written or oral, but all terms of the contract are explicitly stated. In the medical office, some contracts, to be

FIGURE 4-6 Form for Patient Discharged against Medical Advice

Health &
wellness Center

William Smith
1212 Economy Drive
Dallas, Texas
75001

Date _____   Time _____ A.M. / P.M.

_____
Signature of Party Leaving Against Medical Advice

WITNESS: IF PARTY DEMANDING DISCHARGE IS OTHER THAN PATIENT:

_____   _____

Signature of Witness   Signature of Party

Relationship _____

INSTRUCTIONS: This demand for discharge should be signed by the patient or authorized party if he/she insists on leaving the Wellness Medical Center against medical advice. If the patient or authorized party not only demands to leave but also refuses to sign this form the following should be completed: _____
(Name of Party Demanding Discharge)
has not only demanded discharge but also has refused to sign this form documenting his/her demand.

Date _____   Time _____ A.M. / P.M.

_____
Signature of Person Receiving Demand

LO 4.6

Relate how the law of agency and the doctrine of *respondeat superior* apply to health care contracts.

law of agency
The law that governs the relationship between a principal and his or her agent.

Law of Agency and Doctrine of *Respondeat Superior*

By law, employers are liable for the actions of their employees when employees perform said actions as part of their work under the supervision of the employer. This is called the **law of agency**. In performing workplace duties, the employee acts as the agent of the employer.

Agency may be expressed or implied. In the medical office, it is most often implied. Medical office employees act as the physician's agent when they schedule appointments, speak with patients and other individuals, order supplies for the office, or otherwise perform duties ordered by and supervised by the employing physician in the conduct of his or her business.

Under the doctrine of **respondeat superior,** or "Let the master answer," physicians are liable for the acts of their employees performed "within the course and scope" of employment if two elements are present. First, the servant (employee) must be engaged in furtherance of the master's business; and, second, he or she must be acting within the scope of the master's business. If a tortious act (implying or involving a tort) is committed not in furtherance of the employer's business, but rather for purely personal reasons disconnected from the authorized business of the master, the master is not liable under the doctrine of *respondeat superior.*

respondeat superior
Literally, "Let the master answer." A doctrine under which an employer is legally liable for the acts of his or her employees, if such acts were performed within the scope of the employees' duties.

COURT CASE — Case Tried under *Respondeat Superior*

A patient underwent surgery at a hospital during which a sheath was inserted in an artery of his groin. An employee of the hospital was authorized to enter the patient's hospital room alone, check the groin area for complications, and clean the area. Following the surgery, the patient awoke to discover the employee fondling his genitals. The patient and his wife sued the hospital under the doctrine of *respondeat superior* for assault, battery, and loss of consortium.

The trial court granted summary judgment to the hospital on the grounds that an employer was not liable for the sexual misconduct of an employee. The plaintiff appealed, and the appellate court reversed because it found a question of fact existed about whether the deviation from job responsibilities was great enough to affect the hospital's liability. The hospital appealed, and the state supreme court found the hospital could not be held liable because the employee's conduct was for purely personal reasons and did nothing to further the hospital's business.

Piedmont Hospital, Inc. v. Palladino, et al., 276 Ga. 612, 580 S.E.2d 215; 2003 Ga. April 29, 2003.

Chapter Summary

Learning Outcome	Summary
LO 4.1 Discuss the basis of and primary sources of law.	**What is the basis of law in the United States?** • Federal statutes • State statutes • Municipal ordinances • Constitutional law: Law that derives from federal and state constitutions. • Case law: Law established through common law and legal precedent. • Common law: The body of unwritten law developed in England, primarily from judicial decisions based on custom and tradition.

LO 4.2 Discuss the classifications of law.	**How are laws classified?**
	
	• Substantive: The statutory or written law that defines and regulates legal rights and obligations.
	  • Criminal law involves crimes against the state.
	    • A felony is a criminal offense punishable by death or by imprisonment in a state or federal prison for more than one year.
	    • A misdemeanor is a crime punishable by fine or imprisonment in a facility other than a prison for less than one year.
	  • Civil law does not involve crimes, but instead involves wrongful acts against persons. Under civil law, a person can sue another person, a business, or the government.
	• Procedural: Law that defines the rules used to enforce substantive law.

LO 4.3 Define the concept of torts and discuss how the tort of negligence affects health care.	**What are torts, and how do they affect health care practitioners?**
	
	• A tort is a civil wrong committed against a person or property, excluding breach of contract.
	  • Intentional torts involve intentional misconduct.
	  • Unintentional torts are acts that are not intended to cause harm but are committed unreasonably or with a disregard for the consequences. In legal terms, this constitutes negligence, a charge most often alleged against health care practitioners.

LO 4.4 List and discuss the four essential elements of a contract and differentiate between expressed contracts and implied contracts.	**What is a contract, and what are its essential elements?**
	
	• A contract is a voluntary agreement between two parties in which specific promises are made for a consideration. It includes:
	  • The agreement: One party makes an offer, and another party accepts it.
	  • The consideration: Something of value is bargained for as part of the agreement.
	  • Legal subject matter: Contracts are not valid and enforceable in court unless they are for legal services or purposes.
	  • Contractual capacity: Parties who enter into the agreement must be capable of fully understanding all of its terms and conditions.
	
	How do expressed contracts differ from implied contracts?
	
	• Expressed contracts are spoken or written in precise terms.
	• Implied contracts are not spoken or written in precise terms, but are understood.

Learning Outcome	Summary
LO 4.5 Discuss the contractual rights and responsibilities of both physicians and patients.	What are the contractual rights and responsibilities of both physicians and patients? A physician has the right to: • Set up practice within the boundaries of his or her license to practice medicine. A specialist, for instance, does not have to practice outside the area of specialty and, in fact, would be severely criticized for doing so, except in an emergency in which no other physician were available. • Set up an office wherever he or she chooses and establish office hours. • Specialize • Decide which services he or she will provide and how those services will be provided. The physician has the obligation to: • Use due care, skill, judgment, and diligence in treating patients. • Stay informed about the best methods of diagnosis and treatment. • Perform to the best of his or her ability. • Exercise his or her best professional judgment in all cases. • Consider the established, customary treatment administered by members of the medical profession in similar cases. • Abstain from performing experiments on a patient without first securing the patient's complete understanding and approval. • Provide proper instructions for a patient's care to the person responsible for such care. • Furnish complete information and instructions to the patient about diagnosis, options and methods of treatment, and fees for services. • Take every precaution to prevent the spread of contagious disease. • Advise patients against needless or unwise operations. Patients have the right to: • Receive considerate and respectful care. • Receive complete current information concerning his or her diagnosis, treatment, and prognosis. • Receive information necessary to give informed consent prior to the start of any procedure and/or treatment. • Refuse treatment to the extent permitted by law. • Receive every consideration of his or her privacy. • Be assured of confidentiality. • Obtain reasonable responses to requests for services. • Obtain information about his or her health care. • Know whether treatment is experimental and be free to refuse to participate in research projects. • Expect reasonable continuity of care. • Examine his or her bill and have it explained. • Know which hospital rules and regulations apply to patient conduct. • Terminate the physician–patient contract, which includes leaving a hospital/treatment against medical advice. Patients are obligated to: • Follow any instructions given by the physician and cooperate as much as possible. • Give all relevant information to the physician to reach a correct diagnosis. If an incorrect diagnosis is made because the patient fails to give the physician the proper information, the physician is not liable. • Follow the physician's orders for treatment, provided the treatment is similar to that administered by members of the system or school of medicine to which the physician belongs. If a patient willfully or negligently fails to follow the physician's instructions, that patient has little legal recourse. • Pay the fees charged for services rendered.

Learning Outcome	Summary
LO 4.6 Relate how the law of agency and the doctrine of *respondeat superior* apply to health care contracts.	What is the law of agency, and how does the doctrine of *respondeat superior* apply to health care contracts? • The law of agency governs the relationship between a principal and his or her agent. An agent is one who acts for or represents another. In performing workplace duties, for example, the employee acts as the agent, or authorized representative, of the employer. • *Respondeat superior* is Latin for "Let the master answer." Under this doctrine an employer is legally liable for the acts of his or her employees, if such acts were performed within the scope of the employees' duties.

Ethics Issues Law, the Courts, and Contracts

Ethics ISSUE 1:

Advertising by health care providers used to be considered inappropriate and unprofessional. However, now advertising by health care providers is commonplace and accepted by the various professional organizations, as long as there are no false or misleading statements.

Discussion Questions

1. A dentist advertises that he specializes in creating "dazzling smiles." In your opinion, is this an ethical advertisement? Explain your answer.

2. A chiropractor advertises "miracle" treatments to alleviate back pain. In your opinion, is this an ethical advertisement? Explain your answer.

3. Check your local newspaper for advertising by health care providers. Listen carefully to television ads by health care providers. Bring to class at least two ads from the newspaper and notes from the ads you listened to on television. Be sure to sort out ads that are for providers and those that are for prescription or nonprescription drugs. Are those ads misleading? Do they make promises that cannot be kept? Explain your answer.

4. Study the print ads and notes from television ads you collected for the previous exercise. Choose two as examples. What advantages and disadvantages for consumers can you see to the ads?

5. What advantages and disadvantages for health care practitioners can you see to the ads?

Ethics ISSUE 2:

The patient–physician relationship is contractual in nature. That means that either the physician or the patient may terminate the relationship. The physician must abide by certain rules when terminating an established relationship, but the patient is free to terminate the relationship at any time. Physicians may decline to undertake the care of a patient whose medical condition is not within the physician's current competence. Physicians may not decline to accept patients because of race, color, religion, national origin, or sexual orientation, or on any other basis that would constitute individual discrimination.

Discussion Question

1. A dental hygienist refuses to work on a patient because he has revealed that he is HIV positive. Is her decision ethical? Explain your answer.

_____

_____

Ethics ISSUE 3:

While in private practice, physicians may determine that they will not accept certain new patients because of their inability to pay or because they have an insurance plan with a poor reimbursement policy.

Discussion Question

1. Should all physicians be required to accept a certain number of patients who cannot pay their bills? In other words, should physicians be required to do a certain amount of charity care? Explain your answer.

_____

_____

Ethics ISSUE 4:

The first objective and the primary goal of every code of ethics and ethics guideline for health care practitioners is the _welfare of the patient_.

Discussion Question

1. A nursing assistant working under the supervision of a registered nurse in a hospital has witnessed several occasions when the RN behaves abusively to elderly patients. What should the nursing assistant do?

_____

_____

Chapter 4 Review

Enhance your learning by completing these exercises and more at
http://connect.mheducation.com!

Mc Graw Hill Education **connect**®

Applying Knowledge

Answer the following questions in the spaces provided.

LO 4.1

1. List and define three functions a state government _can_ assume.

_____

_____

_____

_____

2. Which governmental functions are reserved strictly for the federal government?

_____

_____

_____

_____

3. Define *common law.*

_____

_____

_____

_____

4. Define *administrative law.*

_____

_____

_____

_____

5. Decisions made by judges in the various courts and used as a guide for future decisions are called what?

_____

_____

_____

_____

Circle the correct answer for each of the following questions.

LO 4.2

6. Substantive law

   a. Defines the legal relationships between people or between people and the state

   b. Is never written down

   c. Is a type of common law

   d. Is created solely by executive order

7. Procedural law

   a. Is the same as substantive law

   b. Defines the rules used to enforce substantive law

   c. Applies only to criminal law

   d. Does not involve penalties for violations

8. Criminal law

   a. Includes financial payment for violations, but never jail time

   b. Never involves health care practitioners

   c. Involves crimes against the state

   d. Allows violators to be tried in civil court

9. Civil law

   a. Includes felonies and misdemeanors

   b. Is the area of law most likely to affect health care practitioners

   c. Does not involve court cases

   d. Involves crimes against the state

10. A civil offense

    a. Is never unethical

    b. Never involves lawsuits

    c. May involve a family matter

    d. Never applies to health care practitioners

11. *Jurisdiction* refers to

    a. The city where a felony occurs

    b. The fines levied for civil offenses

    c. Crimes against people

    d. The court that has the authority to hear and decide a case

LO 4.3

12. Define *tort*.

    a. A tort is a specific type of felony.

    b. A tort is a civil wrong committed against a person or property.

    c. *Tort* is another term for breach of contract.

    d. A tort is none of the above.

13. What is a tortfeasor?

    a. It is the attorney who represents a client in civil court.

    b. It is a person who commits a felony.

    c. It is the person who commits a tort.

    d. It refers to a court's specific jurisdiction.

14. Negligence is

    a. An intentional tort

    b. The same as assault

    c. A criminal matter

    d. An unintentional tort

15. Intentional torts

    a. Include negligence

    b. Always involve jail time when successfully prosecuted

    c. Include assault, battery, and defamation

    d. Are always felonies

16. If a physician examines a patient without consent, he or she could be charged with which of the following offenses?

    a. Breach of contract

    b. Kidnapping

    c. Battery

    d. Defamation of character

LO 4.4

17. A contract

    a. Is breached only if all parties agree

    b. Is valid only if parties on both sides are competent

    c. Can never be broken

    d. Is valid if an illegal act is involved

18. For what are health care practitioners legally liable?

    a. For all unsatisfactory medical outcomes

    b. For actions of their employees, performed in the course of employment

    c. For actions of their employees away from work

    d. For actions of their coworkers, performed on the job

19. What is the *consideration* of a contract?

    a. The fee, if any, that will be charged

    b. Something of value bargained for

    c. The terms of the agreement

    d. None of these

20. A contract may be voidable if

    a. One party leaves town

    b. One party decides to cancel the contract

    c. One party is a minor

    d. One party engages in an illegal act

21. Under what circumstances may breach of contract be charged?

    a. If either party fails to fulfill the terms of a valid contract

    b. If one party becomes angry with the other

    c. If the contract was invalid from the beginning

    d. None of these

22. The Statute of Frauds

    a. Is federal legislation governing health practitioners accused of fraud

    b. Covers both expressed and implied contracts

    c. Is state legislation governing written contracts

    d. Must be revised every 10 years

23. Third-party payer contracts

    a. May be implied

    b. Are legally invalid

    c. Promise, in writing, that a third party will pay a patient's medical bill

    d. Are never used in the medical office

24. Regulation Z of the Consumer Protection Act of 1968 requires that certain financial arrangements be in writing and include

    a. Proof of ability to pay a debt

    b. A finance charge

    c. A minimum of 10 installment payments

    d. Proof that the arrangement is for business purposes

25. Which of the following is an example of an implied limited contract?

    a. A physician in a medical clinic examines a new patient.

    b. A physical therapist meets regularly with a patient and administers range of motion exercises.

    c. A dental hygienist cleans a patient's teeth.

    d. A physician at the scene provides emergency care to a car accident victim.

LO 4.5

26. List 10 items to which a physician is *not* bound contractually in the context of an implied physician–patient contract.

_____   _____

_____   _____

_____   _____

_____   _____

_____   _____

27. List 10 items to which a physician is obligated in an implied physician–patient contract.

_____   _____

_____   _____

_____   _____

_____   _____

_____   _____

28. List five responsibilities borne by the patient in an implied contract.

_____

_____

_____

29. Name four situations in which premature termination of the physician–patient contract may occur.

_____

_____

_____

30. Why must a physician give the patient ample notice when withdrawing from a case?

_____

_____

_____

LO 4.6

31. Briefly explain how the law of agency applies to health care practitioners.

_____

_____

_____

32. How does the doctrine of *respondeat superior* relate to the law of agency?

_____

_____

_____

Case Studies

Use your critical thinking skills to answer the questions that follow each case study.

LO 4.3 and LO 4.5

An internist had a 54-year-old obese patient who smoked and had a stressful job. After he died of a heart attack, an autopsy revealed that the overweight man had coronary artery disease. The patient's family sued the physician for negligence and won a $3.5 million judgment against the internist. During jury deliberations, some jurors who heard testimony in the case argued that the physician did everything possible to try to help the patient, but others maintained that he could have done more.

33. In your opinion, was the internist negligent for not referring this patient to a cardiologist, as the patient's wife claimed in court? Why or why not?

_____

_____

34. In your opinion, does this case show that people need to take more personal responsibility for their health? Explain your answer.

_____

_____

LO 4.4

Dan, a medical office assistant in a busy clinic, is a sympathetic and understanding employee. Therefore, when an elderly patient complained to him that she "felt terrible most of the time," Dan consoled her. "Don't worry, Mrs. Smith," he told the woman. "Dr. Jones will make you feel better in no time."

35. Has Dan, acting as Dr. Jones's agent, created an implied contract with Mrs. Smith? Explain your answer.

_____

_____

36. If so, can Mrs. Smith sue Dr. Jones if he fails to fulfill the "terms" of the contract? Explain your answer.

_____

_____

37. How might you respond to a patient under similar circumstances?

_____

_____

LO 4.5

38. Does a patient have the legal right to leave the hospital, even though his or her physician believes treatment is incomplete? What procedure should be followed if a patient leaves a hospital against medical advice?

_____

_____

39. Does a patient have the right to know if medical treatment is experimental and to refuse to participate in such treatment? Explain your answer.

_____

_____

Internet Activities LO 4.1 and LO 4.2

Complete the activities and answer the questions that follow.

40. Find a Web site that defines the term *affidavit*. Briefly explain the term, and describe a situation in which a health care professional may have to give an affidavit.

_____

_____

_____

_____

41. Visit the Web site for the U.S. House of Representatives. List any health care legislation currently pending before the House that you believe is relevant to the health care profession you will practice.

_____

_____

_____

_____

42. List two additional Web sites where information about health care legislation can be found.

_____

_____

_____

_____

Resources

Hwang, Stephen W. "Discharge against Medical Advice." (May 2005). U.S. Department of Health and Human Services Web site: **www.webmm.ahrq.gov/case**.

Kubasek, Nancy, et al. *Dynamic Business Law.* New York: McGraw-Hill, 2009.

Liuzzo, Anthony L. *Essentials of Business Law.* New York: McGraw-Hill, 2010.

Mitchell, Joyce, and Lee Haroun. *Introduction to Health Care.* New York: Delmar, 2002.

Payne, January W. "Why People Leave the Hospital against Medical Advice." *U.S. News and World Report* (August 27, 2009). **http://health.usnews.com**.

Prickett-Ramutkowski, Barbara, et al. *Medical Assisting: A Patient-Centered Approach to Administrative and Clinical Competencies.* New York: McGraw-Hill, 1999.

PART TWO

Legal Issues for Working Health Care Practitioners

A registered nurse working as a supervisor in a dialysis clinic slipped in a puddle of water on the floor at work and injured her neck and lower back. She had surgical fusions of the cervical and lumbar spine, and she continued to have serious symptoms, including debilitating pain and urinary incontinence, for which she received numerous medications. The neurosurgeon who treated the injured nurse said that he did not think she would be able to return to gainful employment as a registered nurse, even in a sedentary position. The nurse had been earning $100,000 per year, and her employer had not offered her any other position. The trial court found the defendant to be "100 percent disabled," which entitled her to commensurate Worker's Compensation payments. Since Workers Compensation benefits are paid for, in one way or another, for a state's employers, the injured nurse's employer appealed this decision. The appeals court upheld the trial court's decision.

MOUSSEAU v. DAVITA, INC., No. W2010-02612-SC-WCM-WC (Tenn. Aug. 22, 2011).

laws, and with state medical societies to determine safety rules, rights, and responsibilities. A general safety procedure book for medical office workers should include guidelines for the handling of hazardous laboratory wastes and materials.

LO 5.2

Describe the reasonable person standard, standard of care, and duty of care.

standard of care
The level of performance expected of a health care practitioner in carrying out his or her professional duties.

duty of care
The legal obligation of health care workers to patients and, sometimes, nonpatients.

Standard of Care and Duty of Care

Standard of care refers to the level of performance expected of a health care practitioner in carrying out his or her professional duties. **Duty of care** is the obligation of health care workers to patients and, in some case, nonpatients. Physicians have a duty of care to patients with whom they have established a doctor–patient relationship, but they may also be held to a duty of care toward people who are not patients, such as the patient's family members, former patients, and even office personnel. Generally, if actions or omissions within the scope of a health care practitioner's job could cause harm to someone, that person is owed a duty of care.

For example, medical facility custodians are nonpatients to whom a duty of care is owed. Various drugs, equipment, and supplies are used and discarded daily in a medical facility. Procedures for the proper disposal of drugs and potentially hazardous materials should be detailed in a facility's safety manual, so that employees who handle these materials do not accidentally prick themselves with used needles or otherwise injure themselves.

In some instances, depending on the situation and state law, physicians may have a duty under standard of care to warn nonpatients of danger, as in the case of a psychiatric patient who threatens harm to others or in the case of a patient with a communicable disease.

Two court cases, "Therapists Found Guilty of Failure to Warn" (p. 123) and "Sharing a Prescription Drug Proves Costly" (p. 124), show that courts vary widely in establishing a duty of care, according to the laws in the states where lawsuits are adjudicated. In "Sharing a Prescription Drug Proves Costly," wrongful death was also charged, which is discussed in further detail as you progress through this chapter.

reasonable person standard
That standard of behavior that judges a person's actions in a situation according to what a reasonable person would or would not do under similar circumstances.

As mentioned in Chapter 4, we are responsible for our actions (or our failure to act) under the **reasonable person standard.** That is, we may be charged with negligence if someone is injured because we failed to perform an act that a reasonable person, in similar circumstances, would perform or if we committed an act that a reasonable person would not commit. Professionals—individuals who are specially trained to perform specific tasks—are held to a higher standard of care than nonprofessionals (laypersons). If a patient is injured because a health care professional failed to exercise the care and expertise that under the circumstances could reasonably be expected of a professional with similar experience and training, then that professional may be liable for negligence.

PHYSICIANS

A physician in general practice is expected to conform to the standards of other general practitioners in his or her own or a comparable community. A specialist is held to a higher standard of care than that expected of a general practitioner. The standard of care for a specialist is generally the same as that for like specialists, wherever they practice. Similarly, any health care practitioner—nurse, phlebotomist,

---

LANDMARK COURT CASE | Therapists Found Guilty of Failure to Warn

In October 1969, Prosenjit Poddar, a foreign student from Bengal, India, killed Tatiana Tarasoff. Two months before, Poddar had confided his intention to kill Tarasoff to Dr. Lawrence Moore, a psychologist employed by the Cowell Memorial Hospital at the University of California at Berkeley. Poddar told Moore he would kill Tarasoff after she returned from spending the summer in Brazil.

Acting on this information, Moore notified the campus police, who briefly detained Poddar, but determined that Poddar was rational and released him. Upon Poddar's release, Moore's superior, Dr. Harvey Powelson, directed that all of the letters and notes Moore had written while counseling Poddar be destroyed and no further action be taken to detain Poddar in the future.

Soon thereafter, Poddar convinced Tarasoff's brother to share an apartment with him near Tarasoff's residence. When she returned from Brazil, Poddar went to Tarasoff's home and killed her. Tarasoff had not been warned of the possible danger Poddar posed.

Tarasoff's parents sued, arguing that the psychologist had a duty to warn them of Poddar's danger to their daughter, and that the campus police negligently released Poddar without notifying them of their daughter's grave danger. They also argued that the police failed to confine Poddar, under the Lanterman-Petris-Short Act, a California law designed to protect mentally ill and mentally disabled persons from certain abuses, and to guarantee and protect the public interest.

The defendants argued that there was no duty of care toward Tatiana Tarasoff, and that, as employees of the state,

they had governmental immunity. The trial court granted the defendants' motion to dismiss. On the plaintiffs' appeal, the court affirmed dismissals against defendant police on all claims, stating there was no duty to plaintiffs. Dismissals against the defendant therapists were also upheld, holding they were protected by governmental immunity. Plaintiffs appealed to the Supreme Court of California.

The Supreme Court allowed the plaintiffs to amend their appeal to state that the therapists failed to warn Tatiana (rather than her parents, as in the original complaint).

The Supreme Court of California heard the case based on the question "Did defendant therapists have a duty to warn Tatiana Tarasoff?"

Yes, the court determined. It was found that the defendant therapists should have determined that Poddar presented a serious danger to Tarasoff, and they failed to exercise reasonable care to protect her from that danger (i.e., when a therapist determines that a patient poses a danger to another individual, he or she is obligated to use reasonable care to protect that individual). Therefore, defendant therapists breached their duty of care to Tatiana Tarasoff and were negligent by not warning her of the possible danger posed by Poddar.

Tarasoff v. Regents of University of California, 17 Cal.3d 425, 131 Cal. Rptr. 14, 551 P.2d 334 (1976).

Prosenjit Poddar was later convicted of second-degree murder, but the conviction was appealed and overturned, based on the decision that the jury was inadequately informed. No second trial was held, and Poddar was released on the condition that he return to India.

A restaurant worker, Kasey, attended an employee holiday party held at his workplace. Also present were a coworker and her boyfriend, Followill. Kasey brought a narcotic drug to the party, which his doctor had prescribed for his back pain. He gave his coworker eight of the pain pills, who, in turn, gave them to her boyfriend, Followill. Followill died in his sleep that evening, due to a combination of the prescription drug and alcohol in his system. Plaintiff Gipson, Followill's mother, sued defendant, Kasey, for wrongful death.

The issue presented in court was whether persons who were prescribed drugs owed a duty of care, making them potentially liable for negligence, when they improperly give their drugs to others. The defendant contended that because Arizona law does not impose a duty on social hosts who serve alcohol to adults, there should similarly be no duty here.

The supreme court in this case ruled that such a duty was owed, extending not from the relationship between the two workers, but from state statutes that prohibited distributing prescription drugs to persons not covered by the prescription. The Arizona Supreme Court referred the case back to the superior court for further proceedings consistent with the opinion regarding duty of care.

Gipson v. Kasey, 214 Ariz. 141, 150 P.3d 228 (Ariz. 2007).

dental assistant, physician assistant—is expected to conform to the standards of like practitioners in his or her own or a comparable community.

Courts have generally held that informal consultations among physicians do not create a doctor–patient relationship and thus do not create a duty of care, as discussed in the classic case, "Consultation Did Not Establish a Duty of Care, on page 125."

GUIDELINES FOR PHYSICIANS AND OTHER HEALTH CARE PRACTITIONERS

The following guidelines can help all health care practitioners stay within the scope of their practices and operate within the law and the policy of any employing health care facility. All are addressed at length throughout the text.

- Practice within the scope of your training and capabilities.
- Use the professional title commensurate with your education and experience.
- Maintain confidentiality
- Prepare and maintain health records.
- Document accurately
- Use appropriate legal and ethical guidelines when releasing information.
- Follow an employer's established policies dealing with the health care contract.
- Follow legal guidelines and maintain awareness of health care legislation and regulations.
- Maintain and dispose of regulated substances in compliance with government guidelines.
- Follow established risk management and safety procedures.
- Meet the requirements for professional credentialing.
- Help develop and maintain personnel, policy, and procedure manuals.

Consultation Did Not Establish a Duty of Care

The doctrine that informal physician consultations do not create a doctor–patient relationship was established in 1973 in the California decision *Ranier v. Grossman*. Morton Grossman was a professor of gastroenterology who often lectured physicians at their hospitals, then offered to review their cases with them. After one such lecture, a physician presented the X-rays and medical history for a patient who suffered from ulcerative colitis. Grossman advised surgery without examining the patient.

The surgery was subsequently performed, and the patient sued, claiming that the surgery had been unnecessary. Grossman was cited as a codefendant in the patient's lawsuit. An appeals court upheld summary judgment in Grossman's favor, holding that he had no duty to the patient because he had no direct contact with her and had no control over her treating physicians.

Ranier v. Grossman, 107 Cal. Rptr. 469, 31 Cal. App. 3d 539 (1973).

Check Your Progress

1. As employers, physicians have general liability for _____.

Write "T" or "F" in the blank to indicate whether you think the statement is true or false.

_____ 2. *Standard of care* refers to the level of performance expected of a health care practitioner in carrying out his or her professional duties.

_____ 3. *Duty of care* is the obligation of health care practitioners to patients but never applies to nonpatients.

_____ 4. An obstetrician who helps deliver a baby to a woman who happens to be riding with him in a taxicab would be held to the reasonable person standard.

_____ 5. Policies and procedures of the employing medical facility, as well as the law, should be considered when a health care practitioner performs his or her duties.

Laws clearly dictate what a member of a health care profession can and cannot do on the job. However, in addition to knowing the law, a health care practitioner should know what policies and procedures apply specifically to his or her place of employment. Policy and procedure manuals that clearly define a health care practitioner's responsibilities can serve as a valuable guide and as evidence that policies and procedures are in writing if legal suits should arise.

Privacy, Confidentiality, and Privileged Communication

Not only do physicians and other health care professionals owe a duty of care to patients, but it is also their ethical and legal duty to safeguard a patient's privacy and maintain **confidentiality.**

Privileged communication refers to information held confidential within a protected relationship. Attorney–client and physician–patient

LO 5.3

Briefly outline the responsibilities of health care practitioners concerning privacy, confidentiality, and privileged communication.

confidentiality
The act of holding information in confidence, not to be released to unauthorized individuals.

privileged communication
Information held confidential within a protected relationship.

are examples of relationships in which the law, under certain circumstances, protects the holder of information from forced disclosure on the witness stand. Privileged communication statutes vary from state to state, but in most states, patients may sue a physician or any other health care practitioner for breach of confidence if the holder released protected information and damage to the patient resulted. In many states, breach of confidence is grounds for revocation of a physician's license.

Since health care procedures and facilities present numerous opportunities for a breach of confidentiality (as was the case with Samantha in the chapter's opening scenario), health care practitioners must make every effort to safeguard each patient's privacy. Privacy, confidentiality, and privileged communication are such important subjects for health care practitioners that they are discussed separately in Chapter 8.

The following suggestions for maintaining confidentiality of patient health care records can serve as a guide for all health care practitioners who may be asked to provide or release patient information:

- Do not disclose any information about a patient to a third party without signed consent. This extends to insurance companies, attorneys, and curious neighbors, and it includes acknowledging whether or not the person in question is a patient.

- Do not decide confidentiality on the basis of whether or not you approve of or agree with the views or morals of the patient.

- Do not reveal financial information about a patient, since this is also confidential. For instance, be discreet when revealing a patient's account balance so that others in the vicinity do not overhear.

- When talking on the telephone with a patient, do not use the patient's name if others in the room might overhear.

- Use caution in giving the results of medical tests to patients over the telephone to prevent others in the medical office from overhearing. Furthermore, when leaving a message on a home answering machine or at a patient's place of employment, simply ask the patient to return a call regarding a recent visit or appointment on a specific date. No mention should be made of the nature of the call. It is inadvisable to leave a message with a receptionist or coworker on an answering machine for the patient to call an oncologist, an obstetrician-gynecologist, and so forth. If test results are abnormal, usually the physician speaks directly to the patient, and an appointment is made to discuss the results.

- Do not leave medical charts or insurance reports where patients or office visitors can see them. See that confidentiality protocol is duly noted in the office procedures manual, and make sure new employees learn it.

- If a patient is unwilling to release privileged information, the information should not be released. Exceptions include legally required disclosures, such as those ordered by subpoena; those dictated by statute to protect public health or welfare; or those considered necessary to protect the welfare of a patient or a third party.

On October 31, 2006, Nicole Catsouras, 18, was decapitated in an automobile accident. California Highway Patrol officers arrived at the scene, cordoned off the area where the accident occurred, and took control of the decedent's remains. The CHP officers took multiple photographs of Nicole's decapitated corpse. The photographs were downloaded or otherwise transmitted to one or more CHP computers, but they also reached 2,500 Internet Web sites in the United States and the United Kingdom that were not involved in the official investigation of the car crash. Nicole's family members were subjected to malicious taunting by persons making use of the graphic and horrific photographs. For example, Nicole's father received e-mails containing the photographs, including one titled "Woo Hoo Daddy" that said "Hey, Daddy I'm still alive." Some Web sites painted the decedent's life in a false light, including one that described her as "stupid" and a "swinger." As a proximate result of the acts of the defendants, the plaintiffs suffered severe emotional and mental distress.

Nicole's surviving family members filed suit against the CHP. A California appeals court eventually heard the case, deciding that family members have a common law privacy right in the death images of a decedent, subject to certain limitations. The court also held: "We conclude that the CHP and its officers owed plaintiffs a duty of care not to place decedent's death images on the Internet for the purposes of vulgar spectacle." The court found three factors important in the case (freedom of the press was not at issue):

"*foreseeability, moral blame, and the prevention of future harm. It was perfectly foreseeable that the public dissemination, via the Internet, of photographs of the decapitated remains of a teenage girl would cause devastating trauma to the parents and siblings of that girl. Moreover, the alleged acts were morally deficient. We rely upon the CHP to protect and serve the public. It is antithetical to that expectation for the CHP to inflict harm upon us by making the ravaged remains of our loved ones the subjects of Internet sensationalism. It is important to prevent future harm to other families by encouraging the CHP to establish and enforce policies to preclude its officers from engaging in such acts ever again.*"

Accordingly, the court found that the Catsouras family could bring an action for invasion of privacy against the California Highway Patrol.

Catsouras v. Department of California Highway Patrol, 181 Cal. App. 4th 856—Cal: Court of Appeals, 4th Appellate Dist., 3rd Div. 2010.

Confidentiality may be waived under the following circumstances:

- Sometimes when a third party requests a medical examination, such as for employment, and that party pays the physician's fee.

- Generally when a patient sues a physician for malpractice and patient records are subpoenaed.

- When a waiver has been signed by the patient allowing the release of information (see Figure 5-1).

The Tort of Negligence

LO 5.4

Explain the four elements necessary to prove negligence (the four Ds).

The unintentional tort of negligence is the basis for professional malpractice claims and is the most common liability in medicine. When health care practitioners are sued for medical malpractice, the term generally means any deviation from the accepted medical standard of care that causes injury to a patient.

Hospitals have also been found guilty of negligence. Under the theory of corporate liability, hospitals have been found to have an independent duty to patients, including a duty to grant privileges only to competent doctors, to supervise the overall medical treatment of patients, and to review the competence of staff physicians.

FIGURE 5-1
Consent to Release
Information

I authorize:

Name of person or institution _____
(Provider of information)

Street address _____

City, state, Zip code _____

To release medical information to:

Name of person or institution _____
(Recipient of information)

Street address _____

City, state, Zip code _____

Attention _____

Nature of information to be disclosed:

☐ Clinical notes pertaining to evaluation and treatment _____

☐ Other, please specify _____

Purpose of disclosure:

☐ Continuing medical care _____

☐ Second opinion _____

☐ Other, please specify _____

This authorization will automatically expire one year from the date of signature, unless specified otherwise _____

This consent may be revoked at any time by sending written notice to the above-named provider of information. Any release of information made prior to the revocation of this complaint, authorization is not a breach of confidentiality. Disclosed information may be reviewed by contacting the provider of information.

Patient's name _____

Signature of patient or legal guardian _____ Date _____

Complete address _____

Relationship, if not the patient _____ Patient's date of birth _____

Specific consent for release of information protected by state or federal law

Iowa law (and in some cases federal law) provides spacial confidentiality protection to information relating to substance abuse, mental health, and HIV-related testing. In order for information to be released on this subject matter, this specific authorization and the above authorization must be signed:

I authorize release of information relating to:

☐ Substance abuse (alcohol/drug abuse)
Signature of patient or legal guardian _____ Date _____

☐ Mental health (includes psychological testing and mental health counseling)
Signature of patient or legal guardian _____ Date _____

☐ HIV-related information (AIDS-related testing)
Signature of patient or legal guardian _____ Date _____

Date Information is sent _____

Sent by (name) _____

To the recipient of this information: This information has been disclosed to you from records protected by federal confidentiality rules. The federal rules prohibit you from making further disclosure without additional consent.

All medical professional liability claims are classified in one of three ways, based on the root word *feasance*, which means "the performance of an act."

Malfeasance. The performance of a totally wrongful and unlawful act. For example, in the absence of the employing physician, a medical assistant determines that a patient needs a prescription drug and dispenses the wrong drug from the physician's supply. Medical assistants are not licensed to practice medicine, and the wrong drug was dispensed, so the act was totally wrongful and unlawful and could be called malfeasance.

Misfeasance. The performance of a lawful act in an illegal or improper manner. Suppose a physician orders his or her

malfeasance
The performance of a totally wrongful and unlawful act.

misfeasance
The performance of a lawful act in an illegal or improper manner.

Physician Tried for Negligence

In March 2002, Margarita Munoz, who had been suffering from breakthrough bleeding daily for two months, asked her primary care doctor to remove an intrauterine device (IUD). Her physician tried but was unable to remove the IUD. Munoz's primary care doctor referred her to Dr. Gordon B. Clark, who performed a physical exam. At that time, Munoz was mostly asymptomatic, except for dysmenorrhea—painful cramping during menstruation—and abnormal uterine bleeding. Dr. Clark advised Munoz that her pelvic sonogram showed a complex adnexal mass arising from her right ovary, which could be a cyst or could be cancerous. Because of her history of ovarian cysts, Clark said that one alternative treatment for Munoz was the removal of her ovaries through laparoscopic surgery. Munoz chose that alternative.

In August 2002, Clark performed the laparoscopic surgery and thought he had removed Munoz's ovaries, fallopian tubes, and IUD. Clark sent the removed tissues to a pathologist for examination. From the tissue samples, the pathologist determined that Clark had removed mostly uterine tubes, but had only grazed the ovarian surface. Dr. Clark did not contact the pathologist to discuss her findings or conduct any tests that might explain the discrepancy. Instead, he chose to believe he had successfully removed Munoz's ovaries, and he told the patient that he had removed her ovaries, fallopian tubes, and IUD. He started Munoz on hormone replacement therapy to ward off surgically induced menopause.

Unaware of the discrepancy between the pathologist's report and Dr. Clark's remarks to her, Munoz continued her life as usual. During this time, she experienced severe abdominal pain, breakthrough bleeding, and premenstrual headaches. In April 2004, Munoz visited a hospital emergency room. Doctors there conducted an ultrasound exam of her pelvis and ordered a CT scan. Test results showed a large lobulated multicystic mass in Munoz's pelvis, suggestive of an "ovarian neoplasm" (tumor of the ovary).

Munoz consulted an obstetrician-gynecologist, who found that her ovaries contained endometrial tissue. The specialist removed Munoz's uterus and ovaries and sent the removed tissues to a pathologist, who confirmed the removal of those organs and tissues.

In March 2006, Munoz sued Dr. Clark for medical malpractice. The trial court found for Munoz and awarded damages. Dr. Clark appealed, but the trial court's verdict for the plaintiff was upheld. Justice Hill of the appellate court wrote:

Medical malpractice is negligence of a health care professional in the diagnosis, care, and treatment of a patient.

In a medical malpractice case, the plaintiff must prove the following elements: (1) The physician owes the patient a duty of care and was required to meet or exceed a certain standard of care to protect the patient from injury; (2) the physician breached this duty or deviated from the applicable standard of care; and (3) the patient was injured and the injury proximately resulted from the physician's breach of the standard of care.

The elements of negligence are never presumed. Therefore, expert testimony is generally required to establish the appropriate standard of care and causation because such matters are outside the knowledge of the average person without specialized training. In certain medical malpractice claims, expert testimony is not required because the standard of care and causation are within the common knowledge of a layperson. But, the application of the common knowledge exception is extremely limited.

Munoz v. Clark, 2009 Kan. App.; 199 P.3d 1283.

nurse-employee to change a sterile dressing on a patient's burned hand. The nurse changes the dressing but does not use sterile technique, and the patient's burn becomes infected. The nurse is legally authorized to carry out the physician's instructions in dressing the patient's hand, but violated proper procedure in carrying out the physician's order.

Nonfeasance. The failure to act when one should. For example, a newly certified emergency medical technician is first on the scene of a traffic accident. An injured motorist stops breathing and appears to be in cardiac arrest. The EMT, though trained in

nonfeasance
The failure to act when one should.

cardiopulmonary resuscitation, "freezes" and does nothing. The patient dies. In failing to act, the EMT could be guilty of nonfeasance.

There are four elements that must be present in a given situation to prove that a health care professional is guilty of negligence. Sometimes called the "four Ds of negligence," these elements include:

- *Duty*—The person charged with negligence owed a duty of care to the accuser.
- *Dereliction*—The health care provider breached the duty of care to the patient.
- *Direct Cause*—The breach of the duty of care to the patient was a direct cause of the patient's injury.
- *Damages*—There is a legally recognizable injury to the patient.

In this chapter's opening scenario, how does Samantha's act illustrate the four Ds? In your opinion, does her act illustrate malfeasance, misfeasance, or nonfeasance?

When a plaintiff sues a health care practitioner (defendant) for negligence, the burden of proof is on the plaintiff. That is, it is up to the accuser's attorney to present evidence of the four Ds.

State statutes must be consulted for restrictions that apply to actions against health care providers. Some states limit damage awards or mandate procedural rules that must be followed in medical malpractice claims. In some states, for example, medical review panels must screen claims before they are brought to court. The panel examines the facts and then issues a finding of "malpractice" or "no malpractice." Such panels are generally composed of physicians with expertise in the medical specialty in question and sometimes include a neutral attorney.

THE JOINT COMMISSION (TJC)

Avoiding medical mistakes and safeguarding patients while they are being examined or treated are vital issues for health care practitioners, both to ensure excellent patient care and to avoid issues of medical malpractice liability.

While conscientious health care practitioners do their best to avoid making mistakes, they are human, and mistakes do occur. The legal and ethical response when health care mistakes are made is to report the mistake to attending physicians and supervisors and on the patient's medical record, and to tell the patient he or she has been harmed. In fact, health care practitioners and health care facilities that try to cover up mistakes are most likely to be sued, and hospitals and other facilities that fail to disclose mistakes could lose their Joint Commission accreditation.

To further address patient safety, as of January 1, 2004, all TJC-accredited health care organizations are surveyed for implementation of the following requirements:

1. Improve the accuracy of patient identification.
   - Use at least two patient identifiers whenever taking blood samples or administering medications or blood

products. Do not use a hospital patient's room number as an identifier.

- Prior to the start of any surgical or invasive procedure, confirm the correct patient, procedure, and site, using active—not passive—communication.

2. Improve the effectiveness of communication among caregivers.

- Use a process for taking verbal or telephone orders or critical test results that requires a verification read-back by the person receiving the information.

- Standardize abbreviations, acronyms, and symbols used throughout the organization, including a list of all such terms that are *not* to be used.

3. Improve the safety of using high-alert medications.

- Remove concentrated electrolytes (including, but not limited to, potassium chloride, potassium phosphate, and sodium chloride) from patient care units.

- Standardize and limit the number of drug concentrations available in the organization.

4. Eliminate wrong-site, wrong-patient, wrong-procedure surgery.

- Create and use a preoperative verification process, such as a checklist, to confirm that appropriate documents, such as medical records and imaging studies, are available.

- Use procedures to mark the surgical site and involve the patient in the marking process.

5. Improve the safety of using infusion pumps.

- Ensure free-flow protection on all general-use and patient-controlled analgesia intravenous infusion pumps.

6. Improve the effectiveness of clinical alarm systems.

- Use regular preventative maintenance and testing of alarm systems.

- Be sure that alarms are activated with appropriate settings and can be heard over distances and competing noise within a care unit.

7. Reduce the risk of health care–acquired infections.

- Comply with current Centers for Disease Control and Prevention (CDC) hand hygiene guidelines.

- Manage as sentinel events all identified cases of unanticipated death or major permanent loss of function associated with a health care–acquired infection.

TJC established these requirements to help accredited health care organizations address issues of patient safety that can lead to adverse events that, in turn, can result in lawsuits.

RES IPSA LOQUITUR

Res ipsa loquitur is Latin for "the thing speaks for itself." It is also known as the doctrine of common knowledge. It means that the mistake is so obvious—such as leaving a sponge or surgical instrument inside a

res ipsa loquitur
"The thing speaks for itself"; also known as the doctrine of common knowledge. A situation that is so obviously negligent that no expert witnesses need be called.

6. Define *privileged communication*.

_____

_____

7. Is a breach of confidentiality an offense for which a health care practitioner can be sued? Explain your answer.

_____

_____

8. Distinguish among *malfeasance*, *misfeasance*, and *nonfeasance*.

_____

_____

_____

_____

_____

_____

9. Name the four Ds of negligence.

_____

_____

patient after surgery or operating on the wrong body part—that negligence is obvious. The defendant in such a case may argue that the event was an inevitable accident and had nothing to do with his or her responsibility of control or supervision. Traditionally, expert witnesses did not have to be called to testify in a medical malpractice lawsuit alleging *res ipsa loquitur*, but courts have made exceptions in many cases and allowed expert witness testimony. Judicial consideration of this doctrine varies. Generally, for *res ipsa loquitur* to apply, three conditions must exist:

1. The act of negligence must obviously be under the defendant's control.
2. The patient must not have contributed to the act.
3. It must be apparent that the patient would not have been injured if reasonable care had been used.

Cases that fall under the doctrine of *res ipsa loquitur* include:

- Unintentionally leaving foreign bodies, such as sponges or instruments, inside a patient's body during surgery.
- Accidentally burning or otherwise injuring a patient while he or she is anesthetized.
- Damaging healthy tissue during an operation.
- Causing an infection by the use of unsterilized instruments.

No Expert Testimony Needed

In this case, Dr. Smith, a surgeon, was supposed to perform a hysterectomy and a bilateral salpingo oophorectomy, but simply forgot to perform the latter. When the case was appealed, the jury verdict of $75,000 was upheld. In upholding the *medical malpractice* award, the Virginia Supreme Court concluded: "A reasonably intelligent juror did not need an expert to explain why Dr. Smith's negligence was the proximate cause of Webb's damages because the issue of causation was within the common knowledge of laymen."

The Virginia Supreme Court reiterated that "in *medical malpractice* cases, 'expert testimony is ordinarily necessary to establish the appropriate standard of care, to establish a deviation from the standard, and to establish that such a deviation is the proximate cause of the claimed damages.' Exceptions to this rule exist only in 'those rare cases in which a healthcare provider's act or omission is clearly negligent within the common knowledge of laymen.'"

Such a "rare case" involves the *medical malpractice* doctrine of *res ipsa loquitur,* which translates to "the thing speaks for itself."

Webb v. Smith, 276 Va. 305, 661 S.E.2d 457 (Va. 2008).

Check Your Progress

10. *Res ipsa loquitur* means _____ .

11. *Res ipsa loquitur* is also known as the doctrine of _____ .

12. Name two types of cases that fall under the doctrine of *res ipsa loquitur.*

_____

_____

DAMAGE AWARDS AND MEDICAL MALPRACTICE INSURANCE

When a defendant is found guilty of a tort—such as negligence, breach of contract, libel, or slander—the plaintiff is awarded compensation based on the extent of his or her injuries, loss of income, damage to reputation, or other harm that can be proved. This monetary compensation is called **damages.** Table 5-1 explains the various types of damages and how the court determines them.

Physicians and many other professional health care providers carry liability insurance, which pays damage awards in the event of a negligence or malpractice suit up to the limits of the policy (see Table 5-2 for a list of medical specialties most likely to be sued).

Medical groups maintain that high damage awards in tort cases have led to a malpractice insurance crisis for physicians, especially those in high-risk specialties, such as obstetrics-gynecology, orthopedic surgery, and general surgery. Recent studies and news articles have reported that doctors in some states are participating in walkouts and demonstrations, relocating to states where caps have been legislated on medical malpractice damage awards, limiting

damages
Monetary awards sought by plaintiffs in lawsuits.

Table 5-1 Damage Awards

Types of Damages	Purpose	Considered by Court	Award
General Compenstatory	To compensate for injuries or losses due to violation of patient's rights	Physical disability? Loss of earnings? Mental anguish? Loss of service of spouse or child? Losses to date? Future losses?	Specified by court. Dollar value need not be proved; loss must be proved
Special Compenstatory	To compensate for losses not directly caused by the wrong	Additional medical expenses?	Specified by court. Dollar value and loss must be proved
Consequential	To compensate for losses caused indirectly by a product defect	Loss covered by product warranty? Personal injury?	No limit on damages if personal injuries
Punitive	To punish the offender	How serious was the breach of conduct? How much can the defendant afford to pay?	In some cases, amount of damages is set by law
Nominal	To recognize that rights of the patient were violated, though no actual loss was proved	Legal rights of the patient violated? Actual loss proved?	Token award, usually $1

Table 5-2 Medical Specialties Most Likely to Be Sued

According to a 2013 report published in *Physician's Weekly*, the top ten medical specialties sued for malpractice are:

Internal Medicine	15%
Family Medicine	13%
Ob/Gyn	9%
Psychiatry	8%
Cardiology	6%
Pediatrics	5%
Emergency Medicine	4%
Oncology	4%
Anesthesiology	3%
Diabetes & Endocrinology	3%
General Surgery	3%
Orthopedics	3%

Source: *Physician's Weekly*, July 30, 2013 at **www .physiciansweekly.com/malpractice-report-2013/**.

wrongful death statutes
State statutes that allow a person's beneficiaries to collect for loss to the estate of the deceased for future earnings when a death is judged to have been due to negligence.

procedures, performing additional patient tests to cover all liability bases, and even leaving the profession. Furthermore, some hospitals have shut down or threatened to shut down trauma centers, and long-term care facilities have closed.

In an attempt to address rapidly rising premiums for medical malpractice insurance, some states have placed caps on damage awards in medical malpractice cases. Attorney organizations, however, insist that damage caps are unfair to injured patients.

The issue is an important one for both health care practitioners and patients and is not likely to be settled uniformly across the country. As a future or present health care practitioner, you should stay informed on the issues of medical malpractice insurance and tort reform and form your own opinion.

WRONGFUL DEATH STATUTES

Most states have enacted **wrongful death statutes** which allow a patient's beneficiaries to collect from a health care practitioner for loss to the patient's estate of future earnings when a patient's death is judged to have been due to negligence of health care practitioners. In most states, a cap has been placed on the amount of damages that can be recovered in a civil action for wrongful death.

The state may also prosecute a health care practitioner under criminal statutes for the wrongful death of a patient. The following court cases illustrate wrongful death actions.

Medical wrongful death cases do not always involve physicians, as in the next case.

COURT CASE   Hospital Sued in Wrongful Death Case

A wrongful death suit was brought by a woman's husband against a Randolph County, Illinois, hospital following her death. The plaintiff alleged that during the course of treatment for his wife's back pain, the defendant doctor had prescribed too many medications, which led to her wrongful death.

The defendant doctor testified at the Illinois trial that he had in fact prescribed her numerous medications during the two and a half years he treated her. The decedent had previously been diagnosed with a bulging disc in her back and had a history of pain in her back, leg, and abdomen since 1992. However, despite the numerous narcotic medications the doctor prescribed, she continued to suffer pain in her back, abdomen, hip, and knees. The doctor's testimony stated that during the several years he treated the decedent that he never saw any sign of overmedication.

However, the plaintiff's expert's testimony refuted the doctor's claim that the plaintiff could not have been overmedicated and stated that on autopsy it was discovered that she had significantly elevated levels of Percocet and Demerol, both narcotic pain medications, in her system. The expert also testified that these elevated levels of medications contributed to the plaintiff's death.

The Illinois jury returned a verdict in favor of the plaintiff in the amount of $100,000 which was reduced by 50 percent on the basis of the decedent's contributory negligence. That is, even though the jury found the defendant doctor contributed to the plaintiff's death, it also found the decedent contributed to her own death by taking the prescribed medications. (In contributory negligence situations, the verdict amount is reduced by whatever degree the jury finds the plaintiff contributed to his or her own negligence. So in this case, the plaintiff was essentially awarded $50,000 by the jury.)

Even though the plaintiff won in this case, he brought an appeal to a higher court, alleging that the lower court erred by refusing to add to the verdict. The basis of his appeal rested on a claim that the jury award "was manifestly inadequate and contrary to the evidence" (i.e., that the jury award was too little, given the plaintiff's loss and the overwhelming evidence against the defendant doctor). The plaintiff's argument quoted the defendant doctor's attorney, who stated in his closing argument that if there were liability against the doctor, "a fair verdict on damages would be $1 million."

The appellate court rejected the plaintiff's argument, and affirmed the lower court's refusal to add to the verdict award. The appellate court cited the Illinois Wrongful Death Act, stating that under the act it was impossible to measure the propriety of damage awards by comparing the present case with other Illinois wrongful death cases. The appellate court also explained that it did not see any evidence in the court record referring to a specific loss of money or economic loss as a result of the decedent's death. Because the appellate court did not see any clear evidence to demonstrate that the jury or lower court erred in regard to the amount, it deferred to the jury: "It is not within our province to substitute our judgment for that of the jury to determine the monetary value of the loss of society in this case." The appeals court also rejected that part of the plaintiff's argument that was based on the defendant doctor's attorney's closing statements, stating that the commentary by the defense counsel was an opinion and should not be considered a binding judicial admission.

Dobyns v. Chung, 399 Ill. App.3d 272, 926 N.E.2d 847 (Ill. App. 5 Dist. 2010).

COURT CASE   EMTs Follow Protocol

A woman suffered chest pains and the county's fire rescue team was dispatched to her home, where a team member determined she had sustained a heart attack. The patient's daughter asked that she be transported to a hospital where her doctor was waiting for her. However, the rescue team said that because the patient was "critical" and "unstable," written protocol dictated that she be transported to the closest appropriate facility. The patient died shortly after arriving at that hospital.

The patient's estate representative sued for wrongful death, but the suit was dismissed. The plaintiff appealed, and the appeals court determined that there was no breach of duty of care, and that the fire rescue team performed in a reasonably prudent manner. The appeals court affirmed the lower court's decision to dismiss.

Franco v. Miami-Dade County, 32 Fla. L. Weekly D21, 947 So.2d 512 (Fla. App. 3 Dist. 2006).

Elements of a Lawsuit

As indicated in Chapter 4, the type of court that hears a case depends on the offense or complaint. In civil malpractice or negligence cases, the party bringing the action (plaintiff) must prove the case by presenting to a judge or jury evidence that is more convincing than that of the opposing side (defendant).

PHASES OF A LAWSUIT

The typical malpractice or negligence lawsuit proceeds as follows:

1. A patient feels he or she has been injured.
2. The patient seeks the advice of an attorney.
3. If the attorney believes the case has merit, he or she then requests copies of the patient's medical records. The attorney reviews the medical records and the appropriate standard of care to ascertain merits of the case. In some states, before proceeding to a lawsuit, the attorney must obtain an expert witness report stating that the standard of care has been violated. An affidavit to that effect must then be submitted. An affidavit is a sworn statement in writing made under oath. It may also be a declaration before an authorized officer of the court.

Pleading Phase

4. The plaintiff's (injured patient's) attorney files a complaint with the clerk of the court. In this document, the plaintiff states his or her version of the situation and the amount of money sought from the defendant (the practitioner being sued) for the plaintiff's injury.
5. A **summons** is issued by the clerk of the court and is delivered with a copy of the complaint to the defendant, directing him or her to respond to the charges. If the defendant does not respond within the specified time limit, he or she can lose the case by default.
6. The defendant's attorney files an answer to the summons, and a copy of it is sent to the plaintiff. In this document, the defendant presents his or her version of the case, either admitting or denying the charges. The defendant may also file a counterclaim or a cross-complaint.
7. If a cross-complaint is made, the plaintiff files a reply.

Interrogatory or Pretrial Discovery Phase

8. The court sets a trial date.
9. Pretrial motions may be made and decided. For example, the defendant may request that the lawsuit be dismissed, the plaintiff may amend the original complaint, or either side may request a change of venue (ask that the trial be held in another place).
10. Discovery procedures may be used to uncover evidence that will support the charges when the case comes to court. A court order called a **subpoena** may be issued commanding the presence of

summons
A written notification issued by the clerk of the court and delivered with a copy of the complaint to the defendant in a lawsuit, directing him or her to respond to the charges brought in a court of law.

subpoena
A legal document requiring the recipient to appear as a witness in court or to give a deposition.

the physician or a medical facility employee in court or requiring that a **deposition** be taken. A deposition is sworn testimony given and recorded outside the courtroom during the pretrial phase of a case. (See the following section entitled "Witness Testimony.")

An **interrogatory** may be requested instead of or in addition to a deposition. This is a written set of questions requiring written answers from a plaintiff or defendant under oath.

The subpoena commanding a witness to appear in court and to bring certain medical records is called a **subpoena** *duces tecum.* Failure to obey a subpoena may result in contempt-of-court charges. Contempt of court is willful disobedience to or open disrespect of a court, judge, or legislative body. It is punishable by fines or imprisonment.

11. A pretrial conference may be called by the judge scheduled to hear the case. During this conference, the judge discusses the issues in the case with the opposing attorneys. This helps avoid surprises and delays after the trial starts and may lead to an out-of-court settlement. (*Note:* At any point after the complaint is filed before the case comes to trial, an out-of-court settlement may be reached.)

Trial Phase

12. The jury is selected (if one is to be used), and the trial begins.

13. Opening *statements* are made by the lawyers for the plaintiff and the defendant, summarizing what each will prove during the trial.

14. Witnesses are called to testify for both sides. They may be cross-examined by opposing attorneys.

15. Each attorney makes closing *arguments* that the evidence presented supports his or her version of the case. No new evidence may be presented during summation.

16. The judge gives instructions to the jury (if one was chosen), and the jury retires to deliberate.

17. The jury reaches a verdict.

18. The final judgment is handed down by the court. The judge bases his or her decision for judgment on the jury's verdict.

Appeals Phase

19. Posttrial motions may be filed.

20. An appeal may be made for the case to be reviewed by a higher court if the evidence indicates that errors may have been made or if there was injustice or impropriety in the trial court proceedings. During an appeal, the judge has the option of affirming, reversing, or modifying a decision. A judgment is final only when all options for appeal have been exercised.

WITNESS TESTIMONY

An estimated 9 out of 10 lawsuits are settled out of court, but health care practitioners are often asked to give testimony. Testimony may be given in court on the witness stand, or it may be given in an attorney's

deposition
Sworn testimony given and recorded outside the courtroom during the pretrial phase of a case.

interrogatory
A written set of questions requiring written answers from a plaintiff or defendant under oath.

subpoena *duces tecum*
A legal document requiring the recipient to bring certain written records to court to be used as evidence in a lawsuit.

conference room in a pretrial proceeding called a deposition. (See the earlier section entitled "Interrogatory or Pretrial Discovery Phase.") Depositions are of two types:

1. Discovery depositions
2. Depositions in lieu of trial.

Discovery depositions cover material that will most likely be examined again when the witness testifies in court. Since there will be an opportunity for the opposing attorney to question the witness a second time in court, the deposition need not cover every possible question.

Both before a deposition and before in-court testimony, the witness is sworn to tell the truth and then is questioned by attorneys representing both sides. During courtroom testimony, however, a judge is present to rule on objections raised by the attorneys. When an objection is raised, the witness should stop speaking until the judge either *sustains* or *overrules* the objection. If the objection is sustained, the witness need not answer the question. If the objection is overruled, the witness must answer. If in doubt about whether an objection to a question was sustained or overruled, the witness may ask the judge whether a question should be answered. During a deposition, witnesses should take the attorney's advice regarding questions that should be answered.

Depositions in lieu of trial are used instead of the witness's in-person testimony in court. Since the opposing attorney has one opportunity to question the witness, questions are thorough, and the witness should carefully consider his or her answers.

Sometimes depositions in lieu of trial are videotaped, to be played in the courtroom during the trial. Witnesses whose depositions will be videotaped should be informed in advance, so they can dress as though they were appearing in court in person.

Witnesses may offer two kinds of **testimony:** fact and expert. Health care practitioners or laypersons may offer *fact testimony,* and this type of testimony concerns only those facts the witness has observed. For example, regarding testimony in a medical malpractice case, medical assistants, LPNs/LVNs, and registered nurses may testify about how many times a patient saw the physician, the patient's appearance during a particular visit, or similar observations. If asked to give fact testimony, a health care practitioner's powers of observation and memory are more important than his or her professional qualifications. A health care practitioner giving fact testimony is not allowed to give his or her opinion on the facts.

Only experts in a particular field have the education, skills, knowledge, and experience to give *expert testimony.* In medical negligence lawsuits, physicians are usually called as expert witnesses to testify to the standard of care regarding the matter in question. Expert witnesses may, and usually do, give their opinions on the facts. If the defendant/physician is a specialist, the expert witness generally practices or teaches in the same specialty. Acceptable expert witnesses are not coworkers, friends, or acquaintances of the defendant. It is ethical and acceptable for expert witnesses to set and accept a fee commensurate with time taken from regular employment and time spent preparing their expert testimony.

testimony
Statements sworn to under oath by witnesses testifying in court and giving depositions.

COURTROOM CONDUCT

Most health care practitioners will never have to appear in court. If you should be asked to appear, however, the following suggestions can help:

- Attend court proceedings as required. If you were subpoenaed but fail to appear, you could be charged with contempt of court. (If either the plaintiff or the defendant fails to appear, that person forfeits the case.)

- Find out in advance when and where you are to appear, and do not be late for scheduled hearings.

- Bring the required documents to court, and present them only when requested to do so.

- Before testifying, refresh your memory concerning all the facts observed about the matter in question, such as dates, times, words spoken, and circumstances.

- When testifying, speak slowly, use layperson's terms instead of medical terms whenever possible, and do not lose your temper or attempt to be humorous.

- Answer all questions in a straightforward manner, even if the answers appear to help the opposing side.

- Answer only the question asked, no more and no less.

Check Your Progress

13. Name the four phases of a typical medical professional liability lawsuit, and describe how a medical assistant might be involved in each trial phase.

_____

_____

14. A subpoena *duces tecum* is issued during which trial phase?

_____

_____

15. The complaint is filed during which trial phase?

_____

_____

16. During which trial phase is the court's judgment handed down?

_____

_____

17. A judgment is final only when

_____

_____

18. Distinguish between *deposition* and *interrogatory*.

_____

_____

- Because you are testifying about what you recall, be careful of broad generalizations, such as "That is all that took place." A better answer might be, "As I recall, that is what took place."

- Your attorney may help you prepare your testimony, but do not discuss your testimony with other witnesses or others outside the courtroom. Answer truthfully if asked whether you discussed your testimony with counsel.

- Appear well groomed, and dress in clean, conservative clothing.

Alternative Dispute Resolution

Alternative dispute resolution (ADR), also known as appropriate dispute resolution, consists of techniques for resolving civil disputes without going to court. As court calendars have become overcrowded in recent years, ADR has become increasingly popular. Several alternative methods of settling legal disputes are possible, including mediation, arbitration, and a combination of the two methods called med-arb.

Some states require mediation and/or arbitration for certain civil cases, while in other states alternative dispute resolution methods are voluntary. *Mediation* is an ADR method in which a neutral third party listens to both sides of the argument and then helps resolve the dispute. The mediator does not have the authority to impose a solution on the parties involved.

Arbitration is a method of settling disputes in which the opposing parties agree to abide by the decision of an arbitrator. An arbitrator is either selected directly by the disputing parties or chosen in one of the following two ways:

1. Under the terms of a written contract, an arbitrator is chosen by the court or by the American Arbitration Association.

2. If no contract exists, each of the two involved parties selects an arbitrator, and the two arbitrators select a third.

In an informal proceeding, each side presents evidence and witnesses. In the alternative dispute resolution method called med-arb, the mediator resolves the dispute if the two parties are unable to reach agreement after mediation.

Advocates of alternative dispute resolution claim that these methods are faster and less costly than court adjudication. Critics claim that medical malpractice cases are best decided when all the factual information is brought out, as in pretrial judicial discovery procedures. Critics also argue that selecting arbitrators acceptable to both parties can take weeks, months, even years, and that attorneys' fees and damage awards can be as costly as in court-tried cases. Figure 5-2 illustrates a sample arbitration agreement to be signed by the patient and physician involved in a dispute.

Professional liability and medical malpractice are major concerns for all health care practitioners. However, the individual who is aware of the risks and how to avoid them, yet practices competently within the law and within his or her scope of practice, can enjoy a long, successful, and satisfying career without ever facing malpractice charges.

FIGURE 5-2 Sample Patient—Physician Arbitration Agreement

Article 1: It is understood that any dispute as to medical malpractice, that is as to whether any medical services rendered under this contract were unnecessary or unauthorized or were improperly, negligently, or incompetently rendered, will be determined by submission to arbitration as provided by California law, and not by a lawsuit or resort to court process except as California law provides for judicial review of arbitration proceedings. Both parties to this contract, by entering into, are giving up their constitutional right to have such dispute decided in a court of law before a jury, and instead are accepting the use of arbitration.

Article 2: I understand and agree that this arbitration agreement binds me and anyone else who may have a claim arising out of or related to all treatment or services provided by the physician, including any spouse or heirs of the patient and any children, whether born or unborn at the time of the occurrence giving rise to any claim. This includes, but is not limited to, all claims for monetary damages exceeding the jurisdictional limit of the small claims court, including, without limitation, suits for loss of consortium, wrongful deaths, emotional distress or punitive damages. I further understand and agree that if i sign this agreement on behalf of some other person for whom I have responsibility, then, in addition to myself, such person(s) will also be bound, along with anyone else who may have a claim arising out of the treatment or services rendered to that person. I also understand agree that this agreement relates to claims against the physician and any consenting substitute physician, as well as the physician's partners, associates, association, corporation or partnership, and the employees, agents, and estates of any of them. I also hereby consent to the intervention or joinder in the arbitration proceeding of all parties relevant to a full and complete settlement of any dispute arbitrated under this Agreement, as ser forth in the CA/HHS/CMA Medical Arbitration Rules.

Article 3: I understand and agree that I will be bound by this arbitration agreement and that this agreement will be valid and enforceable for any and all treatment provided by the physician in the future regardless of the length of time since my last visit to this physician, and regardless of the fact that the patient -physician relationship between myself and the physician may be interrupted for any reason and then recommenced.

Article 4: I understand that i do not have to sign this agreement to receive the physician's services, and that if i do sign the agreement and change my mind within 30 days of today, then i may cancel this agreement by giving written notice to the undersigned physician within that time stating that i want to withdraw from this arbitration agreement.

Article 5: On behalf of myself and all others bound by this agreement as set forth in Article 2, agreement is hereby given to be bound by the Medical Arbitration Rules of the California Association of Hospitals and Health Systems (CAHHS) and the California Medical Association (CMA), as they may be amended from time to time, which are hereby incorporated into this agreement, A copy of these rules is included in the pamphlet in which this agreement is found. Additional copies of the Rules are available from the California Medical Association, P.O. Box 7690, San Francisco, Ca. 94120-7690, Attention: Arbitration Rules, I understand that disputes covered by this Agreement will be covered by California law applicable to actions against health care providers, including the Medical Injury Compensation Reform Act of 1975 (including any amendments thereto).

Article 6: Optional: retroactive effect
If I intend this agreement to cover services rendered before the date it is signed (for example, emergency treatment), I have indicated the earlier date I intend this agreement to be effective from and initialed below.

Earlier effective date:_____   Patient's initials:_____

Article 7: I have read and understood all the information in this pamphlet, including the explanation of the Patient-Physician Arbitration Agreement, this Agreement, and the rules. I understand that in the case of any pregnant woman, the term "patient" as used herein means both the mother and the mother's expected child or children.

If any provision of this arbitration agreement is held invalid or unenforceable, the remaining provisions shall remain in full force and shall not be affected by the invalidity of any other provision.

Notice: By signing this contract you are agreeing to have any issue of medical malpractice decided by neutral arbitration and you are giving up your right to a jury or court trial. See article 1 of this contract.

_____   Dated: _____
(Patient, Parent, Guardian or Legally Authorized Representative of Patient)

If signed by other than patient, indicate relationship: _____

Physician's agreement to arbitrate:

In consideration of the foregoing execution of this Patient-Physician Arbitration Agreement, I likewise agree to be bound by the terms set forth in this agreement and in the rules specified in Article 5 above.

_____   Date:_____
(Physician or Duly-Authorized Representative)

_____   _____
   Title—e.g., Partner, President, etc.   Print name of Physician, Medical Group, Partnership or Association

Chapter Summary

Learning Outcome	Summary
LO 5.1 Identify three areas of general liability for which a physician/employer is responsible.	What are the three areas of general liability for which a physician/employer is responsible? • The practice's building and grounds. • Automobiles used as part of employees' duties. • Employee safety
LO 5.2 Describe the reasonable person standard, standard of care, and duty of care.	What are the differences among the reasonable person standard, standard of care, and duty of care? • Under the reasonable person standard, individuals may be charged with negligence if someone is injured because he or she failed to perform an act that a reasonable person, in similar circumstances, would perform, or if he or she committed an act that a reasonable person would not commit. • Standard of care is the level of performance expected of a health care practitioner in carrying out his or her professional duties. • Duty of care is the legal obligation of health care workers to patients and, sometimes, nonpatients.
LO 5.3 Briefly outline the responsibilities of health care practitioners concerning privacy, confidentiality, and privileged communication.	What are the responsibilities of health care practitioners concerning privacy, confidentiality, and privileged communication? • Health care practitioners have a legal and ethical obligation to safeguard a patient's privacy and maintain confidentiality, which is the act of holding information in confidence, not to be released to unauthorized individuals. • Privileged communication refers to information held confidential within a protected relationship, such as the physician–patient relationship, and patients may sue for breach of confidence if protected information is released and results in damage to the patient.
LO 5.4 Explain the four elements necessary to prove negligence (the four Ds).	What are the four Ds of negligence? • *Duty*—The person charged with negligence owed a duty of care to the accuser. • *Dereliction*—The health care provider breached the duty of care to the patient. • *Direct Cause*—The breach of the duty of care to the patient was a direct cause of the patient's injury. • *Damages*—There is a legally recognizable injury to the patient.
LO 5.5 Outline the phases of a lawsuit.	What are the phases of a lawsuit? • Pleading phase • Interrogatory or pretrial discovery phase • Trial phase • Appeals phase What is the difference between testimony by deposition and interrogatory testimony? • A deposition is sworn testimony given and recorded outside the courtroom during the pretrial phase of a case. An interrogatory is a written set of questions requiring written answers from a plaintiff or defendant under oath.
LO 5.6 Name two advantages to alternative dispute resolution.	What is alternative dispute resolution? • Settlement of civil disputes between parties using neutral mediators or arbitrators without going to court. • Such settlements can save time and money.

Ethics ISSUE 1:

As citizens and as professionals with special training and experience, health care practitioners are ethically obligated to assist in the administration of justice. If a patient who has a legal claim requests a health care practitioner's assistance, he or she should furnish medical evidence, with the patient's consent, to secure the patient's legal rights.

Medical experts should have recent and substantive experience in the area in which they testify and should limit testimony to their sphere of medical expertise.

Discussion Questions

1. An orthopedic surgeon who has been retired from practice for 15 years and is a friend of the plaintiff's has been called to testify in the plaintiff's suit alleging damage to his hip joint sustained in a car accident. In your opinion, is it ethical for the physician described previously to testify? Explain your answer.

_____

_____

2. In your opinion, is it ever ethical for a health care practitioner to testify against another health care practitioner in a medical malpractice lawsuit? Explain your answer.

_____

_____

3. As a health care practitioner, do you consider it ethical to charge for your services to testify as an expert witness? Explain your answer.

_____

_____

4. Are there circumstances when you might consider it unethical to charge for your services as an expert witness? Explain your answer.

_____

_____

Ethics ISSUE 2:

Health care practitioners are ethically bound to respect the patient's dignity and to make a positive effort to secure a comfortable and considerate atmosphere for the patient, in such ways as providing appropriate gowns and drapes, private facilities for undressing, and clear explanations for procedures.

Discussion Questions

1. An adolescent male patient is visibly uncomfortable as a female physician begins a physical examination. What actions might the physician and/or her attending certified medical assistant take to make the patient more comfortable?

_____

_____

2. A hospital patient who is mentally disabled becomes extremely agitated and violent. She disrobes and runs through the hallways. Nurses and other employees are unable to calm the woman, and security officers arrive. Other patients and employees in the area stand around watching the woman as the officers attempt to subdue her. As a health care practitioner in the immediate vicinity, what, if anything, might you do to protect the woman's privacy?

_____

_____

relevant literature is readily accessible to physicians. As required by the Occupational Safety and Health Administration (OSHA), employees should have access to Material Safety Data Sheets (MSDS) for each hazardous chemical in use in the medical facility. (See Chapter 10 for more information about OSHA medical workplace requirements.)

WHY DO PATIENTS SUE?

From a medical/legal standpoint, several studies conducted over the last decade have identified seven recurring reasons for medical malpractice lawsuits:

1. Cancer misdiagnosis, failure to diagnose, or a delay in diagnosis.
2. Birth injury or negligent maternity care.
3. Wrong diagnosis and misdiagnosis of negligent fracture or trauma.
4. Delay in diagnosis or failure to consult in a timely manner.
5. Medication errors or medication malpractice resulting from negligent drug treatment.
6. Malpractice resulting from a physician's negligent procedures or surgical errors.
7. Failure to obtain informed consent.

Studies have consistently found additional reasons when patients were asked directly why they sued physicians. The first major study to determine why patients sue hospitals and health care practitioners and what might prevent an injured patient or his or her family members from filing a lawsuit was conducted in 1992 by Gerald B. Hickson and others. This study looked at factors that prompted parents to file medical malpractice suits after a perinatal injury. (*Perinatal* refers to the period immediately before and after a child's birth.)

According to Hickson and his colleagues, there are six common reasons for patients suing for medical malpractice, as shown in Table 6-1.

Table 6-1 Hickson and Colleagues' Reasons for Patient Lawsuits

Reason	Percentage of Respondents
Plaintiffs advised by knowledgeable acquaintances to sue	33
Recognized a cover-up	24
Needed money	24
Recognized that the child would have no future	23
Needed information about what had happened	20
Wanted revenge or to protect others from harm	19

Source: Adapted from Gerald B. Hickson et al., "Factors That Prompted Families to File Medical Malpractice Claims Following Perinatal Injuries," *Journal of the American Medical Association* 267 (1992), p. 1359.

In a separate, equally well-known study, Charles Vincent and others examined why patients and their relatives sue physicians, and also investigated which actions might have prevented litigation. Study participants were given a list of 13 statements and asked whether they agreed or disagreed with each one. Table 6-2 lists the results.

Just over 41 percent of the respondents in the Vincent study said that certain actions after their injuries might have prevented litigation. In order of frequency, such actions included:

1. An explanation and apology. (However, a 2013 Medscape Malpractice Report found that 93 percent of physicians who had been sued for malpractice said an apology would have made no difference.)

2. Correction of the mistake.

3. Financial compensation

4. Correct treatment at the time.

5. An admission of negligence.

6. Listening to the patient.

7. Disciplinary action against medical personnel involved.

8. Honesty

9. Investigation by the hospital.

Table 6-2 Vincent and Colleagues' Findings on Why Patients Sue

Why Injured Patients Sued	Percentage Who Agreed with Statement
Prevent injury from happening to anyone else	91
To receive an explanation	91
Wanted the doctors to realize what they had done	90
To get an admission of negligence	87
To make the doctor realize how I felt	68
My feelings were ignored	67
Wanted financial compensation	66
I was angry	65
Didn't want the doctor to get away with it	54
Wanted the doctor to be disciplined	48
Allowed me to cope with my feelings	46
Because of the staff's attitude afterward	43
To get back at the doctor	23

Source: Adapted from Charles Vincent et al., "Why Do People Sue Doctors? A Study of Patients and Relatives Taking Legal Action," *The Lancet* 343 (1994), pp. 1609, 1611.

testing or the examination of a rape victim, evidence may need to be collected in a certain manner to be admissible in court. When in doubt about what documentation to make, you should contact legal authorities for advice.

Physicians should keep records that clearly show what treatment was done and when it was done. It is important that they be able to demonstrate that nothing was neglected and that the care given fully met the standards demanded by law. Physicians should also document all referrals to other physicians, withdrawals from cases, and cases in which patients refuse to follow their advice. Today's health care environment requires complete documentation of actions taken and, in many cases, actions not taken. Medical facility employees should pay particular attention to the following:

Referrals. Make sure the patient understands whether the referring physician's staff will make the appointment and notify the patient or whether the patient must call to set up the appointment. Make notations that the patient has been referred, and follow up with telephone calls to verify that an appointment was scheduled and kept. Note whether or not reports of the consultation were received in your office, and document all recommendations from the referring physician concerning further care of the patient.

Missed Appointments. At the end of each day, a designated person in the medical office should gather all patient records of those who missed or canceled appointments without rescheduling. Charts and electronic or handwritten schedule books should be dated, stamped, and documented "no show" or "canceled, no reschedule," respectively. The treating physician should review these records and note whether or not follow-up is indicated. If follow-up occurs, it should be documented as completed.

Dismissals. To avoid charges of abandonment, the physician must formally withdraw from a case or formally dismiss the patient. Be sure that a letter of withdrawal or dismissal has been filed in the patient's records.

Treatment Refusals. A patient's decision to decline treatment, evaluation, or testing should be documented in the patient record. "Informed refusal" should be obtained with respect to any treatment or procedure which could have either diagnostic or therapeutic consequences. "Informed refusal" should be obtained in writing or, at the very least, noted in the patient's medical record.

All Other Patient Contact. Patients' records should include reports of all tests, procedures, and medications prescribed, including refills. Make sure all necessary informed-consent papers have been duly signed and filed in a patient's record. Keep a record of all telephone conversations with the patient. Remember that correct documentation requires the initials or signature of the person making a notation on the patient's medical record, as well as the date and time. Remember the rule, "If it wasn't documented, it wasn't done."

Check Your Progress

1. Name and briefly define the four Cs of medical malpractice prevention.
2. Briefly describe how practicing effective communication skills can help prevent a medical malpractice lawsuit.
3. If a patient refuses treatment, what legal options remain for the health care practitioner in charge?
4. Name five reasons often cited for the suing of health care practitioners by patients and their families.

Types of Defenses

When, in spite of all the best efforts to avoid litigation, a medical malpractice lawsuit is filed, the physician or other health care professional must defend himself or herself against the charges.

LO 6.2
Describe the various defenses to professional liability suits.

DENIAL

Denial of wrongdoing, or the assertion of innocence, may be used as a defense in professional liability suits. If some of the alleged facts are true, defendants may not claim innocence. Instead, they should claim that the charge or charges do not meet all of the elements of the theory of recovery. In other words, the charge may be missing one of the four Ds of negligence.

denial
A defense that claims innocence of the charges or that one or more of the four Ds of negligence are lacking.

AFFIRMATIVE DEFENSES

Affirmative defenses that may be used by the defendant in a medical professional liability suit allow the accused to present factual evidence that the patient's condition was caused by some factor other than the defendant's negligence.

affirmative defenses
Defenses used by defendants in medical professional liability suits that allow the accused to present factual evidence that the patient's condition was caused by some factor other than the defendant's negligence.

Contributory Negligence When the defense claims **contributory negligence,** this alleges that the patient or complaining party, through a "want of ordinary care," caused or contributed to his or her own injury. The physician may deny that he or she committed a negligent act and claim the patient was totally responsible for the damage or injury. Alternatively, the physician may admit negligence but claim that the patient was also somehow at fault and so contributed to the injury.

contributory negligence
An affirmative defense that alleges that the plaintiff, through a lack of care, caused or contributed to his or her own injury.

In some states, damages are apportioned according to the degree to which a plaintiff contributed to the injury. This is called **comparative negligence.** For instance, if the court decides that a patient, through his or her own negligence, contributed 20 percent toward the injury and the physician contributed 80 percent, the patient's damage award may be reduced by 20 percent.

comparative negligence
An affirmative defense claimed by the defendant, alleging that the plaintiff contributed to the injury by a certain degree.

In hearing cases alleging contributory negligence, the court will consider the patient's ability to comprehend and carry out the physician's instructions. Minors or adults who are unconscious, mentally disabled, insane, or otherwise incompetent may be judged unable to have contributed to a negligent act.

Patient Can Contribute to Negligence

A man who was a detainee at a county jail was taken to a county hospital emergency room when he complained of pain in his lower abdomen, nausea, and vomiting of blood for two weeks. An RN took the man's vital signs, finding his blood pressure to be 159/106 and his pulse to be fast. The nurse also drew blood and ordered initial lab work. A physician saw the patient and ordered that a nasogastric tube be inserted to check for blood in the stomach. The nurse tried to insert the tube, but the patient complained that it was extremely painful and said he did not want the tube inserted. The nurse explained why the tube was necessary, but the patient declined, insisting that his problems were due to his appendix. He signed a form indicating that he was refusing medical treatment against medical advice. The man was returned to the jail, where he died one week later of gastrointestinal hemorrhaging.

Blood test results that came back after the patient left the hospital were abnormal, indicating a life-threatening condition. Since the patient had signed himself out of the hospital, and the hospital claimed it no longer had a duty to him, his test results were not forwarded to the physician who examined the patient or to the patient.

The administrator of the patient's estate filed a malpractice suit against the nurse and the hospital. A trial jury found for the defendants, under the defense of contributory negligence. The administrator appealed, but the appellate court affirmed the lower court's judgment.

Margaret Lyons as the administratrix of the estate of Kenneth Cook, deceased v. Walker Regional Medical Center, Inc., and Laurie Hunter, 868 So.2d 1071 Supreme Court of Alabama, 2003.

assumption of risk
A legal defense that holds that the defendant is not guilty of a negligent act because the plaintiff knew of and accepted beforehand any risks involved.

Assumption of Risk **Assumption of risk** is a defense based on the contention that the patient knew of the inherent risks before treatment was performed and agreed to those risks. Informed consent (see Chapter 7) is vital to this defense, since the defendant must show that the patient was fully informed of the risks prior to treatment and that the risks inherent in the treatment were the cause of the patient's injury.

For example, in one lawsuit in which the defendant used the assumption of risk defense, it was held that a physician was not liable for injuries suffered by a chronically ill woman when she fell in the examining room while attempting to undress without assistance. Because she had refused assistance, the woman had assumed the risk of injury.

In other cases, it has been held that individuals submitting to X-ray treatment assume the risk of burns from a proper exposure to X-rays but not the risk of negligence in the application of the treatment.

emergency
A type of affirmative defense in which the person who comes to the aid of a victim in an emergency is not held liable under certain circumstances.

Emergency If services were provided during an **emergency**, this may also be used as an affirmative defense. The health care practitioner who comes to the aid of a victim in an emergency would not be held liable under common law if the defense established that:

1. A true emergency situation existed and was not caused by the defendant.

2. The appropriate standard of care was met, given the emergency situation.

Health care professionals who provide assistance in emergencies may also be protected from liability under Good Samaritan Acts, which are discussed in Chapter 7.

Assumption of Risk Defense Denied

A physician treated a patient for Crohn's disease (a painful inflammation of the small intestine of indeterminate cause). To treat the patient's pain, the physician prescribed Percocet and Tylenol #3 with codeine. The patient developed an addiction to the drugs and was forced to undergo extensive drug rehabilitation. The plaintiff patient sued the physician, alleging that he negligently prescribed dangerous and addictive narcotic drugs and failed to recognize her addiction to them. A trial court granted a directed verdict to the physician on the basis of the plaintiff's assumption of risk. The patient appealed.

The appellate court agreed that the doctor was negligent in failing to fully consider the possibility that the patient could become addicted to the drugs he prescribed. Testimony indicated that errors in the patient's medical record could have interfered with the physician's ability to effectively monitor the patient's drug use. The appellate court found that the patient's classic drug-addicted behavior, in attempting to acquire additional narcotics, did not automatically relieve the physician from his duty to monitor her for signs of abuse or relieve the doctor from any liability for continuing to prescribe narcotics. Insofar as addiction is a compulsive behavior, the court could not find that the patient voluntarily acquiesced to the risks involved with taking excessive medication.

The judgment of the trial court was reversed, and the case was returned to the trial court for a new trial.

Conrad-Hutsell v. Colturi, 2002 Ohio 2632; 2002 Ohio App.

TECHNICAL DEFENSES

When defenses to liability suits are based on legal technicalities, instead of on factual evidence, they are called **technical defenses.** Technical defenses include those that claim the statute of limitations has run out, there is insufficient evidence to support the plaintiff's claim of negligence, and the assertion that the plaintiff has no standing to sue.

technical defenses
Defenses used in a lawsuit that are based on legal technicalities.

Release of Tortfeasor A tortfeasor is one who is guilty of committing a tort. Suppose a third party causes injury to a person as in an automobile accident, and a physician treats the injured person. In most states, the party who caused the accident (the tortfeasor) is liable both for the victim's injury and for any medical negligence by the physician who treats the injured victim. This is the basis for the **release of tortfeasor** defense.

If the injured party sues the tortfeasor, settles the case, and then releases the tortfeasor from further liability, the injured party cannot also sue the physician unless the victim expressly reserved that right in the release. If the victim's settlement with the tortfeasor provided compensation for all medical expenses, the release of tortfeasor is usually an absolute defense.

Laws governing release of tortfeasor contain many modifiers, which must be applied in individual cases.

release of tortfeasor
A technical defense that prohibits a lawsuit against the person who caused an injury (the tortfeasor) if he or she was expressly released from further liability in the settlement of a suit.

Res Judicata Under the doctrine of *res judicata*, "The thing has been decided," a claim cannot be retried between the same parties if it has already been legally resolved. For example, if a patient sues a physician for negligence and loses, the patient cannot then sue the physician for breach of contract based on evidence presented in the trial for negligence. If a patient refuses to pay a physician's fees on the grounds

res judicata
"The thing has been decided." Legal principle that a claim cannot be retried between the same parties if it has already been legally resolved.

groups that routinely employ or contract with health care providers. Credentialing usually consists of the following:

1. A provider fills out an application and attaches copies of his or her medical license, proof of malpractice insurance coverage, and other requested credentials.

2. The listed sources are asked to verify the information.

3. Medicare and Medicaid sanctions and malpractice history are checked via the National Practitioner Data Bank.

4. The findings are presented to a credentialing committee.

5. A peer review process completes the credentialing procedure.

Check Your Progress

Circle the correct answer for each of the following questions.

8. Risk management has become a necessary health care practice component because
   a. Liability insurance is often unavailable.
   b. Liability is a major factor in health care delivery.
   c. Patients with bad outcomes always sue.

9. Methods used to manage risk are part of
   a. The provisions in liability insurance policies
   b. Every health care provider's practice
   c. Quality improvement or quality assurance

10. Which of the following activities help health care providers avoid litigation?
    a. Vocal disclaimers before procedures are performed
    b. Medical record charting
    c. Issuing written denials in response to accusations of wrong-doing

11. Which of the following is *not* a duty of a medical practice's quality improvement and risk manager?
    a. Credentialing
    b. Checking compliance with health care regulatory agencies' requirements
    c. Scheduling patient appointments

12. Credentialing consists of
    a. Publishing health care provider job vacancies
    b. Filing health care employees' credentials with state agencies
    c. Verifying health care providers' credentials before hiring

LO 6.4

Discuss five different types of medical liability insurance.

liability insurance
Contract coverage for potential damages incurred as a result of a negligent act.

Professional Liability Insurance

Because costs for defending a medical malpractice lawsuit can be high, **liability insurance** may be purchased to cover the costs up to the limits of the policy. For example, if a medical professional liability insurance policy covers an insured physician up to $10 million, in the event that he or she loses a malpractice suit and must pay damages, the insurance company will not pay more than that amount.

The cost of liability insurance premiums for a physician is based on the physician's specialty and the dollar amount covered by the policy. Insurance for those physicians in the least risky insurance risk class (for example, family practitioners and specialists who do not perform surgery) is generally less costly than insurance for those in specialties considered riskier (for example, orthopedic surgeons and obstetricians). States vary regarding those medical specialties considered to carry the highest risk of liability and, therefore, are subject to the highest liability insurance premiums.

Some physicians drop liability insurance coverage when rates become too high. However, this can adversely affect a physician's practice, since most hospitals require proof of coverage up to a predetermined minimum amount to grant hospital privileges. In addition, managed care organizations require physicians to provide proof of liability insurance coverage as a prerequisite for entering into a contractual agreement and as a component of their credentialing process.

There are two main types of medical malpractice insurance:

1. **Claims-made insurance** covers the insured only for those claims made (not for any injury occurring) while the policy is in force. With this kind of insurance, the determining factor is when the claim is made, not when the injury occurs. For example, a policy in force during a previous year would cover only those claims made during that year.

2. **Occurrence insurance** (also known as claims-incurred insurance) covers the insured for any claims arising from an incident that occurred or is alleged to have occurred while the policy is in force, regardless of when the claim is made. For example, suppose an alleged incident of negligence by a physician occurred in September 2013, while the physician's occurrence insurance policy was in effect with XYZ Insurance Company. If a patient files a claim against the physician in January 2016, after the policy period has passed, the physician is covered under the terms of the occurrence insurance policy.

There are three types of insurance that health care practitioners can purchase to extend coverage of a canceled claims-made policy or for claims-made coverage when the insured switches to a different insurance carrier:

Tail coverage. When a claims-made policy is discontinued, tail coverage (sometimes called a reporting endorsement) is an option available to health care practitioners from their former carriers to continue coverage for those dates that claims-made coverage was in effect. Once a claims-made policy is canceled, coverage does not continue in the future for any claims that might be reported unless tail coverage or prior acts coverage is secured at the time the policy is canceled. If neither is purchased, any future claims that might arise from services performed during the policy period will no longer be covered.

Prior acts insurance coverage. This is a supplement to a claims-made policy that health care practitioners can purchase from a new carrier when they change carriers. Prior acts coverage, also

claims-made insurance
A type of liability insurance that covers the insured only for those claims made (not for any injury occurring) while the policy is in force.

occurrence insurance
A type of liability insurance that covers the insured for any claims arising from an incident that occurred, or is alleged to have occurred, during the time the policy is in force, regardless of when the claim is made.

tail coverage
An insurance coverage option available for health care practitioners: When a claims-made policy is discontinued, it extends coverage for malpractice claims alleged to have occurred during those dates that claims-made coverage was in effect.

prior acts insurance coverage
A supplement to a claims-made insurance policy that can be purchased from a new carrier when health care practitioners change carriers.

known as "nose" coverage, covers incidents that occurred prior to the beginning of the new insurance relationship but have not yet been brought to the insured's attention as a claim. Prior acts coverage is an alternative to a reporting period endorsement (also known as tail coverage), which is purchased from the original carrier when a change in carriers is made. Companies typically require the new insured to purchase either tail or nose coverage to protect against claims arising from prior acts.

Self-insurance coverage. As medical malpractice insurance premiums have continued to rise, self-insurance coverage has become an option for health care practitioners in some states. It works like this: An insurance company writes a policy with a limit of $X, and the insured parties contribute to a trust fund up to a limit of $X to be used in paying potential medical malpractice awards. The insurance company charges fees for managing the fund. One advantage to self-insurance coverage is that premiums are considerably lower than with traditional types of medical malpractice insurance. A disadvantage is that state laws regulating insurance do not always allow such plans, and even in states where such coverage is allowed, hospitals must agree to accept self-insurance plans for those physicians who apply for hospital privileges.

Physicians and other health care practitioners should notify their insurance companies immediately if advised of the possibility of a malpractice lawsuit. Insurance companies almost always provide legal representation for covered physicians, and some insurance contracts require that the insurance company's attorneys represent the insured physician.

Once a lawsuit seems imminent, the health care practitioner and/or his or her employees should not mention the suit on the telephone or in correspondence unless the insurance company's legal counsel approves such a reference.

self-insurance coverage
An insurance coverage option whereby insured subscribers contribute to a trust fund to be used in paying potential damage awards.

Check Your Progress

13. If a health care practitioner covered by medical malpractice insurance receives notice of a lawsuit, he or she should first notify _____.

14. Claims-made insurance pays for _____.

15. Occurrence insurance pays for _____.

16. Name two types of insurance that, in certain circumstances, extend coverage of claims-made insurance. _____

17. Explain how physicians might insure themselves.

_____

In short, few patients sue health care practitioners they like and trust. If patients perceive health care providers as cold, uncaring, or rude, however, they may be more inclined to sue if something goes wrong, and patients who feel ignored, deserted, or who suspect that there is a medical "coverup" may also be more inclined to sue.

Learning Outcome	Summary
LO 6.1 List and define the four Cs of medical malpractice prevention.	**What are the four Cs of medical malpractice prevention?**
	• Caring
	• Communication
	• Competence
	• Charting
	Why do patients sue?
	• Unrealistic expectations
	• Poor rapport and poor communication.
	• Greed
	• Lawyers and our litigious society.
	• Poor quality of care—either in fact or in perception.
	• Poor outcome
	• Failure to understand patients' and families' perspectives and devaluing their point of view.
	What general categories of information should be documented for legal purposes?
	• What treatment was performed and when.
	• Referrals
	• Missed appointments
	• Dismissals
	• Treatment refusals
	• All other patient contact.
LO 6.2 Describe the various defenses to professional liability suits.	**What types of defense may be used in a medical malpractice lawsuit?**
	• Denial
	• Affirmative
	• Contributory negligence
	• Comparative negligence
	• Assumption of risk
	• Emergency
	• Technical
	• Release of tortfeasor
	• *Res judicata*
	• Statute of limitations
LO 6.3 Explain the purpose of quality improvement and risk management within a health care facility.	**What purpose does risk management serve?**
	• Helps minimize liability
	• Quality improvement (QI) or quality assurance.
	• Verifies credentials
LO 6.4 Discuss five different types of medical liability insurance.	**What types of professional liability insurance are available to medical providers?**
	• Claims-made
	• Tail coverage
	• Prior acts coverage
	• Occurrence
	• Self-coverage

Requests for release of records may ask for records concerning a specific date or time span. Records may also be requested for a specific diagnosis, symptom, or body system, or for results of certain diagnostic tests. Medical records personnel should not send unsolicited records. They should carefully review the signed release form to ensure that the correct records are sent.

When medical records are requested for use in a lawsuit, a signed consent for the release of the records must be obtained from the patient, unless a court subpoenas the records. In this case, the patient should be notified in writing that the records have been subpoenaed and released.

ROUTINE RELEASE OF INFORMATION

Medical information about a patient is often released for the following purposes:

Insurance Claims. The medical office supplies specific requested information, but does not usually send the patient's entire medical record. An authorization to release information, signed by the patient, is required before records may be released, but most health care providers incorporate the release into the patient registration form so that information can be provided in a timely manner.

Transfer to Another Physician. The physician may photocopy and send all records, or may send a summary. The patient must sign an authorization to release records.

Use in a Court of Law. When a subpoena *duces tecum* is issued for certain records (the subpoena commands a witness to appear in court and to bring certain medical records), the patient's written consent to release the records is waived.

The court case, "Not Guilty of Breach of Confidentiality," illustrates that physicians who produce patients' medical records for use in court, or those who testify in court as expert witnesses, are not liable for breach of confidentiality.

As illustrated in the chapter's opening scenario, individuals responsible for releasing medical information must follow procedure to protect against unauthorized release, even in the previous situations where medical records are routinely requested.

The court case, "Breach of Confidentiality Declared—Damages Upheld," determined that damages were properly awarded to the plaintiff in a suit against a nurse who released confidential medical information without authorization.

fiduciary duty
A physician's obligation to his or her patient, based on trust and confidence.

COURT CASE Not Guilty of Breach of Confidentiality

A physician cannot be sued for breach of confidentiality when required to produce a patient's medical records for use in court testimony.

A patient (Cruz) sued a physician (Agelides) for breach of fiduciary duty. (**Fiduciary duty** is a physician's duty to his or her patient, based on trust and confidence.) In a previous malpractice action brought by Cruz against another

physician, Agelides had given a sworn pretrial affidavit and video deposition in favor of the defending physician. The court held that Agelides was immune from any civil liability action as a result of his testimony as a witness in the previous trial.

Cruz v. Agelides, 574 So 2d 278 (Fla. App. 3 Dist., 1991).

Breach of Confidentiality Declared— Damages Upheld

A 20-year-old unmarried woman who lived with her parents decided to terminate her pregnancy at the Long Island Surgi-Center. Because her parents strongly disapproved of premarital sex and were implacably opposed to abortion, she did not tell them of her decision. When she arranged for the procedure, the woman provided her cell phone number, but told the clinic never to call her at home. Nevertheless, a day after the abortion one of the clinic's nurses telephoned the young woman at home and spoke with a person she knew to be the woman's mother. Because blood test results had been received at the center that morning, but had not been entered in the patient's medical record, the nurse called the patient's home to determine (1) information about the patient's blood type, and (2) if the

patient was experiencing vaginal bleeding. The nurse did not explicitly tell the patient's mother that her daughter had undergone an abortion, but the mother deduced the truth from the nurse's questions. The patient's relationship with her parents was irreparably damaged, and she sued the clinic, charging breaches of confidentiality, privacy, and fiduciary duty, and seeking compensatory and punitive damages. The center conceded liability, and the matter proceeded to trial on the question of damages. The jury awarded the plaintiff $65,000 for past and future emotional distress and $300,000 in punitive damages. The Surgi-Center appealed the damages awarded, but the appeals court upheld the awards.

Randi A. J. v. Long Is. Surgi-Ctr., 2007 NY Slip Op 06953; 46 A.D. 3d 74.

While Michael, Sally, and Teresa, medical records employees, are explicitly aware of the dangers of releasing confidential medical information, all health care practitioners, like the nurse in the court case, "Breach of Confidentiality Declared—Damages Upheld," also need to be constantly aware of protecting confidentiality of patients' medical records.

Physicians receive subpoenas for patient medical records for a variety of reasons, including accidents involving patients, workers' compensation claims, and other nonmedical-liability reasons. When this occurs, the medical office sends a photocopy of the patient's medical records to the attorney who issued the subpoena.

When a physician is sued for medical malpractice, however, responsibility to comply with a subpoena to produce specified medical records in court may fall to the medical office employee in charge of medical records. In that case, the person in charge of medical records should follow these guidelines:

- Check the subpoena to be sure the name and phone number of the issuing attorney and the court docket number of the case are listed.

- If a copy of the subpoena is received, verify with the issuing attorney that it is the same as the original in every way.

- Verify that the patient named was a patient of the physician named.

- Verify the trial date and time as listed on the subpoena.

- Notify the physician that a subpoena was received, and then notify the physician's insurance company or attorney, if so directed.

- Check all subpoenaed records to be sure they are complete, but never alter them in any way.

- Document the number of pages in the record and itemize its contents. Make a photocopy of the original to be submitted, if permitted by state law and the court.

- Offer sworn testimony regarding the record, if so instructed by the court.

Confidentiality of Alcohol and Drug Abuse, Patient Records
A federal statute that protects patients with histories of substance abuse regarding the release of information about treatment.

Some state laws specifically address the release of confidential medical information, especially as it pertains to treatment for mental or emotional health problems, HIV testing, and substance abuse. In addition, the federal statute **Confidentiality of Alcohol and Drug Abuse, Patient Records** protects patients with histories of substance abuse regarding the release of information about treatment. Under no circumstances should information of this type be released without specific, written permission from the patient to do so. The patient also has the right to rescind (cancel) consent to release information, in which case the information should not be released.

The following rules for authorizations for the release of medical records can serve as a general guide for medical assistants, health information technicians, and other health care practitioners:

- Authorizations should be in writing.
- Authorizations should include the patient's name, address, and date of birth.
- The patient should sign authorizations, unless he or she is not a legal, competent adult. In that case, parents or guardians should sign authorizations.
- Only the information specifically requested should be released.
- Requests for information coming into the medical office from insurance companies, physicians, or other sources should be witnessed and dated and include the complete name, address, and signature of the party requesting the information, as well as that of the party asked to release the information.
- Include a specific description of the information that is needed. List the purpose for which the data will be used and the date on which the consent expires.

CONSENT

consent
Permission from a person, either expressed or implied, for something to be done by another.

By giving **consent,** the patient gives permission, either expressed (orally or in writing) or implied, for the physician to examine him or her, to perform tests that aid in diagnosis, and/or to treat for a medical condition. When the patient makes an appointment for an examination, that patient has given implied consent for the physician to perform the exam. Likewise, when he or she cooperates with various diagnostic testing procedures, implied consent for the tests has been given.

Informed Consent For surgery and for some other procedures, such as a test for HIV, implied consent is not enough. In these cases, it is important to ask the patient to sign a consent form, thereby documenting informed consent (see Figure 7-1).

doctrine of informed consent
The legal basis for informed consent, usually outlined in a state's medical practice acts.

The **doctrine of informed consent** is the legal basis for informed consent and is usually outlined in a state's medical practice acts. Informed consent implies that the patient understands

- Proposed modes of treatment.
- Why the treatment is necessary.
- Risks involved in the proposed treatment.
- Available alternative modes of treatment.
- Risks of alternative modes of treatment.
- Risks involved if treatment is refused.

13. Name three reasons a medical office might be requested to release a patient's medical records.

14. In which of the three situations named for question 13 might a patient's written consent to release records be waived?

15. What is needed before the medical office can send a patient's medical record to the insurer?

16. If an insurance company submits a request for medical records pertaining to an enrolled patient's outpatient foot surgery and you are responsible for sending the records, should you send the patient's entire file to be on the safe side? Why or why not?

17. As the person who reviews requests for patients' medical records, do you need to know the purpose for which the data will be used? Explain your answer.

INFORMED CONSENT for SURGERY and PROCEDURES

1. I hereby authorize staff physicians and resident staff at _____ to perform upon
(Name of Hospital or Facility)
_____ , such treatment, procedures and/or operations necessary to treat or diagnose the
(Name of patient)
condition(s) which appear indicated.

2. The operation(s) or procedure(s) necessary to treat and/or diagnose my condition and the risks, benefits/alternatives and options associated with them have been explained to me by_____ , and I understand the operation(s) or
(Name of Physician or provider)

procedure(s) to be: _____

3. Different Provider: ☐ Not Applicable
I understand and approve that a different provider other than the physician named above may actually perform the procedure.

4. Operative Side: ☐ Not Applicable   ☐ Left   ☐ Right

5. Sedation & Local Anesthetics: I authorize the administration of sedation and the use of local anesthetics, drugs and medicines as may be deemed appropriate. If they will be used, the risks and benefits/alternatives of sedation have been explained to me by the procedural physician.

6. Blood and Blood Products: ☐ Not Applicable
I understand certain surgeries, procedures, or illnesses may result in loss of blood. I authorize the administration of blood and/or blood components during the procedure as well as during the course of my hospital stay. If blood will be used, the risks, benefits/alternatives have been explained to me by the physician.

Patient Initials: _____

7. No Blood Products: ☐ Not Applicable
I request that No blood derivative be administered to me. I hereby release the hospital, its personnel, the attending physician and its agents from any responsibility whatsoever for unfavorable reactions or any untoward results due to my refusal to permit the use of blood or its derivatives. The possible risks and consequences of such refusal on my part have been fully explained and I fully understand such risks and consequences may occur as a result of my refusal.

Signature of Patient/Responsible Person: _____   Relationship: _____

8. Unforeseen Conditions: It has been explained to me that during the course of the operation(s) or procedure(s) unforeseen conditions may be revealed that necessitate an extension of the original procedure(s) or different procedure(s) than those set forth above. I am aware that the practice of medicine is not an exact science and I acknowledge that no guarantees have been made to me concerning the result of the operation(s) or procedure(s).

9. Photography: I consent to the use of photography, closed circuit television recording and to use the photographs and other materials for study, educational and scientific purposes, in accordance with ordinary practices of the facility.

10. I consent to have my procedure/operation observed, for educational purposes, by individual(s) other than those assisting the physician during the procedure/operation.

Physician or Provider Signature	Patient's Signature (if competent)	Witness	Date	Time
Signature of Interpreter (if applicable)	Date Time	Signature of Person Responsible Relationship	Date	Time
Witness (Telephone consent) Date Time		Second Physician or Provider Signature for Emergencies for incompetent patient and No family	Date	Time

Physician must initial faxed copy

FIGURE 7-1
A Sample Consent Form

Informed consent involves the patient's right to receive all information relative to his or her condition and then to make a decision regarding treatment based on that knowledge. Documents establishing that the patient gave informed consent prove that the patient was not coerced into treatment.

Adults of sound mind are usually able to give informed consent. Those individuals who cannot give informed consent include the following:

Minors, Persons under the Age of Majority. Exceptions include:

- Emancipated minors—those who are living away from home and responsible for their own support. A minor becomes "emancipated" through a court hearing where evidence is presented that the minor should be emancipated, and a judge makes a determination that the minor has met certain criteria. The minor is then declared "emancipated" and can consent to his or her health care treatment just as any adult of sound mind determines his or her health care treatment.

- Married minors

- Mature minors—those who, through the doctrine of mature minors, have been granted the right to seek birth control or care during pregnancy, treatment for reportable communicable diseases, or treatment for drug- or alcohol-related problems without first obtaining parental consent.

Persons Who Are Mentally Incompetent. Individuals judged by the court to be insane, senile, mentally challenged, or under the influence of drugs or alcohol cannot give informed consent. In these cases, a competent person may be designated by the court to act as the patient's agent.

Persons Who Speak Limited or No English. When a patient does not speak or understand English, an interpreter may be necessary to inform the patient and obtain his or her consent for treatment.

The rights of emancipated minors, married minors, and mature minors to consent to their own health care are discussed further in Chapter 11.

Other problems in obtaining informed consent may arise in situations such as when foster children need medical attention or a spouse seeks sterilization or an abortion. In each case, health care practitioners must determine who is legally able to give informed consent for treatment. When in doubt, seek legal advice.

Patient education is vital to the issue of informed consent. Stocking the medical office with brochures about various medical problems is not sufficient if the physician does not review the material with the patient. Patients who sue have successfully claimed lack of informed consent because they did not read the consent form they signed or did not read brochures handed to them. Health care personnel should be sure that patients understand all forms and all treatments/surgeries to be performed before signing.

Before proceeding with treatment, health care practitioners must determine whether or not patients are competent to give informed consent.

In 1970 a single woman in Texas became pregnant. She had difficulty finding work because of her pregnancy and feared the stigma of an illegitimate birth. Under the fictitious name "Jane Roe," the woman sued Henry Wade, the district attorney in Dallas County, Texas, claiming that she had limited rights to an abortion and sought an injunction against the Texas statute prohibiting abortion except to save a woman's life.

It took three years for the case to reach the U.S. Supreme Court, which struck down the Texas statute.

The ruling came too late for Jane Roe to have the abortion she originally sought, of course, but it affected the rights of all women who would seek abortions from that time on. The Court held that the constitutional right to privacy includes a woman's decision to terminate a pregnancy during the first trimester (three months), but that states could impose restrictions and regulate abortions after that.

Roe v. Wade, 410 U.S. 113, 144 "n 39" (1973).

Informed Consent and Abortion Law In *Planned Parenthood v. Casey,* U.S. 833 (1992), the U.S. Supreme Court upheld a 24-hour waiting period, an informed consent requirement, a parental consent provision for minors, and a record-keeping requirement for women seeking an abortion. At the same time, the Court struck down the spousal notice requirement of a Pennsylvania statute, in addition to other specific requirements. *Casey* and *Webster v. Reproductive Health Services* before it (1989) upheld *Roe v. Wade,* the 1973 Supreme Court decision that legalized abortion in the United States (see the above case, "Case Legalizes Abortion"), but allowed state regulation of abortion. A number of state legislatures took the cue and passed new abortion restrictions.

Among a long list of state-imposed abortion restrictions are laws that specify certain changes in informed consent. For example, some states require that a woman seeking an abortion be clearly informed of all alternatives to abortions and be told of all risks associated with such surgeries before she can give informed consent to the abortion. In addition, before a woman can consent to an abortion in many states, she must wait a certain length of time (usually 24 hours) before actually signing a consent form.

A more recent court case, "Case Allows State Regulation" on the next page, upheld *Roe v. Wade,* and also allowed a state to regulate abortion.

Technically, abortion is legal in all 50 states, but state legislatures have added many restrictions.

Since abortion law is constantly changing, health care practitioners must stay informed about current abortion laws in their respective states. A good Web site for finding abortion laws in your state is statelaws.findlaw.com/family-laws/abortion.html.

HIV and Informed Consent State public health law varies for human immunodeficiency virus (HIV) testing, but, generally, health care practitioners must consider the following factors:

Can a minor (aged less than 18 in some states, 21 in others) consent to his or her own HIV test? Informed consent law for minors vary, but this determination may sometimes be made without regard to age, depending on the minor's situation:

- Infants and young children do not have the capacity to consent, because they do not yet have the ability to make informed decisions. The person legally designated to make health care decisions

The Pennsylvania legislature amended its abortion control law in 1988 and 1989. Among the new provisions, the law required informed consent and a 24-hour waiting period prior to the procedure. A minor seeking an abortion required the consent of one parent (the law allowed for a judicial bypass procedure). A married woman seeking an abortion had to indicate that she notified her husband of her intention to abort the fetus. These provisions were challenged by several abortion clinics and physicians. A federal appeals court upheld all the provisions except the husband notification requirement.

The question in this case was, can a state require women who want an abortion to obtain informed consent, wait 24 hours, and, if minors, obtain parental consent

without violating their right to abortions as guaranteed by *Roe v. Wade?* In a bitter 5-to-4 decision, the Court again reaffirmed *Roe*, but it upheld most of the Pennsylvania provisions. For the first time, the justices imposed a new standard to determine the validity of laws restricting abortions. The new standard asks whether a state abortion regulation has the purpose or effect of imposing an "undue burden," which is defined as a "substantial obstacle in the path of a woman seeking an abortion before the fetus attains viability." Under this standard, the only provision to fail the undue-burden test was the husband notification requirement.

Planned Parenthood v. Casey, 505 U.S. 833 (1992).

for the child has the right to decide whether the child should be tested for HIV.

- Married minors, emancipated minors, and minor parents may have the right to give consent for HIV testing, depending on state law.

Can an HIV-infected minor consent to his or her treatment? Generally, parental or guardian consent is required for a physician to treat a minor for HIV/AIDS, including treatment in school-based clinics. Married, emancipated, and mature minors can usually consent to their own care.

When Consent Is Unnecessary In emergency situations, when the patient is in immediate danger, the physician is not expected to obtain consent before proceeding with treatment.

All 50 states have passed **Good Samaritan acts.** These acts were intended to protect physicians and, in some states, other health care practitioners and laypersons from charges of negligence or abandonment if they stop to help the victim of an accident or other emergency, provided they:

Good Samaritan acts
State laws protecting physicians and sometimes other health care practitioners and laypersons from charges of negligence or abandonment if they stop to help the victim of an accident or other emergency.

- Give such care in good faith.
- Act within the scope of their training and knowledge.
- Use due care under the circumstances.
- Do not bill for their services. (If a physician treats a patient as a "Good Samaritan" and later bills the patient for services, he or she may be held as having established a physician–patient relationship and may not have the immunity from civil damages that a Good Samaritan law would otherwise provide.)

While some states offer immunity to Good Samaritans, sometimes the act of rescuing an accident victim can result in a legal claim of negligent care if the injuries or illness were made worse by the volunteer's actions. Statutes typically don't exempt a Good Samaritan who acts in a wilful and wanton or reckless manner in providing emergency care, advice, or assistance. Furthermore, Good Samaritan laws usually don't apply to a person rendering emergency care, advice, or assistance during the course of regular employment, such as services rendered by a health care provider to a patient in a health care facility.

Good Samaritan in legal terms refers to someone who renders aid in an emergency to an injured person on a voluntary basis. Usually, if a volunteer comes to the aid of an injured or ill person who is a stranger, the person giving the aid owes the stranger a duty of being reasonably careful. A person is not obligated by law to do first aid in most states, unless it's part of a job description. However, some states will consider it an act of negligence if a person doesn't at least call for help. Generally, where an unconscious victim cannot respond, a Good Samaritan can help on the grounds of implied consent. However, if the victim is conscious and can respond, a person should first ask permission to help.

If a person helps a victim in an emergency and is later sued, whether or not the defendant can use a state Good Samaritan law for his or her defense may depend on the court's definition of the state's law, as shown in the case, "Good Samaritans Can Be Liable for Damages to Person Injured during Rescue Attempt."

COURT CASE   Good Samaritans Can Be Liable for Damages to Person Injured during Rescue Attempt

Good friends Alexandra Van Horn and Lisa Torti spent the evening partying in a bar; then each woman left the bar in her own car. Van Horn drove away first, and crashed into a curb and streetlight standard at 45 mph. Torti, behind Van Horn in the second car, saw the accident and, afraid the wrecked car was about to "blow up," she removed Van Horn. As a result, Van Horn was paralyzed.

Van Horn sued Torti. Torti's defense was based on California's Good Samaritan law, Health & Safety Code section 1799.102, which provides: "No person who in good faith, and not for compensation, renders emergency care at the scene of an emergency shall be liable for any civil damages resulting from any act or omission. The scene of an emergency shall not include emergency departments and other places where medical care is usually offered."

Based on this statute, the trial court granted summary judgment for the defendant. The plaintiff appealed, and the case eventually reached the California Supreme Court, where justices interpreted the state's Good Samaritan law to apply strictly to *medical* care, because the statute appears in the Health & Safety Code, in the division entitled "Emergency Medical Services." (A statute providing broad immunity would likely appear in the Civil Code.) Torti did not render emergency medical care; she merely pulled Van Horn from her crashed car, and, therefore, she was found potentially liable. This ruling meant that Van Horn could take her case to a jury.

Common law principles applied were that the defendant's broad interpretation of Health & Safety Code 1799.102

would undermine established common law regarding liability for assisting others. There is no general duty to give assistance, but under the common law, a person who undertakes to help others has a duty to exercise due care. Nothing in the statute overcomes the judicial presumption that the legislature does not intend to overrule established common law principles when it enacts legislation. A broad interpretation, the court held, would also render superfluous other California "Good Samaritan" statutes, such as Govt C. 50086 (immunity for a person trained in first aid who is summoned by authorities and renders emergency services) and Harb. & Nav C. 656(b) (immunity for a person who assists at scene of vessel collision) (45 C 4th 333).

As a result of the ruling, the California legislature changed the state's Good Samaritan law. Health and Safety Code section 1799.102 now reads in part: "No person who in good faith, and not for compensation, renders emergency medical or nonmedical care or assistance at the scene of an emergency shall be liable for civil damages resulting from any act or omission other than an act or omission constituting gross negligence or wilful or wanton misconduct."

Trial Court: *Van Horn v. Watson* (2008) 45 C 4th 322, 86 C.R. 3d 350, 197 P 3d 164. California Supreme Court: *Alexandra Van Horn, Plaintiff and Appellant, v. Anthony Glen Watson et al., Defendants and Respondents; Anthony Glen Watson, Cross-complainant and Appellant, v. Lisa Torti, Cross-defendant and Respondent,* Supreme Court of California, Dec. 18, 2008. Rehearing Denied Feb. 11, 2009.

18. Who may give informed consent?

19. Who may not give informed consent?

20. Must consent to perform routine medical care, such as a physical examination, always be in writing? Explain your answer.

21. In which health care situations is implied consent not sufficient?

22. What consequences generally ensue if a legally competent adult is treated without consent and an adverse event occurs?

LO 7.4

Describe the necessity for electronic medical records and the efforts being made to record all medical records electronically.

health information technology (HIT)
The application of information processing, involving both computer hardware and software, that deals with the storage, retrieval, sharing, and use of health care information, data, and knowledge for communication and decision making.

Health Information Technology (HIT)

According to the U.S. Department of Health and Human Services, **health information technology (HIT)** is "the application of information processing involving both computer hardware and software that deals with the storage, retrieval, sharing, and use of health care information, data, and knowledge for communication and decision making." The broad category *health information technology* also includes telemedicine and use of the Internet for health information purposes. A central component of HIT is the patient's medical file, and as electronic medical records become more widely adopted, confidentiality and privacy concerns must be addressed.

As of 2004, President George W. Bush had set a 10-year goal for the broad adoption of **electronic medical records** in the United States. President Barack Obama, who took office January 1, 2009, continued to urge health care providers to convert records to electronic form. In fact, under the Patient Protection and Affordable Care Act signed into law in 2010, physicians could receive up to $44,000 from the government to help with the cost of converting to electronic records.

Government-initiated steps toward broad adoption of electronic health information include the following:

1. **The Health Insurance Portability and Accountability Act (HIPAA).** Passed in 1996 and implemented in stages through 2005, HIPAA addresses privacy of health information and mandates certain procedures and standards for the electronic transmission and storage of health care information.

2. **Executive Orders.** In April 2004, President George W. Bush signed an executive order establishing the position of National Coordinator for Health Information Technology. The coordinator was charged with the development, maintenance, and oversight of a plan for nationwide adoption of health information technology.

    In August 2006, a second executive order stated that all federal agencies would utilize, where available, health information technology systems and products meeting certain "recognized" standards. These HIT systems and products "shall be used for implementing, acquiring, or upgrading health information technology systems used for the direct exchange of health information between agencies and with nonfederal entities." The order further stipulated that federal agencies shall require in contracts or agreements with health care providers, health plans, or health insurance issuers that, where available, health information technology systems and products meeting recognized standards shall be used.

3. **Adoption of the Health Information Standards Developed by Health and Human Services (HHS).** As part of this effort, HHS has negotiated and licensed a comprehensive medical vocabulary and made it available to everyone in the United States at no cost. The results of these projects include standards for the following types of information:

- Transmitting X-Rays over the Internet: Today, a patient's chest X-ray can be sent electronically from a hospital or laboratory and read by the patient's doctor in his or her office.

- Electronic Laboratory Results: Laboratory results can be sent electronically to the physician for immediate analysis, diagnosis, and treatment, and could be automatically entered into the patient's electronic health record if one existed. For example, a doctor could retrieve this information for a hospitalized patient from his or her office, ensuring a prompt response and eliminating errors and duplicative testing due to lost laboratory reports.

- Electronic Prescriptions: Patients save time because prescriptions can be sent electronically to their pharmacists. By eliminating illegible handwritten prescriptions, and because the technology automatically checks for possible allergies and harmful interactions with other drugs, standardized electronic prescriptions help avoid serious medical errors.

4. **Use of the Federal Government to Foster the Adoption of Health Information Technology.** As one of the largest buyers of health care—in Medicare, Medicaid, the Affordable Care Act, the Community Health Centers program, the Federal Health Benefits program, veterans' medical care, and programs in the Department of Defense—the federal government can create incentives and opportunities for health care providers to use electronic records.

The federal government maintains that the broad use of health information technology will improve individual patient care by:

- Improving health care quality
- Preventing medical errors
- Reducing health care costs
- Increasing administrative efficiency
- Decreasing paperwork
- Expanding access to affordable care

The previous benefits can be seen in the following examples:

- When arriving at a physician office, new patients do not have to enter their personal information, allergies, medications, or medical history, since these facts are already available.

- A parent, who previously may have had to carry a large folder containing the child's medical records and X-rays by hand when seeing a new physician, can now keep the most important medical history on a keychain, or simply authorize the new physician to retrieve the information electronically from previous health care providers.

- Arriving at an emergency room, an elderly patient with a chronic illness and memory difficulties can authorize his or her physicians to access her medical information from a recent hospitalization at another hospital—thus avoiding a potentially fatal drug interaction between the planned treatment and the patient's current medications.

Public health benefits will include:

- Early detection of infectious outbreaks around the country. For example, three patients experience unusual sudden-onset fever and cough that would not individually be reported. They show up at separate emergency rooms, and through access to electronic health information, the trend is instantly reported to public health officials, who alert authorities of a possible disease outbreak or bioterror attack.
- Improved tracking of chronic disease management.
- Evaluation of health care based on comparisons of price and quality.

When Hurricane Katrina hit the Louisiana and Mississippi coasts on August 29, 2005, the destruction that resulted included the loss of countless paper medical records. As a result, many of the survivors couldn't remember the names of lost prescriptions, or when they had last been immunized against tetanus and other diseases. In addition, storm victims who reported to physicians had no medical records health care providers could use as a basis for treatment, and reconstruction, if even possible, would take valuable time.

By contrast, when Hurricane Sandy struck the East Coast on October 29, 2012, many health care providers had already converted paper files to digital files as part of HIPAA-mandated disaster planning. In fact, for most of the providers who suffered through Sandy, the process of compliance began long before the storm. Those providers that had disaster plans in place and had practiced them to be sure they worked were in the best position to ride out the storm without loss of critical data and services. And those providers who had duplicated all necessary electronic data at off-site data centers were also able to function during the storm or to restore function more quickly after the storm hit. For example, AtlantiCare, a health care system in New Jersey with a large regional medical center and 70 other locations throughout the state, made it through Sandy with few disruptions, thanks to advance disaster planning.

THE HIPAA DISASTER RECOVERY PLAN

A HIPAA disaster recovery plan for health care providers is a document that specifies the resources, actions, personnel and data that are required to protect and reinstate health care information in the event of a fire, vandalism, natural disaster or system failure.

A HIPAA-compliant disaster recovery plan must state how operations will be conducted in an emergency and which workforce members are responsible for carrying out those operations. The plan must explain how data will be moved without violating HIPAA standards for privacy and security. It must also explain how confidential data and safeguards for that data will be restored. Although HIPAA doesn't specify exactly how to do this, it does note that failure to adequately recover from a disaster could lead to noncompliance, exposing officers of the organization to fines or even jail time.

TECHNOLOGICAL THREATS TO CONFIDENTIALITY

Increasingly, as the federal government mandates and encourages health information technology, modern health care facilities rely on technology for creating, maintaining, and transporting patients' medical information. HIPAA imposes penalties for breaches of confidentiality regarding medical records that identify patients by name. The following guidelines can help ensure that confidentiality is not breached when employees use photocopiers, fax machines, computers, and printers to reproduce and send medical records.

Photocopiers

- Do not leave confidential papers anywhere on the copier where others can read the information.
- Do not discard copies in a shared trash container; shred them.
- If a paper jam occurs, be sure to remove from the machine the copy or partial copy that caused the jam.

Fax Machines

- Always verify the telephone number of the receiving location before faxing confidential material.
- Never fax confidential material to an unauthorized person.
- Do not fax confidential material if others in the room can observe the material.
- Do not leave confidential material unattended on a fax machine.
- Do not discard fax copies in a shared trash container; shred them.
- Use a fax cover sheet that states, "Confidential: To addressee only. Please return if received in error."

Check Your Progress

23. How does an electronic medical record differ from one kept on paper?
24. Define *health information technology.*
25. Name two measures the federal government has taken to speed the adoption of electronic medical records.
26. According to the federal government, what are two ways the use of electronic records might improve patient care?
27. You are photocopying a patient's medical record and an employee from the clinic's accounting department is reading over your shoulder while he waits to use the copier. What should you do?

Computers

- Locate the monitor in an area where others cannot see the screen.
- Do not leave a monitor unattended while confidential material is displayed on the screen.
- Because it is difficult to ensure the privacy of e-mail messages, sending confidential patient information via e-mail is not recommended.
- When computers are sold or otherwise recycled, it's vital that hard drives be erased or removed and destroyed.

Printers

- Do not print confidential material on a printer shared by other departments or in an area where others can read the material.
- Do not leave a printer unattended while printing confidential material.
- Before leaving the printing area, check to be sure all computer disks containing confidential material and all printed material have been collected.
- Be certain that the print job is sent to the right printer location.
- Do not discard printouts in a shared trash container; shred them.

Since medical records are legal documents, and their confidentiality is protected by law, health care practitioners must take every precaution to properly enter information into medical records and to keep that information confidential.

Chapter Summary

Learning Outcome	Summary

LO 7.1 Explain the purpose of medical records and the importance of correct documentation.	**What purposes do medical records serve?**
	• They are required by licensing authorities and provide a format for tracking, documenting, and maintaining a patient's communication data, both inside and outside a health care facility.
	• They provide documentation of a patient's continuing health care, from birth to death.
	• They provide a foundation for managing a patient's health care.
	• They serve as legal documents in lawsuits.
	• They provide clinical data for education, research, statistical tracking, and assessing the quality of health care.
	
	What information is entered into a patient's medical record?
	• Contact and identifying information.
	• Insurance information
	• Driver's license information
	• Person responsible for payment and billing.
	• Emergency contact information
	• Patient's health history
	• Dates and times of appointments.
	• Descriptions of patient's symptoms and reasons for appointments.
	• Examinations performed
	• Physician's assessment, diagnosis, recommendations, treatment, progress notes, prescriptions, and instructions to patient.
	• X-rays and all test results.
	• Notations for telephone calls.
	• Notations of copies made.
	• Documentation of informed consent.
	• Names of guardians or legal representatives if patient unable to give informed consent.
	• All other documentation
	• Condition of patient at time of termination of treatment.
	
	What are the five Cs of entries in medical records?
	• Concise
	• Complete
	• Clear
	• Correct
	• Chronologically ordered
	
	What is the accepted manner for correcting errors in a paper medical record?
	• Draw a line through the error.
	• Write correct information above or below original line.
	• Note why correction was made.
	• Enter the date, time, and initial the correction.
	• Ask a coworker to witness and intial the correction when it is made.
	
	What is the accepted method of correcting an electronic medical record?
	• Follow policy for software used to create the electronic medical record.
	• If an addendum is added to record, be sure it includes:
	  • Patient name
	  • Date of service
	  • Account number
	  • Medical record number
	  • Original report to which the addendum is to be attached.
	  • Date and time of the addendum and the electronic signature of the person creating the addendum.

COURT CASE — HIPAA Preempts State Law in Certain Instances

In July 2013, the U.S. Court of Appeals for the Eleventh Circuit ruled that HIPAA preempts state law in certain instances. The case centered on a Florida statute that allowed nursing homes to release medical records of a current or former resident to "spouse, guardian, surrogate, proxy or attorney in fact" of the individual. However, many Florida nursing homes refused to disclose records to surviving spouses who had not been designated as the personal representative by the probate courts. The Florida Agency for Health Care Administration (AHCA) ordered the various nursing homes to release the information stating the surviving spouses were equal to personal representatives. OPIS Management

Resources, an owner of several nursing homes in Florida filed suit against AHCA, claiming that HIPAA standards were higher and thus the state law conflicted. The Court of Appeals held the state statute was fatally flawed and "authorizes sweeping disclosures, making a deceased (nursing home) resident's protected health information available to a spouse or other enumerated party upon request, without any need for authorization, for any conceivable reason, and without regard to the authority of the individual making the request to act in a deceased resident's stead."

OPIS Management Resources LLC v. Secretary Florida Agency for Health Care Administration, No. 12-12593 (11th Cir. Apr. 9, 2013).

Table 8-1 Major Federal Privacy Laws

Date Enacted	Law	Purpose
1986	Electronic Communications Privacy Act (ECPA)	Provides privacy protection for new forms of electronic communications, such as voice mail, e-mail, and cellular telephone
1994	Computer Abuse Amendments Act	Amends the 1984 act to forbid transmission of harmful computer code such as viruses
1996	Health Insurance Portability and Accountability Act (HIPAA)	Guarantees that workers who change jobs can obtain health insurance. Increases efficiency and effectiveness of the U.S. health care system by electronic exchange of administrative and financial data. Improves security and privacy of patient-identifying information. Decreases U.S. health care system transaction costs
1999	Gramm-Leach-Bliley Act	Requires all financial institutions and insurance companies to clearly disclose their privacy policies regarding the sharing of nonpublic personal information with affiliates and third parties
2005	Patient Safety and Quality Improvement Act (PSQIA)	Helps assess and resolve patient safety and health care quality issues, encourages reporting and analysis of medical errors, authorizes HHS to impose civil money penalties for violations of patient safety confidentiality
2009	American Recovery and Reinvestment Act (ARRA), commonly called the Stimulus Bill	Title XIII, the Health Information Technology for Economic and Clinical Health (HITECH) Act, makes substantive changes to HIPAA, including privacy and security regulations, changes in HIPAA enforcement, provisions about health information held by entities not covered by HIPAA, and other miscellaneous changes
2010	Patient Protection and Affordable Care Act (PPACA) commonly called the Affordable Care Act or ACA	Deals mostly with the availability of health insurance coverage for all Americans, but also reinforces privacy regarding protected health information
2010	Health Care and Education Reconciliation Act (HCERA)	A federal law that adds to regulations imposed on the insurance industry by PPACA

Check Your Progress

1. Does the Constitution provide specifically for the protection of privacy? Explain your answer.
2. What was the first federal law to deal explicitly with the privacy of medical records?
3.–6. Name four considerations for protecting privacy when federal and/or state legislation is written.

Since HIPAA is the federal legal standard for privacy and security of electronic health information throughout the health care industry, health care employees must follow the law's provisions, which are contained within four standards:

Standard 1. Transactions and Code Sets. A transaction refers to the transmission of information between two parties to carry out financial or administrative activities. A code set is any set of codes used to encode data elements, such as tables of terms, medical concepts, medical diagnostic codes, or medical procedure codes.

Required code sets for use under Standard 1 include Current Procedural Terminology (CPT) and International Classification System of Diseases; Clinical Modifications 10th Edition (ICD-10-CM); and International Classification System of Diseases—Procedure Coding System 10th Edition (ICD-10-PCS) (Since the publication of ICD-10 has been delayed to 2015, some coders may still be using ICD-9.).

Standard 2. Privacy Rule. Policies and procedures health care providers and their business associates put in place to ensure confidentiality of written, electronic, and oral protected health information.

Standard 3. Security Rule. Security refers to those policies and procedures health care providers and their business associates use to protect electronically transmitted and stored PHI from unauthorized access.

Standard 4. National Identifier Standards. Provide unique identifiers (addresses) for electronic transmissions.

By now all four sets of HIPAA standards have been implemented, and most health care practitioners are familiar with the language and rules that make up the requirements for compliance. Anyone needing a refresher course can visit **www.hipaa.com** for specific information.

Of special concern in this chapter are Standard 2, the Privacy Rule and Standard 3, the Security Rule.

HIPAA's Requirements for Disclosing Protected Health Information

LO 8.2

Explain HIPAA's special requirements for disclosing protected health information.

HIPAA's Standard 2, the Privacy Rule says that **protected health information (PHI)** must be protected against unauthorized disclosure, whether it is written, spoken, or in electronic form. PHI refers to information that contains one or more patient identifiers and can, therefore, be used to identify an individual. Information that includes one or more of the following makes a patient's health care information identifiable:

protected health information (PHI)
Information that contains one or more patient identifiers.

- Name
- Zip code or other geographic identifier, such as address, city, or county.

- For essential government functions.
- In claims for Workers' Compensation.

6. Limited data set. A **limited data set** is protected health information from which certain specified, direct identifiers of individuals and their relatives, household members, and employers have been removed. A limited data set may be used and disclosed for research, health care operations, and public health purposes, provided the recipient enters into an agreement promising specified safeguards for the PHI within the limited data set.

The HIPAA Privacy Rule does not give patients the express right to sue. Instead, the person must file a written complaint with the secretary of Health and Human Services through the Office for Civil Rights. The HHS secretary then decides whether or not to investigate the complaint. Patients may have other legal standings to sue under state privacy laws. (See Court Case, "EMT Liable for Violating Patient's Privacy.") See Table 8-3 on page 222 for a list of patients' rights under the HIPAA Privacy Rule.

COURT CASE   EMT Liable for Violating Patient's Privacy

An EMT employed by a volunteer fire department provided emergency treatment to a female patient for a possible drug overdose. The unresponsive patient was transported to a hospital. The EMT returned home and later spoke to a friend, telling her that she had assisted in taking a specific patient to the hospital emergency room for treatment for a possible drug overdose.

Prior to the emergency, the EMT had never met the patient. However, about two weeks prior to the incident, the EMT had heard about the patient and her medical problems at a social event. The woman who spoke about the patient was apparently a friend, and it was this person whom the EMT telephoned, after the patient's overdose.

The patient sued the EMT and her insurance company, alleging that she had defamed her and violated her privacy by publicizing information concerning her medical condition and making untrue statements indicating that she had

attempted suicide. The patient claimed that she had been and was continuing to undergo medical care due to illness, and that the apparent overdose she suffered was a "reaction to medication."

The insurance company claimed the EMT's actions were within the scope of her employment. The EMT argued that she had not acted recklessly or unreasonably in contacting the patient's friend regarding her care.

The EMT offered to settle for $5,000, but the plaintiff refused and the matter went to a jury trial. The jury found that the EMT had violated the plaintiff's right of privacy, as alleged. The jury also awarded the plaintiff/patient $37,909.86 in compensatory damages and attorney fees.

The EMT and her insurance company appealed. An appeals court upheld the judgment of the lower court.

Pachowitz v. Ledoux, 2003 WL 21221823 (Wis. App., May 28, 2003).

Check Your Progress

7. Define *protected health information*.

8. Define *de-identify*.

9. Which law usually prevails, federal or state, if a state law provides greater privacy protection than a federal law? Explain your answer.

10. What is the process illustrated in question 9 called?

11. One can only legally release PHI under six HIPAA-defined _____.

Laws Implemented to Protect the Security of Health Care Information

LO 8.3

Discuss laws implemented to protect the security of health care information as health records are converted from paper to electronic form.

As listed in Table 8-1, the American Recovery and Reinvestment Act (ARRA), commonly called the Stimulus Bill, made substantive changes to HIPAA, including privacy and security regulations, changes in HIPAA enforcement, provisions about health information held by entities not expressly covered by HIPAA, and other miscellaneous changes. The ARRA also mandated a deadline—January 1, 2014—for all public and private health care providers and other eligible professionals across the country to have adopted and demonstrated "meaningful use" of electronic medical records (EMR) in order to keep their existing Medicare and Medicaid reimbursement levels. ("Meaningful use" is explained below.)

First, note the difference between electronic medical records (EMR) and electronic health records (EHR), because, according to **www.healthit.gov,** an online source of information about information technology in the health industry, the two terms are not interchangeable. The **electronic medical record (EMR)** is the electronic form of a patient's medical history from just one practice. It lets health care providers in one facility:

electronic medical record (EMR)
Contains all patient medical records for one practice.

- Track data over time.

- Identify with a glance which patients are due for screenings or check-ups.

- Check patients' progress within certain parameters, such as blood pressure, cholesterol and blood sugar readings, and vaccinations.

- Monitor and improve overall patient care within the practice.

By contrast, the **electronic health record (EHR)** is a more comprehensive electronic patient history, focusing on the total health of the patient and including a broader view of a patient's care. This more detailed record allows for:

electronic health record (EHR)
A more comprehensive record than the EMR, focusing on the total health of the patient and traveling with the patient.

- A record that travels with the patient, so that emergency department clinicians who see a patient in his home city or traveling across the country will know about any life-threatening allergies, or clinicians treating people injured in a disaster will know which medications the patient is taking.

- The opportunity for the patient to log on to her own record and see trends in lab results over time, which can help her plan for staying healthy.

- Specialists to see what tests, X-rays, and other procedures have already been done on a patient, thus avoiding unnecessary duplication when possible.

- Notes from any hospital stays that can help inform discharge instructions and follow-up care for the patient and can let patients move smoothly from one care setting to another.

"Meaningful use" of electronic health records, as defined by HealthIT .gov, consists of using digital medical and health records to achieve the following:

- Improve quality, safety, and efficiency of health care, and reduce health disparities.

- Engage patients and family in comprehensive health care plans.
- Improve care coordination and the health of populations and also improve public health practices.
- Maintain the privacy and security of patient health information.

HIPAA'S SECURITY RULE

HIPAA's Standard 2, the Privacy Rule, details procedures for maintaining the privacy of protected health information. The act's Standard 3, the Security Rule, explains the requirements for maintaining the security of electronic health records, both in transmission and storage. Lack of compliance with HIPAA security measures can lead to substantial fines and in extreme cases even loss of medical licenses. According to **www.hipaa.com,** medical practices can follow 5 steps to ensure compliance to HIPAA standards and to avoid data breaches. (A **breach** is any unauthorized acquisition, access, use, or disclosure of personal health information which compromises the security or privacy of such information.)

1. **Run a complete risk assessment of the medical practice.** There are many electronic health recording systems, but practices need to use a system that meets HIPAA guidelines and standards. A risk assessment against HIPAA guidelines can reveal those areas where changes are needed, and should include evaluating how well each person protects passwords. Passwords should not be posted for anyone to see, should not be unnecessarily divulged to others, and should be changed regularly, and **firewalls** should be in place to protect against outside intrusion (see Figure 8-1). Are security measures reasonable and appropriate for the health care practice and are they periodically reviewed? Have security breaches occurred in the past? If so, what caused the breaches and have causes been remedied? Are internal sanctions in place for security breaches, and have staff members been informed of such sanctions?

2. **Be prepared for a disaster.** One of the best ways to ensure against loss or corruption of medical data is to back up all data regularly. Data is most safely backed up in offsite locations, so that fires, water leaks, and other incidents at the practice site do not threaten

breach
Any unauthorized acquisition, access, use, or disclosure of personal health information which compromises the security or privacy of such information.

firewalls
Hardware, software, or both designed to prevent unauthorized persons from accessing electronic information.

FIGURE 8-1
How Breaches Happen

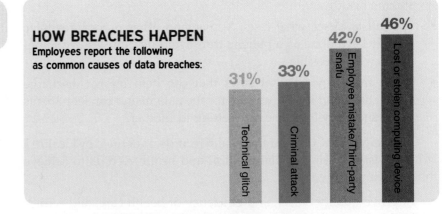

Source: Data from ProPublica: **http://www.propublica.org/**

data. Antivirus programs should also be installed on all computers and regularly updated so that computer viruses and hackers are not a threat to data.

3. **Train all employees in proper computer use.** Access controls such as passwords and PIN numbers, are HIPAA Security Rule requirements, and **encryption** systems provide an additional level of security. Encrypting stored information means that PHI cannot be read or understood except by someone who can decrypt it using a special decryption key provided only to authorized individuals. A medical practice can have a secure encryption system, but if employees don't use their passwords to securely access records and files, the encryption system is useless, and records are open to unauthorized intrusion. Training should be ongoing, so that new employees are informed and long-term employees are reminded of proper use.

encryption
The scrambling or encoding of information before sending it electronically.

4. **Buy products with security compliance and compatibility in mind.** When purchasing any new medical computer software or other medical products, check to be sure the new purchase meets HIPAA security rules and will be compatible with other products already in use.

5. **Collaborate with all compliance-affected parties.** All departments within a practice are affected when compliance changes are made, and employees should be informed and consulted.

ProPublica data reveals that new technology trends threaten patient data in that 91 percent of hospitals surveyed are using cloud technology (Internet, off-medical-facility-site storage capability) to store data, yet 47 percent of these hospitals were not confident they could keep the data secure in the cloud. In addition, 81 percent of organizations let employees use their own mobile devices (BYOD), yet 46 percent of these organizations don't ensure that employee devices are secure (see Figure 8-2).

ProPublica estimates that data breaches have cost the health care industry $7 billion to date, both in fraudulent schemes and in identity theft, where criminals use health care data to assume a person's identity and make unauthorized purchases in that person's name.

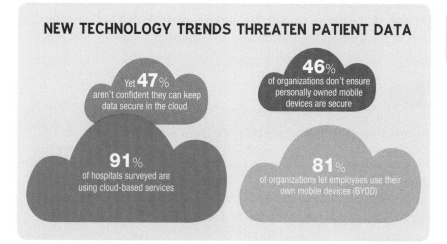

NEW TECHNOLOGY TRENDS THREATEN PATIENT DATA

Yet **47**% aren't confident they can keep data secure in the cloud

46% of organizations don't ensure personally owned mobile devices are secure

91% of hospitals surveyed are using cloud-based services

81% of organizations let employees use their own mobile devices (BYOD)

FIGURE 8-2
New Technology Trends Threaten Patient Data

Source: Data from ProPublica: **http://www.propublica.org/**

Health Information Technology
for Economic and Clinical Health
Act (HITECH)

A section of the American Recovery
and Reinvestment Act (ARRA) that
strengthened certain HIPAA privacy
and security provisions.

American Recovery and
Reinvestment Act (ARRA)

A 2009 act that made substantive
change to HIPAA's privacy and
security regulations.

HITECH RULE

The **Health Information Technology for Economic and Clinical Health (HITECH) Act,** part of the **American Recovery and Reinvestment Act (ARRA)** of 2009, strengthened the privacy and security protections for health information established under HIPAA. Provisions under HITECH carried a September 23, 2013 enforcement date.

The HITECH Rule strengthens privacy and security by:

- Extending compliance with HIPAA privacy and security rules to business associates and their subcontractors.

- Prohibiting the sale of protected health information without appropriate authorization.

- Expanding individual rights to electronically access one's protected health information (PHI).

- Prohibiting the use of genetic information for insurance underwriting purposes.

- Finalizing breach notification requirements.

- Expanding individuals' rights to obtain restrictions on certain disclosures of protected health information to health plans if services are paid for out of pocket.

- Establishing new limitations on the use and disclosure of protected health information for marketing and fund-raising purposes.

- Providing easier access to immunization records by a school.

- Removing HIPAA Privacy Rule protections for PHI of an individual deceased for more than 50 years.

A provision of the law states that breaches must be reported, not just to the Office of Civil Rights (OCR), which has federal enforcement authority, but also to the media. A quick search of the Internet will reveal that breaches occur frequently. Since October 2009 through November 2013, there have been 768 complaints alleging a violation of the Security Rule. The HHS/OCR closed 579 complaints after investigation and appropriate corrective action and as of November 30, 2013 had 254 open complaints and compliance reviews.

While maintaining privacy and security of PHI are vital considerations in today's health care environment, fraud is claiming a huge portion of the health care dollar, and has necessitated federal intervention in the form of legislation and anti-fraud measures.

Check Your Progress

12.–13. Briefly distinguish between the electronic medical record (EMR) and the electronic health record (EHR).

14. What is a *breach* of PHI?

15.–17. If you use computers in the course of your daily work, what are three important rules for you to remember, in order to protect the security of electronic medical records?

18. Briefly explain the purpose of HITECH.

Controlling Health Care Fraud and Abuse

LO 8.4
Discuss the federal laws that cover fraud and abuse within the health care business environment and the role of the Office of the Inspector General in finding billing fraud.

According to the following figures, as published by *The Sentinel*, for fiscal year 2011 (the latest FY for which statistics were available) estimates for dollar losses, including fraud, abuse, and waste in all health care arenas included:

- $1.2 trillion a year, based on a 2008 report by Pricewaterhouse-Coopers' Health Research Institute.

- $600 to $850 billion a year, according to a Thomson Reuters report that broadly defined "waste" as "healthcare spending that can be eliminated without reducing the quality of care."

- $64.8 billion in improper payments by Medicare and Medicaid for FY 2011, according to the Government Accounting Office (GAO). ("Improper" meaning the care was not necessary or the bill was wrong. Improper payments may include fraudulent claims, but not all improper payments are fraudulent. Improper payments may be due to honest mistakes.)

- $28.8 billion in improper payments were made to Medicare fee-for-service (Original Medicare) providers in 2011, according to GAO.

- $21.9 billion in improper Medicaid payments in 2011, according to GAO.

- $2.4 billion in health care fraud judgments and settlements were won or negotiated in 2011, according to the 2011 Health Care Fraud and Abuse Control Program report by the Department of Health and Human Services (HHS) and Department of Justice (DOJ).

- $1.2 billion in Medicare and Medicaid audit disallowances (findings of unallowable costs), according to the HHS Office of Inspector General (OIG).

Source: Aldrich, Nancy & Benson, Bill, **The_Sentinel_May2012_HBABCs_Fraud_Estimates.pdf**

Medicare fraud is not easy to estimate, because:

1. Fraudulent spending is not always separated from total health care dollars spent when records are kept.

2. Dollar amounts spent in a single incident of fraud are increasing, so statistics from prior years are not always reliable, thus effecting more current estimates.

3. Fraud is often undetected, and therefore difficult to count.

Clearly the health care dollar is far from well spent. The health care system no doubt loses enough money each year to pay for insurance for the uninsured, keep premiums from rising, and improve the health of every American—all on the taxpayers' dime.

While much of the deliberate health care fraud and abuse is committed by legitimate health care providers, because of the huge profits possible, organized crime has also become involved. "Organized crime has figured out that it is much safer to defraud the government in a variety of health care scams then to sell illegal drugs," said an investigator in the Office of Inspector General in June 2012 who wishes to remain anonymous.

In 2013, ProPublica, an independent, nonprofit newsroom that produces investigative journalism in the public interest, released a series of critical articles about fraud in Medicare Part D, the prescription drug plan. For their investigation the ProPublica staff used the Freedom of Information Act to obtain data on the drugs prescribed by every provider in the Part D program for 5 years. No patient information was released, just prescribing patterns of physicians. The investigation, which was ongoing into 2014, revealed that physicians sometimes did not know that prescriptions were being filled for patients they did not even see, due to unscrupulous business managers and accountants. As a result, both Congress and the Obama administration have indicated that targeting organized crime for health care fraud and abuse will be a priority.

THE FRAUD PATROL

Since its 1976 establishment, the Office of Inspector General (OIG) of the U.S. Department of Health & Human Services (HHS) has been charged with fighting waste, fraud, and abuse in Medicare, Medicaid and more than 300 other HHS programs. The OIG has many offices across the country, which create a nationwide network of auditors, investigators and evaluators. The OIG oversees enforcement of all federal laws related to health care fraud and abuse, including the following major federal statutes outlined in Table 8-2 and discussed further after.

THE FEDERAL FALSE CLAIMS ACT

Federal False Claims Act
A law that allows for individuals to bring civil actions on behalf of the U.S. government for false claims made to the federal government, under a provision of the law called *qui tam* (from Latin meaning "to bring an action for the king and for oneself").

The **Federal False Claims Act** allows for individuals to bring civil actions on behalf of the U.S. government for false claims made to the federal government, under a provision of the law called *qui tam* (from Latin meaning "to bring an action for the king and for oneself"). These individuals, commonly known as whistle-blowers, are referred to as *qui tam relators* and can share in any court-awarded damages.

Suits brought under the False Claims Act are most often related to the health care and defense industries. The act prohibits:

- Making a false record or statement to get a false claim paid by the government.

- Conspiring to have a false claim paid by the government.

Table 8-2 Major Federal Health Care Fraud and Abuse Laws

Date Enacted	Law	Purpose
1863—significantly amended in 1986 and several times since.	False Claims Act	Provides for civil penalties for persons knowingly making false claims to the federal government for payment.
1972	Anti-Kickback Statute	Criminal law that prohibits giving, soliciting, accepting or arranging items of value as a reward for referrals of services paid for by the government health care system.
1989—Expanded in 1995.	Stark Law, or Physician Self-Referral Law	Physicians or members of their immediate families cannot refer patients to health care facilities they own if the government is to pay for the care.
Unknown—Part of the U.S. Code, 18, Section 1347	Criminal Health Care Fraud Statute	Makes it a criminal offense to knowingly defraud a health care benefit program.

- Withholding government property with the intent to defraud or willfully conceal it from the government.

- Making or delivering a receipt for government property that is false.

- Buying government property from someone who is not authorized to sell it.

- Making a false statement to avoid or deceive an obligation to pay money or property to the government.

- Causing someone else to submit a false claim by giving false information.

The opportunity for fraud and abuse under the Federal False Claims Act is great. The Justice Department secured $3.8 billion in settlements and judgments from civil cases involving fraud during fiscal year 2013. From January 2009 through the end of the 2013 fiscal year, the Justice Department used the False Claims Act to recover $12.1 billion in federal health care dollars. Most of these recoveries relate to fraud against Medicare and Medicaid.

THE FEDERAL ANTI-KICKBACK LAW

In effect since 1972 and amended many times since then, the **Federal Anti-Kickback Law** states that anyone who knowingly and willfully receives or pays anything of value to influence the referral of federal health care program business, including Medicare and Medicaid, can be held accountable for a felony. Violations of the law, which excludes from prosecution some designated "safe harbor" arrangements, are punishable by up to 5 years in prison, fines from $25,000 to $50,000, and exclusion from participation in federal health care programs.

Federal Anti-Kickback Law Prohibits knowingly and willfully receiving or paying anything of value to influence the referral of federal health care program business.

COURT CASE | University Overbilled Medicare and Medicaid for Patients Enrolled in Clinical Trial Research

Major universities often do clinical trials and treat Medicare and Medicaid patients during those trials. The clinical trial sponsor pays for the medical care and services. In this case, Emory University was also billing Medicare and Medicaid for the same services.

A lawsuit was filed by Elizabeth Elliot under the *qui tam*, or whistle-blower, provisions of the False Claims Act, which allow private citizens to bring civil actions on behalf of the United States and share in any recovery obtained. The Office of Inspector General of Health and Human Services investigated and the FBI investigated the claims and found that Emory had billed, and in some cases received payment from Medicare or Medicaid, for services the clinical trial sponsor had already paid.

The United States Attorney's Office for the Northern District of Georgia announced a settlement in August 2013 with Emory University. Emory agreed to pay $1.5 million to settle claims that it violated the False Claims Act by billing Medicare and Medicaid for clinical trial services that were not permitted by the Medicare and Medicaid rules.

Ms. Elliot received a share of the settlement payment that resolves the *qui tam* suit that she filed. However, the claims settled in the civil settlement are allegations only, and there has been no determination of liability.

United States of America and State of Georgia ex rel. Elizabeth Elliott v. Emory University, et al., Civ. No. 1:09-cv-3569-AT (N.D. Ga. Dec. 18, 2009).

9

Key Terms

administer

Amendments to the Older Americans Act

autopsy

Child Abuse Prevention and Treatment Act

Controlled Substances Act

coroner

dispense

Drug Enforcement Administration (DEA)

federalism

Food and Drug Administration (FDA)

forensics

medical examiner

National Childhood Vaccine Injury Act

National Vaccine Injury Compensation Program (VICP)

prescribe

Smallpox Emergency Personnel Protection Act (SEPPA)

Unborn Victims of Violence Act

vital statistics

Physicians' Public Duties and Responsibilities

LEARNING OUTCOMES

After studying this chapter, you should be able to:

LO 9.1 List at least four vital events for which statistics are collected by the government.

LO 9.2 Discuss the procedures for filing birth and death certificates.

LO 9.3 Explain the purpose of public health statutes.

LO 9.4 Cite examples of reportable diseases and injuries, and explain how they are reported.

LO 9.5 Discuss federal drug regulations, including the Controlled Substances Act.

FROM THE PERSPECTIVE OF. . .

JASON, RN, BSN, is a public health nurse working for sections of three counties in the rural Northwest. "My duties range from home visits for parenting education, to foster child care, to the mainstays of public health—communicable disease investigation and reporting—and everything in between. In fact, once during a home visit I even delivered a baby—it was a boy," Jason says. "I enjoy the autonomy I have in my job, and I've established good rapport with the families I see regularly."

The ability to establish rapport is important, Jason explains, when he contacts individuals who have been diagnosed with a reportable disease, such as a sexually transmitted disease (STD), also referred to as a sexually transmitted infection (STI) and their contacts. "We have a fairly high percentage of STIs in my area, and I'm often persuading people to give me the names of those with whom they have been intimate, so I can let those individuals know that they should see a doctor."

The information is kept confidential, of course, Jason continues, "but it's still a hard subject to approach. Most people are cooperative, but there are a few who don't want to talk to me. That's when my job really becomes difficult."

From Jason's perspective, his job involves helping keep families within his practice area healthy, and also helping hold down the spread of a contagious infection or disease once patients are diagnosed. His investigative work as a public health nurse is mandated by state law, but the process can be difficult and can feel intrusive. Nevertheless, Jason does his best to see that the people in his area are protected.

From the perspective of Jason's patients who learn they have a reportable, contagious condition, his visit is probably stressful. Those who are concerned for loved ones or others with whom they have had contact, however, are generally willing to provide names of individuals he can contact.

From the perspective of public health authorities, nurses like Jason not only see patients in their homes, where health problems often arise, but they also keep contagious diseases from becoming epidemic, and they help get vital treatment to those who have been exposed to infectious diseases.

Vital Statistics

To assess population trends and needs, state and federal governments collect **vital statistics.** Vital events for which statistics are collected include live births, deaths, fetal deaths, marriages, divorces, induced terminations of pregnancy, and any change in civil status that occurs during an individual's lifetime. Health care practitioners help in gathering this information and in filling out forms for filing with the appropriate state and federal agencies.

The information provided through the reporting of vital statistics is useful to educational institutions, governmental agencies, research scientists, private industry, and many other organizations and individuals. For example, the recording of vital statistics allows for tracking population composition and growth, measuring educational

LO 9.1

List at least four vital events for which statistics are collected by the government.

vital statistics
Numbers collected for the population of live births, deaths, fetal deaths, marriages, divorces, induced terminations of pregnancy, and any change in civil status that occurs during an individual's lifetime.

standards, and monitoring communicable diseases and other community and environmental health problems. Health care practitioners play an important role in collecting and recording valuable health data required by law; therefore, it is important that they know the correct methods and procedures for reporting public health information.

Records for Births and Deaths

LO 9.2

Discuss the procedures for filing birth and death certificates.

Birth and death certificates are permanent legal records, and a copy of a person's birth certificate is required to obtain certain government documents, such as a passport, driver's license, voter registration card, or Social Security card. Guidelines for completing the forms are as follows:

- Type or legibly print all entries. In some states, only black ink may be used.
- Leave no entries blank. Each state has specific requirements for recording information.
- Avoid corrections and erasures.
- Where requested, provide signatures. Do not use rubber stamps or initials in place of signatures.
- File only originals with state registrars.
- Verify the spelling of names.
- Avoid abbreviations, except those recommended in instructions for specific items.
- Refer any problems to the appropriate state officials.

BIRTHS

All live births must be reported to the state registrar. Figure 9-1 illustrates a sample birth certificate. In some states, separate birth and death certificates must be filed for stillbirths, while in others there are special forms for stillbirths that include both birth and death information. Generally, birth and death certificates are not required for fetal deaths in which the fetus has not passed the 20th week of gestation.

Hospitals file birth certificates for babies born to mothers who have been admitted as patients. The attending physician must verify all medical information. For nonhospital births, the person in attendance is responsible for filing the birth certificate. (Jason, the public health nurse in the chapter's opening scenario, filed the birth certificate for the birth he attended.)

DEATHS

After a person is pronounced dead, the attending physician must complete the medical portion of the certificate of death, which generally includes the following information:

- Disease, injury, and/or complication that caused the death and how long the decedent was treated for this condition before death occurred.
- Date and time of death.
- Place of death.

FIGURE 9-1 A Sample Birth Certificate

U.S. STANDARD CERTIFICATE OF LIVE BIRTH

LOCAL FILE NO.

BIRTH NUMBER:

C H I L D

1. CHILD'S NAME (First, Middle, Last, Suffix)	2. TIME OF BIRTH (24 hr)	3. SEX	4. DATE OF BIRTH (Mo/Day/Yr)

5. FACILITY NAME (If not institution, give street and number)	6. CITY, TOWN, OR LOCATION OF BIRTH	7. COUNTY OF BIRTH

M O T H E R

8a. MOTHER'S CURRENT LEGAL NAME (First, Middle, Last, Suffix)	8b. DATE OF BIRTH (Mo/Day/Yr)

8c. MOTHER'S NAME PRIOR TO FIRST MARRIAGE (First, Middle, Last, Suffix)	8d. BIRTHPLACE (State, Territory, or Foreign Country)

9a. RESIDENCE OF MOTHER-STATE	9b. COUNTY	9c. CITY, TOWN, OR LOCATION

9d. STREET AND NUMBER	9e. APT. NO.	9f. ZIP CODE	9g. INSIDE CITY LIMITS? ☐ Yes ☐ No

F A T H E R

10a. FATHER'S CURRENT LEGAL NAME (First, Middle, Last, Suffix)	10b. DATE OF BIRTH (Mo/Day/Yr)	10c. BIRTHPLACE (State, Territory, or Foreign Country)

CERTIFIER

11. CERTIFIER'S NAME: _____

TITLE: ☐ MD ☐ DO ☐ HOSPITAL ADMIN. ☐ CNM/CM ☐ OTHER MIDWIFE

☐ OTHER (Specify)_____

12. DATE CERTIFIED _____ / _____ / _____ MM DD YYYY

13. DATE FILED BY REGISTRAR _____ / _____ / _____ MM DD YYYY

INFORMATION FOR ADMINISTRATIVE USE

M O T H E R

14. MOTHER'S MAILING ADDRESS: 9 Same as residence, or: State: City, Town, or Location:

Street & Number: Apartment No.: Zip Code:

15. MOTHER MARRIED? (At birth, conception, or any time between) ☐ Yes ☐ No
IF NO, HAS PATERNITY ACKNOWLEDGEMENT BEEN SIGNED IN THE HOSPITAL? ☐ Yes ☐ No

16. SOCIAL SECURITY NUMBER REQUESTED FOR CHILD? ☐ Yes ☐ No

17. FACILITY ID. (NPI)

18. MOTHER'S SOCIAL SECURITY NUMBER:

19. FATHER'S SOCIAL SECURITY NUMBER:

INFORMATION FOR MEDICAL AND HEALTH PURPOSES ONLY

M O T H E R

20. MOTHER'S EDUCATION (Check the box that best describes the highest degree or level of school completed at the time of delivery)

☐ 8th grade or less
☐ 9th - 12th grade, no diploma
☐ High school graduate or GED completed
☐ Some college credit but no degree
☐ Associate degree (e.g., AA, AS)
☐ Bachelor's degree (e.g., BA, AB, BS)
☐ Master's degree (e.g., MA, MS, MEng, MEd, MSW, MBA)
☐ Doctorate (e.g., PhD, EdD) or Professional degree (e.g., MD, DDS, DVM, LLB, JD)

21. MOTHER OF HISPANIC ORIGIN? (Check the box that best describes whether the mother is Spanish/Hispanic/Latina. Check the "No" box if mother is not Spanish/Hispanic/Latina)

☐ No, not Spanish/Hispanic/Latina
☐ Yes, Mexican, Mexican American, Chicana
☐ Yes, Puerto Rican
☐ Yes, Cuban
☐ Yes, other Spanish/Hispanic/Latina

(Specify)_____

22. MOTHER'S RACE (Check one or more races to indicate what the mother considers herself to be)

☐ White
☐ Black or African American
☐ American Indian or Alaska Native (Name of the enrolled or principal tribe)_____
☐ Asian Indian
☐ Chinese
☐ Filipino
☐ Japanese
☐ Korean
☐ Vietnamese
☐ Other Asian (Specify)_____
☐ Native Hawaiian
☐ Guamanian or Chamorro
☐ Samoan
☐ Other Pacific Islander (Specify)_____
☐ Other (Specify)_____

F A T H E R

23. FATHER'S EDUCATION (Check the box that best describes the highest degree or level of school completed at the time of delivery)

☐ 8th grade or less
☐ 9th - 12th grade, no diploma
☐ High school graduate or GED completed
☐ Some college credit but no degree
☐ Associate degree (e.g., AA, AS)
☐ Bachelor's degree (e.g., BA, AB, BS)
☐ Master's degree (e.g., MA, MS, MEng, MEd, MSW, MBA)
☐ Doctorate (e.g., PhD, EdD) or Professional degree (e.g., MD, DDS, DVM, LLB, JD)

24. FATHER OF HISPANIC ORIGIN? (Check the box that best describes whether the father is Spanish/Hispanic/Latino. Check the "No" box if father is not Spanish/Hispanic/Latino)

☐ No, not Spanish/Hispanic/Latino
☐ Yes, Mexican, Mexican American, Chicano
☐ Yes, Puerto Rican
☐ Yes, Cuban
☐ Yes, other Spanish/Hispanic/Latino

(Specify)_____

25. FATHER'S RACE (Check one or more races to indicate what the father considers himself to be)

☐ White
☐ Black or African American
☐ American Indian or Alaska Native (Name of the enrolled or principal tribe)_____
☐ Asian Indian
☐ Chinese
☐ Filipino
☐ Japanese
☐ Korean
☐ Vietnamese
☐ Other Asian (Specify)_____
☐ Native Hawaiian
☐ Guamanian or Chamorro
☐ Samoan
☐ Other Pacific Islander (Specify)_____
☐ Other (Specify)_____

Mother's Name

Mother's Medical Record No.

26. PLACE WHERE BIRTH OCCURRED (Check one)
☐ Hospital
☐ Freestanding birthing center
☐ Home Birth: Planned to deliver at home? 9 Yes 9 No
☐ Clinic/Doctor's office
☐ Other (Specify)_____

27. ATTENDANT'S NAME, TITLE, AND NPI

NAME: _____ NPI:_____

TITLE: ☐ MD ☐ DO ☐ CNM/CM ☐ OTHER MIDWIFE
☐ OTHER (Specify)_____

28. MOTHER TRANSFERRED FOR MATERNAL MEDICAL OR FETAL INDICATIONS FOR DELIVERY? ☐ Yes ☐ No
IF YES, ENTER NAME OF FACILITY MOTHER TRANSFERRED FROM:

_____

REV. 11/2003

- If decedent was female, presence or absence of pregnancy.
- Whether or not an autopsy was performed. An **autopsy** is a postmortem examination to determine the cause of death or to obtain physiological evidence, as in the case of a suspicious death.

In most states, it is against the law for an attending physician to sign a death certificate if the death was:

- Possibly due to criminal causes.
- Not attended by a physician within a specified length of time before death.
- Due to causes undetermined by the physician.
- Violent or otherwise suspicious.

If any of these situations exist, a coroner or medical examiner must sign the death certificate. If a death occurs under suspicious circumstances, permission from next of kin is *not* needed for an autopsy to be performed. If the death did not occur under suspicious circumstances, however, consent from next of kin or a legally responsible party must be obtained for an autopsy to be performed.

When death has occurred under normal circumstances, after authorization has been obtained from the next of kin or from a legally responsible party, the body can be removed to a funeral home. In many states, the death certificate must be signed within 24 to 72 hours. The *mortician* or *undertaker* (person trained to attend to the dead) files the death certificate with the state. (See Figure 9-2 for a sample death certificate.)

If the deceased has not been under a physician's care at the time of death, the appropriate county health officer—usually the coroner or medical examiner—is responsible for completing the death certificate. A **coroner** is a public official who investigates and holds inquests over those who die from unknown or violent causes. He or she may or may not be a physician, depending on state law.

The purpose of a coroner's inquest is to gather evidence that may be used by the police in the investigation of a violent or suspicious death. It is not a trial, but it is a criminal proceeding, in the nature of a preliminary investigation.

Some states employ a medical examiner instead of a coroner. A **medical examiner** is a physician, frequently a pathologist, who investigates suspicious or unexplained deaths in a community. As a physician, the medical examiner can order and perform autopsies.

FORENSIC MEDICINE

Forensics is a division of medicine that incorporates law and medicine and involves medical issues or medical proof at trials having to do with malpractice, crimes, and accidents. Forensic scientists investigate crime scenes and present medical proof at trials and hearings. Crime scene investigators are specifically trained to determine cause of death or injury and to help identify a criminal, a victim, and others involved in crimes. Specialists in forensic medicine study such subjects as forensic pharmacology, doping control, postmortem toxicology, blood spatter interpretation, DNA (deoxyribonucleic acid) analytical techniques, and expert testimony procedures. They work for police departments

FIGURE 9-2 A Sample Death Certificate

U.S. STANDARD CERTIFICATE OF DEATH

LOCAL FILE NO.   STATE FILE NO.

NAME OF DECEDENT — For use by physician or institution

To Be Completed/ Verified By: FUNERAL DIRECTOR:

1. DECEDENT'S LEGAL NAME (Include AKA's if any) (First, Middle, Last)	2. SEX	3. SOCIAL SECURITY NUMBER

4a. AGE-Last Birthday (Years)	4b. UNDER 1 YEAR		4c. UNDER 1 DAY		5. DATE OF BIRTH (Mo/Day/Yr)	6. BIRTHPLACE (City and State or Foreign Country)
	Months	Days	Hours	Minutes		

7a. RESIDENCE-STATE	7b. COUNTY	7c. CITY OR TOWN

7d. STREET AND NUMBER	7e. APT. NO.	7f. ZIP CODE	7g. INSIDE CITY LIMITS? ☐ Yes ☐ No

8. EVER IN US ARMED FORCES? ☐ Yes ☐ No	9. MARITAL STATUS AT TIME OF DEATH ☐ Married ☐ Married, but separated ☐ Widowed ☐ Divorced ☐ Never Married ☐ Unknown	10. SURVIVING SPOUSE'S NAME (If wife, give name prior to first marriage)

11. FATHER'S NAME (First, Middle, Last)	12. MOTHER'S NAME PRIOR TO FIRST MARRIAGE (First, Middle, Last)

13a. INFORMANT'S NAME	13b. RELATIONSHIP TO DECEDENT	13c. MAILING ADDRESS (Street and Number, City, State, Zip Code)

14. PLACE OF DEATH (Check only one: see instructions)

IF DEATH OCCURRED IN A HOSPITAL: ☐ Inpatient ☐ Emergency Room/Outpatient ☐ Dead on Arrival	IF DEATH OCCURRED SOMEWHERE OTHER THAN A HOSPITAL: ☐ Hospice facility ☐ Nursing home/Long term care facility ☐ Decedent's home ☐ Other (Specify):

15. FACILITY NAME (If not institution, give street & number)	16. CITY OR TOWN , STATE, AND ZIP CODE	17. COUNTY OF DEATH

18. METHOD OF DISPOSITION: ☐ Burial ☐ Cremation ☐ Donation ☐ Entombment ☐ Removal from State ☐ Other (Specify):___	19. PLACE OF DISPOSITION (Name of cemetery, crematory, other place)

20. LOCATION-CITY, TOWN, AND STATE	21. NAME AND COMPLETE ADDRESS OF FUNERAL FACILITY

22. SIGNATURE OF FUNERAL SERVICE LICENSEE OR OTHER AGENT	23. LICENSE NUMBER (Of Licensee)

To Be Completed By: MEDICAL CERTIFIER

ITEMS 24-28 MUST BE COMPLETED BY PERSON WHO PRONOUNCES OR CERTIFIES DEATH	24. DATE PRONOUNCED DEAD (Mo/Day/Yr)	25. TIME PRONOUNCED DEAD

26. SIGNATURE OF PERSON PRONOUNCING DEATH (Only when applicable)	27. LICENSE NUMBER	28. DATE SIGNED (Mo/Day/Yr)

29. ACTUAL OR PRESUMED DATE OF DEATH (Mo/Day/Yr) (Spell Month)	30. ACTUAL OR PRESUMED TIME OF DEATH	31. WAS MEDICAL EXAMINER OR CORONER CONTACTED? ☐ Yes ☐ No

CAUSE OF DEATH (See instructions and examples)

32. **PART I.** Enter the chain of events--diseases, injuries, or complications--that directly caused the death. DO NOT enter terminal events such as cardiac arrest, respiratory arrest, or ventricular fibrillation without showing the etiology. DO NOT ABBREVIATE. Enter only one cause on a line. Add additional lines if necessary.

Approximate interval: Onset to death

IMMEDIATE CAUSE (Final disease or condition --------> resulting in death)

a._____ Due to (or as a consequence of): _____

Sequentially list conditions, if any, leading to the cause listed on line a. Enter the **UNDERLYING CAUSE** (disease or injury that initiated the events resulting in death) **LAST**

b._____ Due to (or as a consequence of): _____

c._____ Due to (or as a consequence of): _____

d._____

PART II. Enter other significant conditions contributing to death but not resulting in the underlying cause given in PART I

33. WAS AN AUTOPSY PERFORMED? ☐ Yes ☐ No
34. WERE AUTOPSY FINDINGS AVAILABLE TO COMPLETE THE CAUSE OF DEATH? ☐ Yes ☐ No

35. DID TOBACCO USE CONTRIBUTE TO DEATH? ☐ Yes ☐ Probably ☐ No ☐ Unknown	36. IF FEMALE: ☐ Not pregnant within past year ☐ Pregnant at time of death ☐ Not pregnant, but pregnant within 42 days of death ☐ Not pregnant, but pregnant 43 days to 1 year before death ☐ Unknown if pregnant within the past year	37. MANNER OF DEATH ☐ Natural ☐ Homicide ☐ Accident ☐ Pending Investigation ☐ Suicide ☐ Could not be determined

38. DATE OF INJURY (Mo/Day/Yr) (Spell Month)	39. TIME OF INJURY	40. PLACE OF INJURY (e.g., Decedent's home; construction site; restaurant; wooded area)	41. INJURY AT WORK? ☐ Yes ☐ No

42. LOCATION OF INJURY: State: City or Town:

Street & Number: Apartment No.:   Zip Code:

43. DESCRIBE HOW INJURY OCCURRED:	44. IF TRANSPORTATION INJURY, SPECIFY: ☐ Driver/Operator ☐ Passenger ☐ Pedestrian ☐ Other (Specify)

45. CERTIFIER (Check only one):
☐ Certifying physician-To the best of my knowledge, death occurred due to the cause(s) and manner stated.
☐ Pronouncing & Certifying physician-To the best of my knowledge, death occurred at the time, date, and place, and due to the cause(s) and manner stated.
☐ Medical Examiner/Coroner-On the basis of examination, and/or investigation, in my opinion, death occurred at the time, date, and place, and due to the cause(s) and manner stated.

Signature of certifier:_____

46. NAME, ADDRESS, AND ZIP CODE OF PERSON COMPLETING CAUSE OF DEATH (Item 32)

47. TITLE OF CERTIFIER	48. LICENSE NUMBER	49. DATE CERTIFIED (Mo/Day/Yr)	50. **FOR REGISTRAR ONLY**- DATE FILED (Mo/Day/Yr)

51. DECEDENT'S EDUCATION-Check the box that best describes the highest degree or level of school completed at the time of death.	52. DECEDENT OF HISPANIC ORIGIN? Check the box that best describes whether the decedent is Spanish/Hispanic/Latino. Check the "No" box if decedent ~~is not~~ Spanish/Hispanic/Latino	53. DECEDENT'S RACE (Check one or more races to indicate what the decedent considered himself or herself to be)

and other criminal investigative bureaus, medical examiners' offices, universities, and other facilities and government agencies.

In the case, "Routine Autopsy Overruled," notice how one state law, which mandates when autopsies are routinely performed, is superseded by another protecting religious freedom.

COURT CASE   Routine Autopsy Overruled

When a prisoner was executed in Tennessee on December 2, 2009, an autopsy was scheduled, since Tennessee state law mandates that autopsies be performed for all apparent "homicides" and "unnatural" deaths. The execution was not technically a "homicide," but it was an "unnatural" death, since the prisoner was healthy at the time of execution. Before he was executed, the prisoner had filed a religious objection to autopsy with his religious advisor, and the objection was also stated in

his will. The state claimed it had "a compelling government interest" in performing the autopsy, but the court held for the prisoner's wife, who filed on his behalf under Tennessee's "Preservation of Religious Freedom" statute, asking for an injunction to prevent the autopsy from proceeding. The injunction was granted and the autopsy was not performed.

Johnson v. Levy et al., No. M2009-02596-COA-R3-CV, Tennessee Court of Appeals, Nashville, 2010.

Check Your Progress

1. Define *vital statistics*.

2. Define *autopsy*.

3. Define *coroner*.

4. Define *medical examiner*.

5. Define *forensics*.

6. Where are birth certificates and death certificates filed?

7. Birth certificates must be filed for _____ .
   Requirements vary with states for _____ .

8. Name three circumstances in which an attending physician may not legally complete a death certificate.

LO 9.3

Explain the purpose of public health statutes.

federalism
The sharing of power among national, state, and local governments.

Public Health Statutes

The power of the states to initiate public health statutes is inferred from the Tenth Amendment to the U.S. Constitution, included in the Bill of Rights. The amendment states: "The powers not delegated to the United States by the Constitution, nor prohibited by it to the States, are reserved to the States, respectively, or to the people." In other words, states retain police powers and all other powers not expressively granted to the federal government—a practice referred to as **federalism**—the sharing of power among national, state, and local governments.

In all states, public health statues help guarantee the health and well-being of citizens. As part of public health law, physicians or other health care practitioners must report births, deaths, certain communicable diseases, specific injuries, and child and drug abuse to the appropriate local, state, and federal authorities. Public health statutes vary with states concerning the reporting of fetal deaths and stillbirths, time

eradicated. In the U
peared, and very few
or measles are report

In some states, ce
reported, to allow pu
ment or to otherwis
diseases include car
genital metabolic di
congenital hypothyr
treatment); epilepsy
sciousness (to deterr
poisoning.

COURT CASE

A woman convicted of re
a sexual partner that sh
conviction on grounds th
status before she met hir
newspaper. The plaintiff
he did not know of the
were intimate. Since Gec

COURT CASE

The Plaintiff in this ca
long-term relationship
Following the end of th
discovered that D.D. ha
immunodeficiency virus
and that he had infected
in 2010.

The plaintiff sued se\
treated D.D. and knew (
not notify B.R. Plaintiff a
a duty to her to notify he

THE NATIONAL C ACT OF 1986

Parents usually begir
nicable diseases for
children reach school
children entering the

limits for filing reports, and the manner in which information must be recorded. However, all provide for:

- Guarding against unsanitary conditions in public facilities.
- Inspecting establishments where food and drink are processed and sold.
- Exterminating pests and vermin that can spread disease.
- Checking water quality.
- Setting up measures of control for certain diseases.
- Requiring physicians, school nurses, and other health care workers to file certain reports for the protection of citizens.

Since enforcing public health laws is vital to the health of individuals within communities, the states have enforcement power granted through each state's constitution. For example, the state can:

- Require investigations be conducted in infectious disease outbreaks.
- Make childhood vaccinations a condition for school entry.
- Ban the distribution of free cigarette samples around schools or in areas where children congregate.
- Institute smoking bans or restrictions.
- Involuntarily detain (quarantine) individuals who have certain infectious diseases.
- Seize and/or destroy property to contain the threat of toxic substances.

Table 9-1 shows how laws affect public health issues.

Table 9-1 How Laws Impact Public Health Issues

Law	Public Health Issue	How the Law Works	How the Law Is Enforced
Vaccinations to enter school	Spread of infectious disease	Parental cooperation	Requires proof of vaccination when children register for school.
Smoking bans/restrictions	Diseases caused by exposure to tobacco smoke	Requires behavioral changes	Admonishment or citations for noncompliance.
Child safety seat laws	Accidental injuries/death in children	Requires behavioral changes	Citations for noncompliance.
Fluoridation of public water supply	Dental caries	Requires no action on the part of individuals	Periodic checking of public water supply.
Spraying a community for mosquito control	Spread of infectious disease	Requires no action on the part of individuals	City government orders and pays for spraying.
Requiring pasteurization of milk sold for public consumption	Spread of infectious disease	Requires no action on the part of individuals	Milk is tested for pathogens before it is sold.
Restaurant inspections	Spread of food poisoning or other disease	Requires no action on the part of individuals	Local health department routinely inspects restaurants.
Food supply inspections	Spread of food poisoning or other disease	Requires no action on the part of individuals	FDA inspectors can initiate civil action, as well as criminal prosecution.

Source: Adapted from CDC's Public Health Law 101, Lesson 1, "Key Concepts of U.S. Law in Public Health Practice," PPt Slide 11. **www2.cdc.gov/phlp/phl101/.**

LO 9.4

Cite examples of report
diseases and injuries, an
explain how they are re

The Vaccine Adverse Events Reporting System (VAERS), operated by the FDA and CDC, should be notified of any adverse event by the filing of a VAERS reporting form. Health care providers must report the following events:

- Any event listed in the Vaccine Injury Table, available at the Health Resources and Services Administration Web site and from the Health Resources and Services Administration Bureau of Health Professions, 5600 Fishers Lane, Rockville, MD 20857.

- Any contraindicating event listed in the manufacturer's package insert.

REPORTABLE INJURIES

In all states, physicians must immediately report to law enforcement officials medical treatment of patients whose injuries resulted from certain acts of violence, such as assault, rape, or domestic violence, so that authorities can investigate the incident. (In most states, spousal abuse is reportable only if the patient says his or her injuries are due to spousal abuse.) Reportable acts of domestic violence include child abuse, spousal abuse, and elder abuse.

**Child Abuse Prevention
and Treatment Act**
A federal law passed in 1974 requiring physicians to report cases of child abuse.

Child Abuse To help prevent violence against children, in 1974 Congress passed the **Child Abuse Prevention and Treatment Act,** mandating the reporting of cases of child abuse. All states have enacted legislation making child abuse a crime and requiring that teachers, physicians, and other licensed health care practitioners report child abuse and neglect. The report must immediately be made to the proper authorities—either in person or by telephone—and a written report is generally required within a specified time frame, such as 72 hours. Any individual reporting suspected child abuse is granted absolute immunity from criminal and civil liability resulting from the reported incident. Depending on state law, failure to report suspected cases of child abuse may be a misdemeanor.

Spousal Abuse Unlike cases of child abuse, most state laws do not specifically require a physician to report spousal abuse, unless a spouse

Check Your Progress

9. State public health laws generally provide six areas of responsibility, which are _____.

10. In your opinion, why have most states passed strict antismoking laws?

11. Check the following areas where public health laws can apply:

_____ Public restaurants

_____ Public swimming pools

_____ Public schools

_____ Private homes where residents have communicable diseases

_____ Private schools

12. What provision has the federal government made for people who sue over vaccinations?

13. Why are certain diseases and injuries reportable to state authorities?

states that his or her injuries were the result of spousal abuse. Legal remedies available to battered spouses vary from state to state, but all states have laws protecting victims of domestic abuse. Advocacy programs can explain legal options to victims and can help them cope with the legal system. Courts may issue protective, or restraining, orders, or they may issue injunctions that direct the batterer to stop abusing the victim. In some states, police may be required to arrest batterers under certain conditions. Depending on laws within the jurisdiction and the type of offense committed, a batterer may be criminally prosecuted for assault, battery, harassment, intimidation, rape, or attempted murder.

Elder Abuse The Older Americans Act was signed into law by President Lyndon B. Johnson in 1965. The act created the Administration on Aging and outlined 10 objectives aimed at preserving the rights and dignity of older citizens. The 1987 **Amendments to the Older Americans Act** defines elder abuse, neglect, and exploitation, but does not deal with enforcement. The year 2000 *Amendments to the Older Americans Act* includes a five-year reauthorization for funding, maintains the original 10 objectives, and adds the National Family Caregiver Support Program for addressing the needs of caregivers to elderly individuals. The 2006 amendments to the original Older Americans Act covered a broad range of topics, including aging and disability resource centers, elder justice, elder health, the continuation of a National Family Caregiver Support Program, nutrition, transportation, and other areas of concern for older individuals.

> **Amendments to the Older Americans Act**
> A 1987 federal act that defines elder abuse, neglect, and exploitation but does not deal with enforcement.

For current information about amendments to the Older Americans Act consult this Web site: **www.aoa.gov/aoaroot/aoa_programs/oaa/index.aspx.**

All 50 states and the District of Columbia have enacted legislation instituting reporting systems to identify domestic and institutional elder abuse, neglect, and exploitation. In most states, reporting suspected elder abuse is mandatory for certain professionals, including physicians. (If not mandated by state law, reporting may be voluntary.) Physical, sexual, and financial abuses of elderly people are considered crimes in all states. Some forms of emotional abuse and types of neglect may be considered crimes in some states.

In addition to laws regarding child, spousal, and elder abuse, some states have passed laws protecting vulnerable adults, such as individuals who are mentally ill and mentally challenged. Some states also have statutes dealing with the prevention of fetal abuse stemming from sniffing paint and other chemicals, taking drugs, or drinking alcohol while pregnant.

The Unborn Victims of Violence Act In April 2004, Congress passed and President George W. Bush signed into law the **Unborn Victims of Violence Act,** also called "Laci and Conner's Act," after the December 24, 2002, murder of Laci Peterson, a pregnant woman, and her nine-month-old fetus, Conner. The act provides for the prosecution of anyone who causes injury to or the death of a fetus in utero, in cases where the federal government has jurisdiction. It also states that "the punishment for that separate offense is the same as the punishment provided under Federal law for that conduct had that injury or death occurred to the unborn child's mother." Before this federal law was passed, in most states a person accused of injuring or killing a

> **Unborn Victims of Violence Act**
> Also called Laci and Conner's Act, a 2004 federal law that provides for the prosecution of anyone who causes injury to or the death of a fetus in utero.

pregnant woman was tried for offenses against the mother, but not for injuring or killing her fetus as a separate individual. State law determines whether an unborn fetus is considered a "person" in cases where a pregnant woman is assaulted or otherwise injured and, as a result, her unborn baby dies. For example, read the next case, "Is the Death of an Unborn Baby Always Considered a Homicide?"

Identifying Abuse Health care practitioners should be alert for signs of physical abuse, for purposes both of mandatory reporting and of possible intervention on behalf of the victim. It is imperative, however, that medical personnel not jump to conclusions and make unsubstantiated abuse reports.

Physical signs of abuse may include but are not limited to these:

- Unexplained fractures
- Repeated injuries, especially those in unusual places or those shaped like objects such as electrical cords, hairbrushes, belt buckles, and so forth.
- Burns with unusual shapes (such as a circle, that may have been caused by a cigarette, or the mark of an object such as an iron).
- Friction burns apparently caused by a rope or cord.
- Bite marks
- Signs of malnutrition or dehydration, such as extreme weight loss, dry skin, or red-rimmed, sunken eyes.
- Torn or bloody underwear.
- Pain or bruising in the genital area.
- Unexplained venereal disease or other genital infections.

Behavioral signs of abuse may include the following:

- Illogical or unreasonable explanations for injuries.
- Frequently changing physicians and/or missing medical appointments.
- Attempts to hide injuries with heavy makeup or sunglasses.
- Frequent anxiety, depression, or loss of emotional control.
- Changes in appetite; problems at school or on the job.

Observation of individuals who accompany the patient may also identify a potential abuser. One might suspect abuse, for example, if, in the presence of additional evidence, an alleged victim of abuse is accompanied by someone who smells of alcohol, exhibits pensive or obsessive behavior, seems unusually or inappropriately emotional, or shows aggressive or otherwise suspicious body language toward the patient.

When a health care practitioner suspects abuse, care and tact must be used in eliciting information from patients. Direct, open-ended questions such as "Has someone harmed you?" may encourage a patient to relate what has caused his or her injuries.

Health care practitioners should emphasize to the patient that information offered will be kept confidential, as required by physician–patient confidentiality, except in those cases in which the law mandates reporting abuse. Reporting requirements for abuse should be explained during the patient's first visit. Some sources recommend having patients sign a statement indicating that they understand the reporting requirements and agree with them.

Forcing the issue to encourage an adult to leave a batterer is not always the immediate answer. Similarly, providing hotline numbers, information on safe houses, or handouts about abuse may not be helpful if the batterer is waiting in the reception area for the patient or may later find the material and be further enraged. Instead, many medical facilities have bulletins posted in restrooms, telling patients where to call for help. If tear strips with the telephone number are provided, a victim can tear off the small, easily concealed strip for future reference.

COURT CASE Is the Death of an Unborn Baby Always Considered a Homicide?

In Colorado, a man being pursued by police during a high-speed car chase collided head-on with a car traveling in the opposite direction. The driver of the other car involved in the collision was a woman who was eight and one-half months pregnant. The woman survived her injuries, but the force of the collision caused an 80 percent abruption of her placenta. Her child was born alive, but died shortly thereafter from asphyxia. The death was ruled a homicide, and the defendant was charged with murder, as well as other charges arising from the car chase. The trial court dismissed the homicide charge, based on Colorado's definition of "person," which specifies (1) the individual is a human being; (2) the individual has already been born; and (3) the individual is alive. The prosecutor appealed the trial court's dismissal of the homicide charge, and the appellate court affirmed the dismissal of that charge, but remanded the defendant to be tried for reckless child abuse resulting in death, and vehicular assault, as well as other charges resulting from the high-speed chase.

As of October 2013, 37 states recognized the death of an unborn child, in certain circumstances, as homicide. For the current status of such laws, visit **www.nrlc.org.**

People v. Lage, CO. Ct. App. No. 08CA0617, May 28, 2009.

Check Your Progress

14. You are a medical assistant in a physician office and you suspect a female patient has been abused. What signs might you look for that could indicate abuse?

15. If you see signs of abuse, but the patient does not admit that she has been abused, how might you proceed?

16. What types of injuries are health care practitioners required to report?

17. As a health care practitioner, should you report abuse if a patient asks you not to? Explain your answer.

18. In your opinion, why does the law require medical providers to report suspected abuse?

Drug Regulations

The federal government has jurisdiction over the manufacture and distribution of drugs in the United States. The **Food and Drug Administration (FDA),** an agency within the Department of Health and Human Services, tests and approves drugs before releasing them for public use. This agency also oversees drug quality and standardization.

The FDA also has responsibility for major product recalls—a function vital to maintaining public health. For example, in August 2010 more

LO 9.5

Discuss federal drug regulations, including the Controlled Substances Act.

Food and Drug Administration (FDA)
A federal agency within the Department of Health and Human Services that oversees drug quality and standardization and must approve drugs before they are released for public use.

than a half billion eggs were recalled from stores to prevent the spread of *Salmonella enteritidis* infections linked to the tainted eggs. About 1,500 cases of the infection were reported in the spring of 2010—the largest known outbreak associated with the strain of salmonella found in the eggs. FDA inspectors found widespread food safety violations in the barns of two Iowa egg producers where most of the eggs originated, including flies, maggots, rodents, and overflowing manure pits, and inspectors planned to visit all 600 of the nation's major egg-producing facilities within the following months.

Both federal and state governments regulate the sale and use of certain drugs. At the federal level, the **Drug Enforcement Administration (DEA),** a branch of the Department of Justice, regulates the sale and use of drugs by the authority granted in the Comprehensive Drug Abuse Prevention and Control Act of 1970, commonly called the **Controlled Substances Act.**

General regulations mandated by the Controlled Substances Act require physicians who purchase, **prescribe, dispense,** administer, or in any way handle controlled drugs to follow these procedures:

- Register with the Drug Enforcement Administration through a division office. (A list of division offices is available online at the DEA Web site.) The physician will receive a registration number that must appear on all prescriptions for controlled substances and must be renewed periodically for a specified fee. Each DEA number is issued for a specific physician in a specific location. That location is the only one at which the physician may store controlled substances, including salespeople's samples. If a physician practices in more than one state, he or she needs a DEA number for each state. The physician must notify the appropriate state authorities and the DEA whenever he or she moves from a registered location.

- Keep records concerning the administering or dispensing of a controlled drug on file for two years. Such records must include the patient's full name and address, the reason for use of the drug, the date of the order, the name of the drug, the dosage form and quantity of the drug, and whether the drug was administered or dispensed.

- Note on a patient's chart when controlled substances are administered or dispensed.

- Make a written inventory of drug supplies every two years, and keep such records an additional two years.

- Keep drugs in a locked cabinet or safe, and report any thefts immediately to the nearest DEA office and the local police.

THE CONTROLLED SUBSTANCES ACT

The Controlled Substances Act is a federal law that regulates drugs under five schedules, based on their potential for abuse and their medical usefulness. If a drug has no potential for abuse, it is not listed as controlled. Table 9-3 lists the five schedules for controlled substances.

Drugs included in Schedule II and IIn require a properly executed, manually signed prescription. No refills are permitted on these prescriptions. All other scheduled drugs (Schedules III through V) may be prescribed on written or oral orders, and refills are generally permitted with certain limitations.

Drug Enforcement Administration (DEA)
A branch of the U.S. Department of Justice that regulates the sale and use of drugs.

Controlled Substances Act
The federal law giving authority to the Drug Enforcement Administration to regulate the sale and use of drugs.

prescribe
To issue a medical prescription for a patient.

dispense
To deliver controlled substances in some type of bottle, box, or other container to a patient.

Table 9-3 Drug Schedules for Controlled Substances

Schedule I

Potential for abuse is high and there is no currently accepted medical use of the drug or substance in the United States. Schedule I substances have been used strictly for research. Potential for abuse is determined by the following criteria:

1. There is evidence that individuals are taking the drug or other substance in amounts sufficient to create a hazard to their health or to the safety of other individuals or to the community;

or

2. There is significant diversion of the drug or other substance from legitimate drug channels;

or

3. Individuals are taking the drug or other substance on their own initiative rather than on the basis of medical advice from a practitioner licensed by law to administer such drugs;

or

4. The drug is a new drug so related in its action to a drug or other substance already listed as having a potential for abuse to make it likely that the drug will have the same potential for abuse as such drugs. Of course, evidence of actual abuse of a substance is indicative that a drug has a potential for abuse.

Examples of Schedule I drugs include heroin, lysergic acid diethylamide (LSD), marijuana, and methaqualone (In some states it is legal to use marijuana for medical purposes).

Schedule II

Potential for abuse of these narcotic drugs is high, but there are currently accepted medical uses for the drug or substance in the United States, often with severe restrictions. Severe psychological and physical dependence is possible. Examples of Schedule II drugs include morphine, phencyclidine (PCP), cocaine, methadone, and methamphetamine.

A subdivision of Schedule II, called IIn, refers to nonnarcotic drugs with a high potential for abuse. Examples of such drugs include Dexedrine, Desoxyn, Preludin, Ritalin, and pentobarbital.

Schedule III

The drug or other substance has less potential for abuse than the drugs or other substances in Schedules I and II, and has currently accepted medical uses in the United States.

Abuse of the drug or other substance may lead to moderate or low physical dependence or high psychological dependence. Examples of Schedule III substances include anabolic steroids, codeine and hydrocodone with aspirin or Tylenol, and some barbiturates. Schedule IIIn refers to nonnarcotic central nervous system depressants. These drugs include glutethimide, methyprylon, and barbiturates not listed in other schedules, as well as anorectant agents (suppositories) not listed elsewhere.

Schedule IV

The drug or other substance has a low potential for abuse relative to the drugs or other substances in Schedule III, and has currently accepted medical uses in the United States.

Abuse of the drug may lead to limited physical dependence or psychological dependence. Examples of Schedule IV drugs include Darvon, Talwin, Equanil, Valium, and Xanax.

Schedule V

The drug or other substance has a low potential for abuse relative to the drugs or other substances in Schedule IV, and has a currently accepted medical use in the United States.

Abuse of the drug or other substances may lead to limited physical dependence or psychological dependence relative to the drugs or other substances in Schedule IV. Cough medicines with codeine are examples of Schedule V drugs, as well as antitussive, antidiarrheal, and analgesic drugs.

Whenever prescriptions are written for controlled substances, a copy should be filed with the patient's record. When a physician discontinues practice, he or she must return the registration certificate and any unused order forms (preferably marked "void") to the DEA. When it is necessary to dispose of controlled drugs, the physician or employee charged with disposal should contact the nearest field office of the DEA and the responsible state agency for disposal information.

State laws governing controlled substances may be as strict as or stricter than federal laws. Physicians may be required to register with the appropriate state agency as well as the DEA, and must follow all state and federal requirements in prescribing, dispensing, and administering controlled substances. Whenever state and federal regulations differ, the more stringent regulation must be followed. For example, if federal law requires that records be held for two years and state law specifies five years, the state law takes precedence.

Since violation of a law dealing with a state-controlled and/or federally controlled substance is a criminal offense and can result in fines, jail sentences, and loss of license to practice medicine, physicians, other health care practitioners, and medical office employees should be familiar with all state and federal narcotics laws.

The role of the medical assistant concerning compliance with DEA regulations is to remind the physician of license renewal dates, to keep accurate records for scheduled drugs, to maintain an accurate inventory and inventory records, and to ensure the security of scheduled drugs kept in the office. This is accomplished by:

- Checking to be sure that all controlled substances are kept in a locked cabinet or safe.
- Reminding the physician to keep his or her "black bag" in a safe place.
- Keeping all prescription blanks, especially those used for narcotics, under lock and key.
- Ordering prescription blanks that are serially numbered or otherwise printed to help detect alterations and theft.
- Reporting to the physician any behavior by patients that would suggest an attempt to secure addictive drugs.
- Checking patients' records to verify all prescriptions that may be questioned by a pharmacist.

Physicians and other members of the health care team must be familiar with the laws that govern such threats as communicable disease, physical abuse, and drug abuse because they play a vital role in helping maintain healthy—and ultimately safe—communities.

Check Your Progress

Use these three terms correctly in the sentences that follow: *prescribe, dispense, administer.*

19. Dr. Wellness will _____ the drug to his patient, Mrs. Doe, when he starts an intravenous injection.

20. Under the law, medical assistants may not _____ drugs for patients but may _____ or _____ them under a physician's direct order.

21. When a pharmacist fills a patient's prescription, he or she then will _____ the drug to the patient.

22. What two federal agencies control the manufacture and standardization of drugs and their sale and use?

23. If state and federal regulations differ concerning the abuse of certain drugs, which law will be applied?

Chapter Summary

Learning Outcome	Summary
LO 9.1 List at least four vital events for which statistics are collected by the government.	**What are the vital events for which the government collects statistics?** • Live births • Deaths • Fetal deaths • Marriages • Divorces • Induced terminations of pregnancy. • Any change in an individual's civil status.
LO 9.2 Discuss the procedures for filing birth and death certificates.	**What is the correct procedure for completing a birth certificate?** • Type or legibly print all entries. • Leave no entries blank. • Avoid corrections and erasures. • Where requested, provide signatures. Do not use rubber stamps or initials in place of signatures. • File only originals with state registrars. • Verify the spelling of names. • Avoid abbreviations, except those recommended in instructions for specific items. • Refer any problems to the appropriate state officials. **What information does a death certificate generally include?** • Disease, injury, and/or complication that caused the death and time treated before death. • Date and time of death. • Place of death. • If decedent was female, presence or absence of pregnancy. • Whether or not an autopsy was performed. **When are autopsies performed?** • When a death is suspicious. • To determine cause of death, if cause is unknown. **When is a physician not allowed to sign a death certificate?** • When death is possibly due to criminal causes. • When person is not attended by a physician within a specified length of time before death. • When death is due to causes undetermined by the physician. • In cases of violent or otherwise suspicious deaths.
LO 9.3 Explain the purpose of public health statutes.	**What provisions do all public health statutes have in common?** • Guard against unsanitary conditions in public facilities. • Inspect establishments where food and drink are processed and sold. • Exterminate pests and vermin that can spread disease. • Check water quality. • Set up measures of control for certain diseases. • Require physicians, school nurses, and other health care workers to file certain reports for the protection of citizens.

Learning Outcome	Summary
	What are some examples of the authority states have to enforce public health laws?
	• Require investigations be conducted in infectious disease outbreaks.
	• Make childhood vaccinations a condition for school entry.
	• Ban the distribution of free cigarette samples around schools or in areas where children congregate.
	• Institute smoking bans or restrictions.
	• Involuntarily detain (quarantine) individuals who have certain infectious diseases.
	• Seize and/or destroy property to contain the threat of toxic substances.
LO 9.4 Cite examples of reportable diseases and injuries, and explain how they are reported.	Under public health law, what diseases and conditions are generally reported to public health departments?
	• Diseases that, if left unchecked, could threaten the health and well-being of the population.
	• Infectious diseases
	• Sexually transmitted diseases or infections.
	• Other diseases that may have mandated reporting if a higher than normal incidence occurs.
	Which no-fault federal laws compensate for vaccine injury?
	• National Childhood Vaccine Injury Act of 1986.
	• Established National Vaccine Injury Compensation Program (VICP).
	• Smallpox Emergency Personnel Protection Act of 2003.
	What information must vaccine administrators document in a patient's medical record?
	• The date the vaccine was administered.
	• The vaccine manufacturer.
	• The vaccine lot number.
	• The name, address, and title of the health care provider who administered the vaccine.
	• Any adverse event listed in the Vaccine Injury Table.
	• Any contraindicating event as listed in the manufacturer's package insert.
	What injuries are reportable to the authorities under the auspices of public health?
	• Spousal abuse
	• Child abuse
	• Elder abuse
LO 9.5 Discuss federal drug regulations, including the Controlled Substances Act.	What two federal agencies oversee drugs in the United States?
	• Food and Drug Administration (FDA).
	• Oversees drug quality and standardization and must approve drugs before they are released for public use.
	• Drug Enforcement Administration (DEA).
	• Branch of the U.S. Department of Justice that regulates the sale and use of drugs.
	What are the requirements for physicians who prescribe, dispense, and administer controlled substances?
	• Register with the Drug Enforcement Administration through a division office.
	• Keep records concerning the administering or dispensing of a controlled drug on file for two years.
	• Note on a patient's chart when controlled substances are administered or dispensed.
	• Make a written inventory of drug supplies every two years, and keep such records an additional two years.
	• Keep drugs in a locked cabinet or safe, and report any thefts immediately to the nearest DEA office and the local police.

Learning Outcome	Summary
	What are schedules under which controlled substances are listed?
	• Schedule I—No proven medical use; usually used only for research.
	• Schedule II—Potential for abuse high, but accepted medical uses.
	• Schedule III—Less potential for abuse; have accepted medical uses.
	• Schedule IV—Low potential for abuse compared to other schedules, but may lead to dependency.
	• Schedule V—Low potential for abuse, but may lead to dependency.
	What is the role of the medical assistant regarding controlled substances in the medical facility?
	• Checking to be sure that all controlled substances are kept in a locked cabinet or safe.
	• Reminding the physician to keep his or her "black bag" in a safe place.
	• Keeping all prescription blanks, especially those used for narcotics, under lock and key.
	• Ordering prescription blanks that are serially numbered or otherwise printed to help detect alterations and theft.
	• Reporting to the physician any behavior by patients that would suggest an attempt to secure addictive drugs.
	• Checking patients' records to verify all prescriptions that may be questioned by a pharmacist.

Ethics Issues Physicians' Public Duties and Responsibilities

Two principles are often at odds when health care practitioners must deal with public health issues: the autonomy of each patient and beneficence. As discussed in Chapter 2, *autonomy* refers to the individual's right to make his or her own decisions. *Beneficence* refers to the moral obligation to act in ways that promote the health and welfare of others. As stated in Laurinda Harman's *Ethical Challenges in the Management of Health Information*, "Beneficence and the closely allied principle of nonmaleficence ['first do no harm'] are among the primary justifications supporting public policies that interfere with the autonomy of individuals."

Ethics ISSUE 1:

"Herd immunity" is one of the primary considerations for mandatory vaccinations in the United States. That is, when a large segment of the population is inoculated against certain infectious diseases, individuals—both vaccinated and unvaccinated—benefit, as well as the community as a whole. A true mandate for vaccinating all schoolchildren in the United States has not been enacted since World War I. Today, every state except Mississippi and West Virginia has exceptions that allow parents to exempt their children from state vaccination requirements on the basis of religious or other personal beliefs. Recent epidemics of childhood diseases, such as measles, mumps, and pertussis in the United States indicate that objections to mandatory vaccinations have increased.

Discussion Questions

1. In your opinion, does a parent's failure to vaccinate his or her child constitute a lack of social responsibility? Explain your answer.

---

2. Should one's concern for others supersede objections to vaccination on personal or religious grounds? Explain your answer.

---

3. Should your role as a health care practitioner include encouraging parents to have their children vaccinated? Explain your answer.

_____

_____

4. As a health care practitioner, are you ethically bound to be vaccinated for common contagious diseases?

_____

_____

Ethics ISSUE 2:

A young woman is diagnosed with a sexually transmitted infection and is subsequently reported to the public health department. A public health nurse visits her, but she refuses to name her sexual contacts.

Discussion Questions

1. Should the woman be compelled by law to name her sexual contacts? Why or why not? Does the best interest of the woman's sexual contacts and their contacts supersede the woman's right to privacy? Explain your answer.

_____

_____

2. What values are involved in Ethics Issue 2?

_____

_____

3. What is the first duty of health care practitioners caring for the woman in Ethics Issue 2?

_____

_____

Ethics ISSUE 3:

Laws that require the reporting of cases of suspected abuse of children and elderly persons often create a dilemma for health care practitioners. The parties involved, both the suspected offenders and the victims, will often plead that the matter be kept confidential and not be disclosed or reported for investigation by public authorities.

Discussion Questions

1. Assume you are a member of the health care team that has repeatedly treated a woman for injuries that appear to have been inflicted by another. How might you phrase an opening question to learn whether or not she is the victim of abuse?

_____

_____

2. If the woman protests that she is simply "accident prone," how might you phrase your response? Would you drop the matter at this point or continue to question the woman?

_____

_____

3. What could you do to protect the woman if she does not admit abuse, but you are reasonably sure that she is being abused?

_____

_____

Enhance your learning by completing these exercises and more at
http://connect.mheducation.com!

Applying Knowledge

LO 9.1

1. Four vital statistics that the government collects are _____, _____, _____, and _____ .

2. Of the above, the physician should be concerned with documenting _____ and _____ .

LO 9.2

3. Which of the following is *not* recommended for completing birth and death certificates?

   a. Make entries in ink or in a typewritten form

   b. Use rubber stamps for all signatures

   c. Do not skip any blanks

   d. Check entries for correct spelling

4. Which of the following is *not* included on a death certificate?

   a. Cause of death

   b. Name of attending physician, if any

   c. Time of death

   d. Name of decedent's next of kin

5. Physicians may *not* sign a death certificate in which of the following situations?

   a. Death is suspicious.

   b. Physician was treating the patient.

   c. Death occurred in the home.

   d. Death occurred in the hospital.

6. Which of the following best defines a coroner?

   a. A public official who must be a physician

   b. A public official who is elected by popular ballot

   c. A public official who is appointed by the governor

   d. A public official who investigates and holds inquests over those who die from unknown or violent causes

7. A coroner or medical examiner signs a death certificate if

   a. The death is possibly due to criminal causes or is otherwise suspicious.

   b. The death was not attended by a physician within a specified length of time.

   c. The death is due to causes undetermined by the physician.

   d. All of these

8. State public health laws derive indirectly from _____.

    a. A federal law called U.S. Public Health Law

    b. The Tenth Amendment to the U.S. Constitution

    c. City ordinances

    d. None of these

9. Briefly define the term *federalism.*

    a. Cooperation among federal, state, and local governments.

    b. Federal law is accepted as the law of the land.

    c. State law overrides federal law.

    d. Municipal law overrides state law.

10. Which of the following falls within the supervision of a state's public health department?

    a. Licensing of public health nurses

    b. Admitting cases of infectious disease to hospitals

    c. Mandatory vaccinating of schoolchildren

    d. Prescribing treatment for STIs

LO 9.4

11. Which of the following should be reported to the health department?

    a. Otitis media (middle ear infection)

    b. Strep throat

    c. Influenza

    d. Human immunodeficiency virus (HIV)

12. Which of the following will most likely require notification of the appropriate health agencies?

    a. Auto accident

    b. Staph infection

    c. Strep throat

    d. Phenylketonuria (PKU—a genetic disease sometimes diagnosed in infants)

13. Which no-fault federal law compensates for childhood vaccine injury?

    a. Tenth Amendment to the U.S. Constitution

    b. National Childhood Vaccine Injury Act of 1986

    c. Smallpox Emergency Personnel Protection Act of 2003

    d. None of these

14. Which of the following vaccination information is *not* documented in a patient's medical record?

    a. The date the vaccine was administered

    b. The vaccine manufacturer

    c. The vaccine lot number

    d. The date the vaccine was ordered

15. Which of the following injuries are reportable to law enforcement or to the health department?

    a. A restaurant worker falls off a ladder while changing a lightbulb.

    b. A woman tells her physician that her broken ribs occurred when her husband beat her.

    c. A child is severely injured in an automobile accident.

    d. None of these

LO 9.5

16. Which of the following is *not* the responsibility of the medical assistant working in a facility where physicians prescribe and administer controlled substances?

    a. Checking to be sure that all controlled substances are kept in a locked cabinet or safe

    b. Reminding the physician to keep his or her "black bag" in a safe place

    c. Ordering prescription blanks that are serially numbered or otherwise printed to help detect alterations and theft

    d. Checking with the patient's pharmacist to be sure prescriptions have been filled

17. Prescriptions for which of the following categories of drugs may *not* be renewed?

    a. Schedule I

    b. Schedule II

    c. Schedule IV

    d. Schedule V

18. With one exception, drugs in this category have no accepted medical use and are used for research purposes only.

    a. Schedule V

    b. Schedule II

    c. Schedule I

    d. Schedule III

19. Who must be notified if controlled substances are stolen from a medical facility?

    a. All patients who currently have prescriptions for the stolen drug

    b. The state medical board

    c. The nearest DEA office and the local police

    d. The nearest FDA office

20. A medical facility must keep records concerning the administering or dispensing of a controlled drug on file for

    a. 6 years

    b. 9 years

    c. 10 years

    d. 2 years

21. Which of the following is *not* a requirement for physicians who prescribe, dispense, and administer controlled substances?

    a. Register with the Drug Enforcement Administration through a division office

    b. Note on a patient's chart when controlled substances are administered or dispensed

    c. Make a written inventory of drug supplies every two years, and keep such records an additional two years

    d. Renew permits for prescribing and dispensing controlled substances every six months

Match each definition with the correct term by writing the letter in the space provided.

_____ 22. Tests and approves drugs for public use.

_____ 23. Also known as the Comprehensive Drug Abuse Prevention and Control Act of 1970.

_____ 24. As a branch of the Department of Justice, regulates the sale and use of drugs.

_____ 25. Require reports of communicable diseases and certain injuries, as mandated by state laws.

_____ 26. Mandates reporting of child abuse.

_____ 27. Created a no-fault compensation program for health care practitioners and/or emergency responders injured by the smallpox vaccine.

_____ 28. The federal law that makes killing or injuring a fetus a crime separate from killing or injuring the pregnant mother, in cases where the federal government has jurisdiction.

a. Unborn Victims of Violence Act

b. Drug Enforcement Administration (DEA)

c. Smallpox Emergency Personnel Protection Act of 2003 (SEPPA)

d. Food and Drug Administration (FDA)

e. Amendments to the Older Americans Act

f. Controlled Substances Act

g. Child Abuse Prevention and Treatment Act of 1974

h. Public health statutes

Case Studies

Use your critical thinking skills to answer the questions that follow each case study.

LO 9.4

One of a physician's patients, a well-respected citizen in a small community, saw the doctor with a complaint of blood in his urine (hematuria). The physician asked the patient if he'd had any new sexual partners recently, and the patient admitted that he had. The physician explained to the patient that his urine specimen had been positive for the STI chlamydia. The physician urged the patient to discuss his medical condition with the patient's wife, who was also the physician's patient, but the man was reluctant.

29. If the patient refuses to confide in the wife, what should the physician do?

_____

_____

30. What are the legal issues in this case? What are the ethical issues?

_____

_____

LO 9.5

Barbara, a medical assistant, noticed that her aunt, who suffered chronic pain from a neck injury, carried two bottles of Percodan in her purse. "Two doctors write prescriptions for me," Barbara's aunt confided, "but neither knows about the other. That's the only way I can get enough medication to control my pain."

31. In Barbara's place, would you report your aunt's deception to the physicians named on her prescriptions? Explain your answer.

_____

_____

32. What would you tell your aunt?

_____

_____

33. How can physicians guard against such abuses by patients?

_____

_____

_____

Internet Activities LO 9.1, LO 9.3, and LO 9.4

Complete the activities and answer the questions that follow.

34. Visit the Web site for federal statistics at **www.fedstats.gov.** For what year are the most recent statistics available? How many births and deaths occurred in your state for that year?

_____

_____

35. Search the site for "leading causes of death," and list the top three.

_____

_____

36. Visit the Web site for the National Vaccine Injury Compensation Program (VICP) at **www.hrsa.gov/ vaccinecompensation/.** Who is eligible to file a claim?

_____

_____

37. Find the Web site for your state's department of health. Which communicable diseases must be reported in your state? To whom must you report communicable diseases? What is the process involved? At this Web site, can you tell which diseases are prevalent in your state? How?

_____

_____

Resources

Centers for Disease Control and Prevention, Data & Statistics: **www.cdc.gov/DataStatistics/.**

Centers for Disease Control and Prevention, Health, United States, 2009: **www.cdc.gov/nchs/data/hus/ hus09.pdf#highlights.**

Federal site discussing vaccination (National Vaccine Program Office): **www.hhs.gov/nvpo/law.htm.**

Harman, Laurinda B., and Laurie A. Rinehart-Thompson, eds. _Ethical Challenges in the Management of Health Information_, 2nd ed. Sudbury, MA: Jones & Bartlett, 2006.

Health Resources and Services Administration: **www.hrsa.gov/vaccinecompensation/.**

Federal OSHA authority extends to all private-sector employers with one or more employees, as well as to federal civilian employees. In addition, many states administer their own occupational safety and health programs through plans approved under section 18(b) of the federal OSHA act.

Check Your Progress

15. OSHA provides for _____ in the workplace.

16. The primary source of information for OSHA standards is _____ .

17. What state laws allow employees access to information about toxic or hazardous substances?

18. As an employee in a health care facility, what are your general responsibilities under OSHA standards?

LO 10.3

Discuss the role of health care practitioners in following OSHA standards for infection control in the medical office.

Occupational Exposure to Bloodborne Pathogen Standard An OSHA regulation designed to protect health care workers from the risk of exposure to bloodborne pathogens.

Osha Health Standards and CDC Guidelines

OSHA standards for medical settings and health care workers often are influenced by and/or closely associated with guidelines issued by the Centers for Disease Control and Prevention (CDC). Following are summaries of six OSHA standards and CDC guidelines that most often affect health care practitioners working in medical settings.

1. The Occupational Exposure to Bloodborne Pathogen Standard is an OSHA regulation passed in 1991. The standard is designed to protect workers in health care and related occupations from the risk of exposure to bloodborne *pathogens* (disease-causing organisms) such as the human immunodeficiency virus (HIV) and the hepatitis B virus (HBV). The standard requires posting of safety guidelines, exposure incident reporting, and formulation of a written exposure control plan that outlines the protective measures an employer will take to eliminate or minimize employee exposure to blood and other body fluids. The plan must be available to OSHA inspectors and to employees.

As mandated by the Needlestick Safety and Prevention Act, passed by Congress in 2000, the Occupational Exposure to Bloodborne Pathogen Standard, 29 CFR 1910.1030, was revised in 2001 to include new provisions requiring employers to maintain a sharps injury log and to involve nonmanagerial employees in selecting safer medical devices.

By authority of the Bloodborne Pathogen Standard, OSHA can levy fines for violations leading to employee exposure to bloodborne pathogens, based on guidelines issued by the CDC. The CDC's Guidelines for Universal Precautions for Hospitals apply to any laboratory and include the following:

- Do not contaminate the outside of containers when collecting specimens. All specimen containers should have secure lids.

- Wear gloves when processing patients' specimens, including blood, body fluids containing blood, and other fluids. Masks and goggles should be worn if splashing or aerosolization may occur. Change gloves and wash hands after handling each specimen.

- Use biological safety cabinets for blending and vigorous mixing whenever there is a potential for droplets.

- Do not pipette fluids by mouth. Use mechanical pipetting devices.

- Use extreme caution when handling needles. Do not bend, recap, or remove needles from disposable syringes. Place entire needle assembly in a clearly marked puncture-resistant, leak-proof container.

- Decontaminate work surfaces with a chemical germicide after spills and daily when work is completed. (A clean work surface proved essential in the laboratory scenario at the beginning of this chapter.)

- Clearly and permanently label tissue or serum specimens to be stored as potentially hazardous.

- Never eat, drink, smoke, or apply cosmetics or lip balm in the laboratory.

- Remove protective clothing, and wash hands before leaving the laboratory.

2. The Hazard Communication Standard (HCS) is an OSHA standard that is intended to increase health care practitioners' awareness of risk, improve work practices and appropriate use of personal protective equipment, and reduce injuries and illnesses.

In March 2012, OSHA published the first major revision to the Hazard Communication Standard. The changes aligned the standard with the **United Nations Globally Harmonized System of Classification and Labeling of Chemicals (GHS).** New wording, taken from GHS, was intended to transform the right of employees to know about workplace hazards to the "right to understand" workplace hazards.

GHS established objective criteria for classifying and identifying chemical hazards. The goal was to ensure the safe use of chemicals by providing practical, reliable, consistent, and easy to understand information for workers and students everywhere. For example, to alleviate confusion over "toxicity" as opposed to "toxic," the following phrases are used:

- Fatal if swallowed.

- Toxic if swallowed.

- Harmful if swallowed.

- May be harmful if swallowed.

GHS Pictograms (See Figure 10-1) are used as universal labels, and two single words—Danger! and Warning!—plus specific hazard and cautionary statements denote different levels of risk. (Danger! is the more severe warning.)

Hazard Communication Standard (HCS)
An OSHA standard intended to increase health care practitioners' awareness of risks, improve work practices and appropriate use of personal protective equipment, and reduce injuries and illnesses in the workplace.

United Nations Globally Harmonized System of Classification and Labeling of Chemicals (GHS)
Led to a 2012 revision of the Hazard Communication Standard, in order to transform "right to know" to "right to understand," in line with GHS.

6. OSHA **electrical standards** apply to electrical equipment and wiring in hazardous locations. Special wiring and equipment installation may be required if the facility uses flammable gases.

Every medical and dental workplace must also post the state or federal OSHA poster, explaining employees' rights to a safe workplace.

Medical and dental offices are currently exempt from maintaining an official log of reportable injuries and illnesses (OSHA Form 300) under the federal OSHA record-keeping rule, although they may be required to maintain records in some state plans. Employees in those states that have state OSHA plans should contact the state plan directly for more information. All employers, including medical and dental offices, must report any work-related fatality or the hospitalization of three or more employees in a single incident to the nearest OSHA office. Employees may call (800) 321-OSHA or the relevant state plan for assistance.

At **www.osha.gov**, a guide for medical & dental office compliance with OSHA standards lists basic requirements of the Bloodborne Pathogens Standard:

- Prepare a written exposure control plan, updated annually. Each update should include reference to any changes in technology, such as the use of safer devices to reduce needlesticks, documentation as to why specific devices were chosen, and input from employees regarding the selection of devices.

- Provide for the use of safer needles and other sharps.

- See that employees use the correct personal protective equipment (PPE), such as gowns, gloves, and face and eye protection.

- Require that employees follow universal precautions (Chapter 11).

- Offer no-cost hepatitis B vaccinations for employees at risk of exposure.

- Require medical follow-up after an exposure incident.

- Provide for the proper containment of all regulated waste.

- Identify hazardous waste containers, including sharps disposal boxes, via labels and/or color coding.

- Provide appropriate employee training.

Medical Waste Tracking Act
The federal law that authorizes OSHA to inspect hazardous medical wastes and to cite offices for unsafe or unhealthy practices regarding these wastes.

Medical Waste Tracking Act By authority of the **Medical Waste Tracking Act,** OSHA may inspect hazardous medical wastes and will cite medical facilities for unsafe or unhealthy practices regarding these wastes. Hazardous medical wastes include but are not limited to blood products, body fluids, tissues, cultures, vaccines (live and weakened), sharps, table paper (with body fluids on them), gloves, speculums, cotton swabs, and inoculating loops.

A puncture-proof, leak-proof, approved sharps container must be provided for the disposal of sharp objects. Chemicals should be discarded in a glass or metal container. Flushable chemicals can be washed down the drain with large quantities of water. Other hazardous medical wastes must be contained in plastic, leak-proof biohazard bags. Incineration is often used to dispose of medical wastes.

Reputable, licensed waste handlers should be used to handle this material.

Training Under OSHA standards, each employer must have a written training program detailing how employees will be provided with information and training regarding hazards in the workplace. Training should include information about hazards in the work area, the location of the list of hazards and MSDSs, explanations of MSDSs and the hazardous chemical labeling system, and any measures that employees can take to protect themselves against these hazards. Training logs should be kept, and employees who complete training should sign and date the log.

Current OSHA standards for health care settings may be obtained from the OSHA Web site at **www.osha.gov.**

Centers for Disease Control and Prevention (CDC) Guidelines CDC guidelines have always recommended that health care practitioners wear gloves, eye masks, gowns, and other protective equipment when performing such tasks as capillary puncture, phlebotomy, pelvic exams, minor suturing, and throat culture. Health care workers should also wear protective equipment when performing tasks that do not involve direct contact with blood, body fluids, or tissue, in case accidental exposure occurs. These tasks include urinalysis, blood testing, examination of fecal occult blood, injections, positioning for X-rays, performing ultrasound and ECG tests, and examination of sweat, tears, and nasal secretions.

Most recently, the CDC publishes a comprehensive online guide for all health care workers entitled *Guideline for Isolation Precautions: Preventing Transmission of Infectious Agents in Healthcare Settings,* available at **www.cdc.gov/hicpac/pdf/isolation/Isolation2007.pdf.** The document "is intended for use by infection control staff, health care epidemiologists, health care administrators, nurses, other health care providers, and persons responsible for developing, implementing, and evaluating infection control programs for health care settings across the continuum of care." It contains references to other guidelines and Web sites for more detailed information and for recommendations concerning specialized infection control problems, such as preventing surgical site infections, recommendations for the prevention, treatment, and control of tuberculosis, prevention of intervascular catheter infections, hand hygiene, and so on.

Clinical Laboratory Improvement Act (CLIA)

LO 10.4

Define the role of the Clinical Laboratory Improvement Act (CLIA) of 1988 in quality laboratory testing.

The **Clinical Laboratory Improvement Act (CLIA)** of 1988, also called the Clinical Laboratory Improvement Amendments, replaced 1967 laboratory testing legislation that established standards for Medicare and Medicaid. The act established minimum quality standards for all laboratory testing and has been extensively amended since it was first written. The regulations define a laboratory as any facility that performs laboratory testing on specimens derived from humans for diagnosing, preventing, or treating disease or for assessing health. The law requires that laboratories obtain certification, pay applicable fees,

Clinical Laboratory Improvement Act (CLIA)
Also called Clinical Laboratory Improvement Amendments. Federal statute passed in 1988 that established minimum quality standards for all laboratory testing.

and follow regulations concerning testing, personnel, inspections, test management, quality control, and quality assurance.

The Division of Laboratory Services, within the Survey and Certification Group, under the Center for Medicaid and State Operations (CMSO) has the responsibility for implementing the CLIA program. The Federal Drug Administration has responsibility for some CLIA functions. More information about Clinical Laboratory Improvement Act/Amendments is available online at **www.cms.gov/clia/.**

Check Your Progress

19. For the facility described in this chapter's opening scenario, which OSHA standards, and/or CDC guidelines discussed earlier would apply?

20. What protective gear does the CDC recommend for laboratory employees?

21. What specific health care procedures/facilities does the Clinical Laboratory Improvement Act cover?

22. Are there penalties for violating any of the OSHA standards concerned with safety in the workplace? Explain your answer.

LO 10.5

State the purpose of workers' compensation laws and unemployment insurance.

workers' compensation
A form of insurance established by federal and state statutes that provides reimbursement for workers who are injured on the job.

Workers' Compensation and Unemployment Insurance
WORKERS' COMPENSATION

Federal and state **workers' compensation** laws establish procedures for compensating workers who are injured on the job. The employer pays the cost of the insurance premium for the employee. These laws allow the injured worker to file a claim for compensation with the state or the federal government instead of suing. However, the laws require workers to accept workers' compensation as the exclusive remedy for on-the-job injuries. Federal laws cover the following employees: workers in Washington, DC; coal miners; maritime workers; and federal employees. State laws cover those workers not protected under federal statutes.

Workers who are injured on the job or who contract an occupational disease may apply for five types of state compensation benefits:

• Medical treatment, including hospital, medical and surgical services, medications, and prosthetic devices.

• Temporary disability indemnity, in the form of weekly cash payments made directly to the injured or ill employee.

• Permanent disability indemnity, which can be a lump sum award or a weekly or monthly cash payment.

• Death benefits for survivors, which consist of cash payments to dependents of employees killed on the job.

• Rehabilitation benefits, which are paid for medical or vocational rehabilitation.

Employees who are injured on the job or become ill due to work-related causes must immediately report the injury or illness to a supervisor. An injury report and claim for compensation are then filed with the appropriate state workers' compensation agency. Forms from the attending or designated workers' compensation physician who examines and treats the employee must also be filed with the appropriate agency as proof of the employee's injury or illness.

A medical office employee may be responsible for filing the physician's report with the state workers' compensation agency. Requirements concerning waiting periods and other filing specifics vary with each state. When a claim is filed, all questions must be answered in full and as thoroughly as possible.

UNEMPLOYMENT INSURANCE

Unemployment insurance (sometimes called reemployment insurance) funds are managed jointly by state and federal governments. Under the Federal Unemployment Tax Act (FUTA), employers contribute to a fund that is paid out to eligible unemployed workers. Each state also provides unemployment insurance, and credit is given employers against the FUTA tax for amounts paid to the state unemployment fund. The total cost is borne by the employer in all but a few states.

Out-of-work employees should contact a state unemployment office to determine whether they qualify for unemployment benefits. Former employees are denied unemployment compensation for three main reasons: (1) They quit their jobs without cause, (2) they were fired for misconduct, or (3) they are unemployed because of a labor dispute. Independent contractors and self-employed individuals usually do not qualify for unemployment compensation.

Individuals may file for unemployment benefits at state unemployment offices. A claimant needs:

- A Social Security card.
- W-2 statements for the past 1 to 2 years.
- Other wage records for the past 18 months.
- Employers' names and addresses for the past 18-month employment period.
- A statement of the reasons for leaving the job.
- The employer's unemployment insurance account number, if available.

Hiring and the New Employee

When interviewing for a position or when asked to interview a job applicant, the health care practitioner must know legal boundaries.

INTERVIEWS

Because of federal and state laws against discrimination in hiring, inquiries cannot be made concerning an applicant's

- Race or color.
- Religion or creed.

LO 10.6
Determine the appropriate legal process for hiring employees and maintaining the required paperwork while the person is employed.

- Gender
- Family
- Marital status
- Method of birth control.
- Age, birth date, or birthplace.
- Disability
- Arrest record (with some exceptions in many states).
- Residency duration
- National origin. (However, the Immigration Reform and Control Act of 1986 requires new employees to complete an I-9 form, intended to prevent the employment of illegal aliens.)
- General military experience or discharge.
- Membership in organizations.

Questions concerning one's Social Security number, qualifications (including license or certificate), and job experience are proper, and they should be answered as thoroughly and truthfully as possible. As part of the hiring process, applicants may be asked to take a physical examination.

During a job interview, applicants may refuse to answer a question that is clearly improper or not job-related, but this could cost them the job. The question "May I ask how this relates to the position?" is generally more acceptable than a blunt, "That question is illegal, and I don't have to answer it." Furthermore, the mere asking of an improper preemployment interview question does not in itself give an applicant grounds for a legal challenge if he or she is not hired.

The following guidelines can help those employees who are responsible for conducting preemployment interviews:

- Make a list of questions that relate specifically to the job description of the position to be filled, and stick to them.

- Do not rush the interview, nor let it drag on beyond reasonable time limits.

- General questions that may prove helpful include these: What are your qualifications for this position? Why are you leaving your present position? Why do you want this job? What salary do you expect? When can you begin work? What are your professional strengths? What are your professional goals?

- Remain objective and listen well.

- End the interview on a positive note. Indicate when a decision will be made, and follow through on your promise to inform the applicant of your decision, one way or the other.

BONDING

In some medical offices and other workplace locations where employees are responsible for collecting fees and handling financial matters, prospective employees may be asked whether they are bondable. An employer can purchase a **surety bond** for a specific amount from an insurance carrier. If a bonded employee should embezzle or otherwise abscond with funds, the employer can collect from the insurance carrier up to the amount of the bond. However, the employer must have filed a complaint against the alleged dishonest employee in order to collect on the bond. If the insurance company pays the bond, it will then seek to recover the amount from the offending employee.

surety bond
A type of insurance that allows employers, if covered, to collect up to the specified amount of the bond if an employee embezzles or otherwise absconds with business funds.

EMPLOYMENT PAPERWORK

Once employed, the new worker will be asked to provide certain information so that the employer may comply with federal and state regulations. Complete records for every employee must include:

- Social Security number.
- Number of exemptions claimed.
- Gross salary
- Deductions for Social Security; Medicare; and federal, state, and city taxes.
- Withholding for state disability insurance, state unemployment tax, and health care plans, if applicable.
- Properly completed Form I-9. (This is proof of citizenship or the legal right to work in the United States.)

The law requires employers to withhold specified amounts from employees' pay and to keep records of and send these sums to the proper income tax center. The amount to be withheld is based on the employee's total salary, the number of exemptions he or she claims, marital status, and the length of the pay period involved.

Health care practitioners who are self-employed do not have to deduct withholding, but they must make quarterly city, state, and federal income tax payments. Self-employed individuals must also pay Social Security taxes (FICA), via a self-employment tax percentage that is higher than the rate paid by individuals who are not self-employed. The difference lies in the fact that a self-employed individual is making both the employer and the employee contribution.

Employers must provide each employee with a Form W-2, Wage and Tax Statement, by January 31 of each year. The W-2 shows the following information:

- Employer's tax identification number.
- Employee's Social Security number.
- Total earnings (wages and other compensation) paid by the employer.
- Amounts deducted for income tax and Social Security.
- Amount of advance earned income credit payment, if any.

23. Distinguish between workers' compensation and unemployment insurance.

24. Is it permissible for an employer to ask a job applicant to take a physical exam? Why might such a requirement exist?

25. Place a check mark beside those questions that are considered to be illegal if asked in a preemployment interview.

_____ Why are you leaving your present position?

_____ Do you belong to a church?

_____ What do you hope to achieve over the next five years?

_____ How many children do you have, and how old are they?

_____ Who will watch your children while you work?

_____ Why do you want to work for us?

_____ How many years' experience do you have as a medical assistant/dental assistant/physician assistant/nursing assistant?

_____ Are you married?

_____ Is your husband/wife employed, and if so where?

_____ What nationality are you?

Most employers want the workplace to be as pleasant and safe for employees as it can possibly be. However, it is still the employee's responsibility to know the employment legalities most likely to affect him or her and to work within this legal framework to help ensure a satisfying and productive employer–employee relationship.

Chapter Summary

Learning Outcome	Summary

LO 10.1 Identify how the workplace is affected by federal laws regarding hiring and firing, discrimination, and other workplace regulations.	What issues affected by federal law have traditionally affected employees in the workplace?
	
	• Employment-at-will.
	• Wrongful discharge
	• Just cause
	• Public policy
	
	What categories do federal and state laws generally address, regarding employees in the workplace?
	• Discrimination
	  • Sexual harassment
	  • Physical disability
	  • Pregnancy
	  • Age
	  • Genetic discrimination
	• Wages and work hours.
	  • Equal pay
	  • Retirement income security.
	• Safety and welfare.

LO 10.2 Identify six areas for which standards are mandated by the Occupational Safety and Health Administration (OSHA) for work done in a clinical setting.	What is the role of the health care practitioner following OSHA standards for work done in the clinical setting and for infection control in the medical office? • Right-to-know. • Hazard Communication Standard. • Chemical Hygiene Plan. • Occupational Exposure to Bloodborne Pathogen Standard. • Medical Waste Tracking Act.
LO 10.3 Discuss the role of health care practitioners in following OSHA standards for infection control in the medical office.	What changes were made to comply with the United Nations Globally Harmonized System of Classification and Labeling of Chemicals (GHS)? • Universal warnings (pictograms, Danger! and Warning!) and quantitative, objective criteria. • Chemical Hygiene Plan. • Ionizing Radiation Standard. • Safe and accessible emergency exits. • Electrical wiring • OSHA poster explaining employees' right to a safe workplace. • Medical Waste Tracking Act. • Training
LO 10.4 Define the role of the Clinical Laboratory Improvement Act (CLIA) of 1988 in quality laboratory testing.	What is the role of the Clinical Laboratory Improvement Act (CLIA) in quality laboratory testing? • Established minimum quality standards for all laboratory testing.
LO 10.5 State the purpose of workers' compensation laws and unemployment insurance.	What is the purpose of worker's compensation and unemployment insurance? • Five types of benefits. • Claimant requirements

LO 10.6 Determine the appropriate legal process for hiring employees and maintaining the required paperwork while the person is employed.	What should health care practitioners know about hiring and paperwork for new employees?
	
	• Prohibited questions to ask job applicants.
	• Guidelines for conducting interviews.
	  • Required paperwork
	  • Surety bond

Ethics ISSUE 1:

All ethical guidelines for health care practitioners remind them to be aware that, even though sexually suggestive behavior may not have crossed the line legally, any form of sexual harassment or exploitation between medical supervisors and trainees, employers and employees, coworkers, or medical practitioners and patients is unethical.

Discussion Questions

1. You are a surgical technologist in a large hospital. Whenever you work with a certain surgeon, she tells off-color jokes to you and your coworkers and makes suggestive comments to workers of the opposite sex. One coworker tells you that he might quit his job because he is married, and the surgeon's behavior makes him so uncomfortable that he dreads coming to work. Is the surgeon's behavior illegal or simply in bad taste? Explain your answer.

_____

_____

2. Do you or your coworkers in the previous situation have grounds for a sexual harassment complaint? Explain your answer.

_____

_____

3. If you have determined that you do have a complaint, how would you proceed?

_____

_____

Ethics ISSUE 2:

The *Code of Medical Ethics* for the American Medical Association states: "Sexual contact that occurs concurrent with the patient-physician relationship constitutes sexual misconduct. . . . At a minimum, a physician's ethical duties include terminating the patient-physician relationship before initiating a dating, romantic, or sexual relationship with a patient" (AMA *Code of Medical Ethics,* E-8.14).

Patients are often accompanied by third parties who play an important part in the health care practitioner–patient relationship. The health care practitioner interacts and communicates with these individuals and often is in a position to offer them information, advice, and emotional support. The more deeply involved the individual is in the clinical encounter and in medical decision making, the more troubling sexual or romantic contact with the health care practitioner would be. Key third parties include, but are not limited to, spouses or partners, parents, guardians, and proxies.

Discussion Questions

1. As a medical assistant, you have been present when a young, single father brings his infant in for checkups. The child is seriously ill, and the father begins consulting you about his emotional anguish. You are also single and sense an attraction. When the young man asks you out, should you accept? Explain your answer.

_____

_____

2. Do you believe ethical standards governing such relationships are stricter for health care practitioners than for other professions, such as law professors and students? In your view, is this as it should be? Explain your answer.

_____

_____

Ethics ISSUE 3:

Health care practitioners have legal and ethical responsibilities to follow laws and procedures that protect their safety and patient safety.

Discussion Question

1. Assume you are the medical technologist in the chapter's opening scenario, and you observe that every urine specimen analyzed during a hectic morning has a high leukocyte count. You realize this is unusual, but you don't want to fall behind, and you do not report the anomaly to your supervisor. Have you acted ethically? Explain your answer.

_____

_____

Chapter 10 Review

Enhance your learning by completing these exercises and more at
http://connect.mheducation.com!

Mc Graw Hill Education **connect**®

Applying Knowledge

LO 10.1

1. Under the concept of employment-at-will, who has the right to terminate employment?

   a. The government

   b. Both the employer and the employee

   c. The business owner

   d. The employee's legal representative

2. When might an employee who is fired sue his or her former employer for wrongful discharge?

   a. Never

   b. Only 1 year after the discharge

   c. At any time if the employee was discharged for an illegal reason

   d. Six months after the discharge

3. Which of the following reasons for discharge is *not* illegal under antidiscrimination laws?

   a. The employee is too old.

   b. The employee joined a union.

   c. The employee has been unable to master the requirements of the job.

   d. The employee is too religious.

4. Which of the following common law concepts protects an employee who reports his employer's illegal chemical dumping activities?

   a. Employment-at-will

   b. Public policy

   c. Wages and hour law

   d. Antisexual harassment law

metabolism and respiration.) Mutations in mtDNA may contribute to the loss of neurons in Alzheimer's and Parkinson's disease, and have been associated with diabetes, autism, and a variety of metabolic disorders. Health care practitioners should refer any patient who wants to undergo genetic testing to a **genetic counselor.** Genetic counselors can explain test results and help patients deal with difficult questions concerning those results.

As genetic testing has become more widely available and more reliable, use of test results has become an important issue. For example, if a couple learns through amniocentesis that the fetus the mother is carrying will be born with Down syndrome, should they consider aborting the fetus? Should the young man who learns he has the gene for Huntington's disease opt not to marry, to avoid taking the chance of passing the gene on to offspring? And will the woman in her twenties who learns she has one of two genes known to predispose her to breast cancer live her life any differently than she would have had she not been tested?

Genetic testing has also raised the issue of privacy. For instance, should employers and health and life insurance companies have access to genetic test results? How can individuals be certain that information about their genetic makeup is not shared with unknown sources?

Clearly, advances in genetics and genetic testing have led to difficult ethical, social, and medical questions for patients and their families and for health care practitioners.

GENETIC DISCRIMINATION

With the increased ability to identify genetic differences comes increasing concern for the proper use of such information. The term **genetic discrimination** describes the differential treatment of individuals based on their actual or presumed genetic differences.

Harvard Medical School's Lisa N. Geller and her colleagues conducted a comprehensive and still often-quoted study of genetic discrimination throughout the 1990s. The landmark study found that a number of institutions were reported to have engaged in genetic discrimination, including health and life insurance companies, health care providers, blood banks, adoption agencies, the military, and schools. Geller's study included individuals at risk for or related to people with hemochromatosis, phenylketonuria (PKU), mucopolysaccharidosis (MPS), and Huntington's disease.

Four hundred and fifty-five respondents out of 917 who returned questionnaires for Geller's study said they had experienced genetic discrimination. In one case, a health maintenance organization had covered the medical expenses of a child since birth but refused to pay for occupational therapy after she was diagnosed with mucopolysaccharidosis, claiming that the condition was preexisting.

In another case, a 24-year-old woman was denied life insurance due to her family history of Huntington's disease and the fact that she had not been tested for the presence of the gene. If she agreed to be tested and was found not to carry the gene, the insurance company would issue her a policy.

Geller also reported that in several cases, medical professionals reportedly pressured patients at risk for having children with serious

genetic counselor
An expert in human genetics who is qualified to counsel individuals who may have inherited genes for certain diseases or conditions.

genetic discrimination
Differential treatment of individuals based on their actual or presumed genetic differences.

genetic conditions to undergo prenatal diagnostic testing or to decide against having children.

Partially due to Geller's extensive study, there are now laws in place to prevent genetic discrimination. Many states have laws against genetic discrimination in employment, and the federal Genetic Information Nondiscrimination Act (GINA) of 2008 prohibits discrimination in health insurance and employment based on genetic information. The act defines genetic information as data about an individual's genetic tests and about genetic tests among that individual's family. Provisions within the law also apply to family members' medical histories. The law forbids genetic discrimination in any aspect of employment, and also prohibits harassment in the workplace based on an employee's genetic condition or history. The health insurance aspect of the law prohibits insurance companies from discriminating against clients and their families because of genetic testing results or other information, but in an article for *Science and Engineering Ethics*, Joseph S. Alper and John Beckwith point out that unless legislation addresses the problem of how to distinguish between genetic tests and nongenetic medical tests, it can be severely flawed:

> [W]e argue that much of this legislation is severely flawed because of the difficulty in distinguishing genetic from nongenetic tests. . . . In addition, barring the use by insurance companies of a genetic test but not a nongenetic test (conceivably for the same multifactorial disease) raises issues of fairness in health insurance. These arguments suggest that ultimately the problems arising from genetic discrimination cannot be solved by narrowly focused legislation but only by a modification of the entire health care system.

In addition to state laws against genetic discrimination and GINA at the federal level, the Health Insurance Portability and Accountability Act (HIPAA) passed in 1996 prevents health insurers from denying coverage based on genetic information. HIPAA, however, applies only to individuals moving between group health insurance plans.

The Americans with Disabilities Act (ADA) of 1990, discussed in Chapter 10, also offers some protection against genetic discrimination in the workplace. It protects those who have a genetic condition or disease, or are regarded as having a disability, against discrimination. Under a 1995 ruling by the Equal Employment Opportunities Commission, the ADA applies to anyone who is discriminated against on the basis of genetic information relating to illness, disease, condition, or other disorders. Furthermore, under the ADA, a person with a disability cannot be denied insurance or be subject to different terms or conditions of insurance based on disability alone, if the disability does not pose increased risks.

A major provision of the Patient Protection and Affordable Care Act of 2010 (referred to as ACA) is to establish "guaranteed issue." That is, insurance issuers must provide coverage for all individuals who request it. The law therefore prohibits issuers of health insurance from discriminating against patients with genetic diseases by refusing coverage because of "preexisting conditions." ACA provides additional protections for patients with genetic diseases by establishing that certain health insurance issuers may only vary premiums based on a few specified factors such as age or geographic area, thereby prohibiting the adjustment of premiums because of medical conditions.

genetic engineering
Manipulation of DNA within the cells of plants, animals, and other organisms through synthesis, alteration, or repair to ensure that certain harmful traits will be eliminated in offspring and that desirable traits will appear and be passed on.

Genetic Engineering

Our increased body of knowledge about DNA, chromosome structure, and the basis of heredity has allowed scientists to manipulate DNA within the cells of plants, animals, and other organisms to ensure that certain advantageous traits will appear and be passed on, and that certain harmful traits are eliminated. This is called **genetic engineering.** Because the chemical composition of DNA is nearly identical throughout the plant and animal kingdoms, genes can often be interchanged among plants and animals to transfer desirable characteristics to different species. Through this process, for example, genes from a species of Arctic flounder have been added to strawberry plants to make them better able to withstand cold temperatures. Genetic engineering has also created corn and soybean crops that are resistant to insect-borne diseases, "golden" rice with increased beta-carotene content, and bacteria that can devour oil spilled into oceans.

However beneficial a genetic engineering result may sound, controversy is almost guaranteed as a new project is announced. Objections may be raised on the religious or moral grounds that humans simply should not tamper with the time-honored progression of life as dictated by nature. Or opponents may fear that the process will harm the environment by releasing genetically engineered super-species that may crowd out naturally occurring species and lead to the eventual disappearance of many original organisms. Critics may also fear that the undisclosed addition of genes to plants or animals ingested by humans can have unforeseen effects. For instance, some fear that genes from peanut plants added to a product might cause harmful reactions in unsuspecting consumers who are allergic to peanuts. (In 2013, Congress was considering the Genetically Engineered Right-to-Know Act, which would require the FDA to enforce labeling of all genetically engineered food.)

Clearly, if genetic engineering is to truly benefit society, scientists and governments must consider the objections and fears of concerned individuals and proceed with research in a manner that takes these concerns into account.

LANDMARK COURT CASE

Supreme Court Decides the Issue of Patenting Genes

In June, 2013, the United States Supreme Court decided a case brought by the Association for Molecular Pathology against Myriad Genetics, Inc. Myriad held patents for two of the genes associated with the development of breast cancer—BRCA1 and BRCA2. Ownership of these patents meant that research scientists, and sometimes even physicians and their patients, had to obtain Myriad's permission, and in most cases pay fees, to do research or testing involving the two genes. In its landmark decision, the Supreme Court ruled that genes cannot be patented, because they are "naturally occurring" substances. However, artificial genes may meet requirements for developers to obtain patents.

The decision also emphasized, "[I]t is important to note what is *not* implicated by this decision. First, there are no method claims before this Court. Had Myriad created an innovative method of manipulating genes while searching for the BRCA1 and BRCA2 genes, it could possibly have sought a method patent. But the processes used by Myriad to isolate DNA were well understood and widely used by geneticists at the time of Myriad's patents."

Association for Molecular Pathology v. Myriad Genetics, Inc., 569—Supreme Court, June 13, 2013.

CLONING

One type of genetic engineering that is extremely controversial is cloning. The word **clone** comes from the Latin root meaning "to cut from." A clone is an organism grown from a single cell of the parent, and so it is genetically identical to the parent. In other words, the genes and chromosomes found in each cell's nucleus are the same in clone and parent. Identical twins are clones. So are all the cells in our bodies except for eggs and sperm: Somatic (body) cells divide to produce clones or exact replicas of themselves. Therefore, cells within the liver and other organs, within walls of blood vessels and arteries, within the skin, and so on are exactly like the cells that divided to produce them.

The term **cloning** was thrust into the public consciousness with the birth of Dolly, a Finn Dorset sheep, in July 1996 (Figure 11-2). Dolly was the product of scientists at the Roslin Institute near Edinburgh, Scotland, and was the only lamb born of 277 attempts. Her birth was controversial because she was the world's first mammal cloned from an adult parent cell. That is, Dolly was not the product of a union of egg and sperm, but was created from a single cell scraped from the inside of her 6-year-old mother's udder. Scientists used a process called nuclear transfer to clone Dolly from the udder cell.

Dolly lived until February 2003, when she was put down to prevent further suffering from a progressive lung disease. She had also developed arthritis, leading to speculation that she aged more quickly than normal. Since normal sheep live to 11 or 12 years, Dolly's death at 6 ½ years fueled intensive debate about the health and longevity of cloned animals.

Scientists have continued to clone cattle, goats, mice, monkeys, pigs, and sheep. One objective of the cloning of farm and laboratory animals is to breed genetically identical animals that can produce substances useful in medicine, such as insulin and growth hormone. Another objective in cloning farm animals is the consistent production of prime, low-fat meat.

Some cloned animals have lived normal life spans while others, like Dolly, have died young, suffering from conditions usually associated with aging.

A third objective of animal cloning is to clone animal tissues and organs for human medical use. Because pigs are similar to humans in organ size and other biological aspects, an objective in cloning them is to grow a potential source of organs and tissue for transplanting into human patients. Transplanting animal tissues and organs into humans is called **xenotransplantation.** Research in this area is continuing, but at least two major difficulties make the process problematic. Animal cells produce a sugar that human cells do not, causing a severe immune rejection reaction in humans when animal tissues are transplanted. In addition, scientists have found that human cells can be infected with some viruses that exist in animals.

Many animal rights proponents object on ethical grounds to using animals in this way. They argue that animals should be allowed to exist in nature without being subjected to experiments for the benefit of humankind. Furthermore, other groups object to introducing animal cells into humans on ethical grounds and on grounds that the animal tissue can harm people.

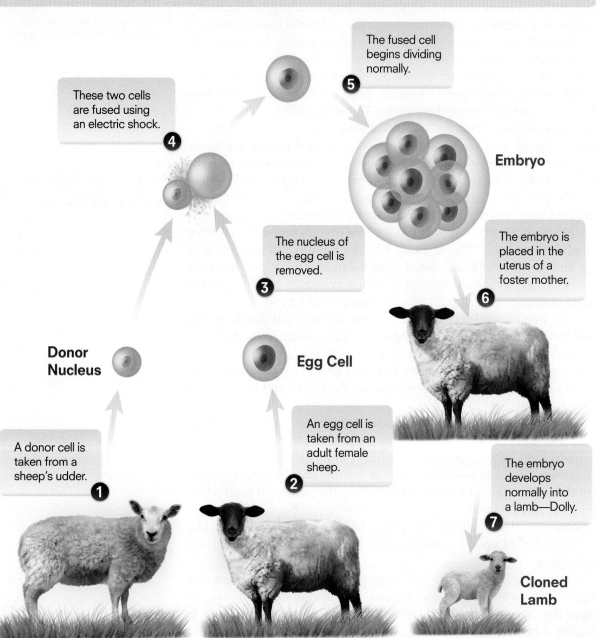

These two cells are fused using an electric shock.
④

The fused cell begins dividing normally.
⑤

Embryo

The nucleus of the egg cell is removed.
③

The embryo is placed in the uterus of a foster mother.
⑥

Donor Nucleus

Egg Cell

A donor cell is taken from a sheep's udder.
①

An egg cell is taken from an adult female sheep.
②

The embryo develops normally into a lamb—Dolly.
⑦

Cloned Lamb

Objections against animal cloning are sometimes also based on grounds that such experiments could lead to the cloning of human beings—for several reasons a frightening prospect:

1. To date, animal cloning does not always yield viable offspring, with only 1 or 2 healthy animals resulting from approximately every 100 experiments.

2. Not only do most attempts to clone mammals fail; about 30 percent of clones born alive are affected with "large-offspring syndrome" and other debilitating conditions. Large-offspring syndrome occurs primarily in cloned lambs and calves which are the result of embryo manipulation. The process often creates oversized offspring due to

deactivation of insulinlike growth factor 2 receptors which would normally block the growth of cells at a certain point. When the receptor is deactivated, the embryos grow too large. Other symptoms can include enlarged hearts, immature lungs, and damaged kidneys.

3. Scientists do not yet understand the processes involved in reproductive cloning well enough to ensure success, and a large failure rate in human clones is unacceptable.

4. Like Dolly the sheep, many cloned animals have died prematurely from infections and other complications. The same problems would be expected to occur in human cloning.

5. Scientists do not know how cloning could impact mental development. While factors such as intellect and mood may not be important for a cloned cow or mouse, they are crucial for the development of healthy humans.

With so many unknowns concerning reproductive cloning, many scientists and physicians believe the attempt to clone humans at this time is potentially dangerous and ethically irresponsible.

Congress has made several attempts to pass legislation banning human cloning research in the United States, but to date no such laws have been passed. Most states have laws banning the cloning of humans.

HUMAN STEM CELL RESEARCH

Early-stage human embryos, called *blastocysts*, consist of about 20 cells and are considered valuable for research because they are composed of **stem cells.** These early embryonic cells have the potential to become any type of body cell. Interest in this type of research—the *therapeutic use* of stem cells—remains intense because stem cells have shown promise for treating patients with a wide variety of medical problems. For example, stem cells that develop into neuronal tissue could be used to treat patients with Parkinson's and Alzheimer's diseases, as well as patients with strokes, spinal cord injuries, and other neurological disorders. Stem cells that become pancreatic islet cells might help those with diabetes. Skin tissue grown from stem cells could replace burned tissue, and cultivated cardiac tissue might help damaged arteries and hearts.

Most embryos used in stem cell research in the United States are the frozen products of in vitro fertilization that were not used to produce a pregnancy and are destined to eventually be destroyed. In 2001, President George W. Bush ordered that federal financing could be allowed only for stem cell research using cells grown from human embryos destroyed before August 9, 2001. By 2004, in contrast, England, Australia, Israel, and Portugal actively supported stem cell research without such restrictions.

In March 2009, President Barack Obama issued an executive order that reversed George W. Bush's order, stating he would "vigorously support scientists who pursue this research." Obama's order allowed the National Institutes of Health (NIH) to fund scientists working on embryonic stem cell research. The order was blocked and reinstated more than once, until the U.S. Supreme Court finally ruled in January 2013 that federal funding of embryonic stem cell research could resume.

Opponents to human embryonic stem cell research of any kind argue that regardless of how the embryos were created, they are human

stem cells
Cells that have the potential to become any type of body cell.

beings with inherent rights to ethical and legal protection. Others argue that since the embryos are not growing within a uterus, they are not subject to the same protection as fetuses, and since most would be destroyed anyway, the good that could come from such research far outweighs any downside. To date, the U.S. government can fund embryonic stem cell research. Some state governments such as California, Connecticut, Illinois, Maryland, Massachusetts, New Jersey, New York, and Wisconsin have funded embryonic stem cell research, but many states prohibit funding all or certain aspects of the research.

Partly because of the controversy over using human embryonic cells in research, scientists are searching for other sources of stem cells. They have discovered that some adult human body tissues, such as bone marrow and fat, also contain cells that can function as stem cells. Adult stem cells are **multipotent,** however, which means they can become only a limited number of types of tissues and cells in the body. For example, adult blood-forming stem cells (found in bone marrow) have been used successfully to treat only blood-based diseases such as leukemia and lymphoma. Embryonic stem cells have greater potential to treat a wider variety of diseases because they are **pluripotent**—they can become almost all types of tissues and cells in the body. A breakthrough development in 2010 offered the possibility that within a year, peripheral blood drawn from adult donors could be used to culture pluripotent stem cells.

Stem cells are found in small quantities in adult tissues and in umbilical cord blood, but scientists have found they do not have the same capacity to produce diverse tissues or to multiply as do embryonic stem cells. If a patient receives an adult stem cell transplant from a donor, the patient's body might reject it—a problem that researchers anticipate could be overcome with therapeutic cloning. Furthermore, adult stem cells may have more genetic abnormalities, which occur naturally during the aging process and with exposure to harmful agents.

Some scientists are exploring the possibility that adult stem cells are more flexible than previously thought, but many questions remain about the potential of adult stem cells, and much more research is required to answer them.

Amniotic stem cells are another possibility as a source for researchers. Amniotic stem cells are found in the fluid that surrounds a fetus. Scientists recently showed that they can be induced to create more cell types than was previously thought. However, the research is not intended as a replacement for embryonic stem cell research.

Some individuals within the scientific community agree that both adult and embryonic stem cell research show great potential to revolutionize the practice of medicine and that both types of research should be pursued.

GENE THERAPY

Gene therapy is rapidly becoming an effective tool for correcting and preventing certain diseases. In fact, therapy for genetic disease is often very similar to therapy for other types of disorders, as in the following cases:

- Special diets can eliminate compounds that are toxic to patients. This applies to such diseases as phenylketonuria (PKU) and homocystinuria.

multipotent stem cells
Stem cells that can become a limited number of types of tissues and cells in the body.

pluripotent stem cells
Stem cells that can become almost all types of tissues and cells in the body.

gene therapy
Treating harmful genetic diseases or traits by eliminating or modifying the harmful gene.

- Vitamins or other agents can improve a biochemical pathway and thus reduce toxic levels of a compound. For example, folic acid reduces homocysteine levels in a person who carries the 5,10-methylenetetrahydrofolate reductase polymorphism gene.

Gene therapy may involve replacing a deficiency or blocking an over-active pathway. For instance, a fetus can sometimes be treated by treating the mother (e.g., corticosteroids for congenital virilizing adrenal hypoplasia) or by using in utero (inside the uterus) cellular therapy (e.g., bone marrow transplantation). Similarly, a newborn with a genetic disease may be a candidate for treatment with bone marrow or organ transplantation.

Genetic therapy may also involve the insertion of normal copies of a gene into the cells of persons with a specific genetic disease (this is called somatic gene therapy). Such somatic gene therapy has been undertaken for severe genetic disorders such as adenosine deaminase deficiency, an immunodeficiency that usually results in death during the first few months of life.

Germ-line gene therapy involves the correction of an abnormality in the genes of sperm or egg but is presently considered an inappropriate way to deal with genetic diseases because of ethical issues, cost, lack of research in humans, lack of knowledge about whether or not changes would be maintained in the growing embryo, and the relative ease of treating the pertinent conditions somatically when needed.

Gene therapy could also involve turning off genes before their harmful properties can be expressed. For example, if the gene for Huntington's disease could be turned off before carriers reached adulthood, theoretically the disease could not develop.

Check Your Progress

6. List five possible uses for genetic testing.

7. The process of manipulating the DNA of organisms to produce desired results is called
_____.

8. Define *genetic discrimination*.

9. Define *cloning*.

10. Distinguish between multipotent and pluripotent stem cells.

11. What are the foremost objections to embryonic stem cell research?

12. Name and briefly define five methods of gene therapy.

Conception and the Beginning of Life

Fortunately, most couples who decide to have a child are able to conceive naturally, and most pregnancies proceed without problems. However, it is estimated that about 10 to 15 percent of reproductive-age couples in the United States will have difficulty conceiving. Of this percentage, either husband or wife will experience **infertility**—that is, the failure to conceive for a period of 12 months or longer due to a deviation from or interruption of the normal structure or function of any reproductive part, organ, or system.

LO 11.4

Discuss three possible remedies for couples experiencing infertility problems.

infertility
The failure to conceive for a period of 12 months or longer due to a deviation from or interruption of the normal structure or function of any reproductive part, organ, or system.

INFERTILITY

When couples have reproductive difficulties and consult physicians who specialize in infertility problems, diagnoses are made and appropriate treatment recommended. Several options for infertile couples exist, depending on the type of fertility problem. Here are a few of the most common:

- **In vitro fertilization (IVF).** In this process, eggs and sperm are brought together outside the body in a test tube or petri dish. When fertilization takes place, the resulting embryo can then be frozen in liquid nitrogen for future use or implanted in the female uterus for pregnancy to occur.
- **Artificial insemination.** This process involves the mechanical injection of viable semen into the vagina. If a man's sperm cells are used to fertilize a woman's eggs, the process is called **homologous artificial insemination.** If the partner's sperm cells are not viable, a donor's sperm may be used to fertilize the woman's eggs. This is called **heterologous artificial insemination.**
- **Surrogacy.** If a woman cannot carry an embryo to term, the couple may elect to contract with a surrogate mother.

in vitro fertilization (IVF)
Fertilization that takes place outside a woman's body, literally "in glass," as in a test tube.

artificial insemination
The mechanical injection of viable semen into the vagina.

homologous artificial insemination
The process in which a man's sperm is mechanically injected into a woman's vagina to fertilize her eggs.

heterologous artificial insemination
The process in which donor sperm is mechanically injected into a woman's vagina to fertilize her eggs.

surrogate mother
A woman who becomes pregnant, usually by artificial insemination or surgical implantation of a fertilized egg, and bears a child for another woman.

SURROGACY

A **surrogate mother** is a woman who agrees to carry a child to term for a couple, often for a fee. If the surrogate is not genetically related to the embryo, the type of surrogacy is called *gestational* surrogacy. If the surrogate contributes eggs to produce the embryo or is related to either partner in the relationship, the type of surrogacy is called *traditional* surrogacy. (In one much-publicized case in the United States, a woman carried her own grandchild to term for her married daughter who was born without a uterus.) Traditional surrogacy differs from gestational surrogacy in that a traditional surrogate is genetically related to the fetus she carries.

Infertility treatments can cost several thousand dollars, with no guarantee of success. Most insurance plans do not cover expenses for infertility treatments or for contracting with a surrogate mother to bear a child. The law has been slow to catch up with technology, but many states have passed legislation regulating infertility clinics and

---

LANDMARK COURT CASE Baby M—First Surrogacy Case

In 1985, a woman signed a contract agreeing to serve as a surrogate for a couple who could not conceive. She was then medically inseminated with the husband's sperm and a pregnancy resulted. When the child was born in March 1986, the surrogate mother refused to give up the infant. The genetic father sued for violation of the surrogacy contract. The contract specified that the genetic father and his wife held custody and that the surrogate would terminate her parental rights. The trial court, considering the best interests of the child, affirmed the validity of the contract. In March 1987, an appellate court terminated the surrogate mother's parental rights and gave full custody of the then 1-year-old Baby M to her genetic father and his wife. The genetic father's wife legally adopted the baby.

In re Baby M, 537 A.2d 1227, 109 N.J. 396 (1988).

surrogacy. Health care practitioners dealing with infertility should check state laws for current regulations.

Surrogacy is a relatively new concept in reproductive technology; thus, there is not a large volume of case law. The two cases, "Baby M—First Surrogacy Case" and "Gestational Surrogacy Contract Held Valid," however, have contributed to establishing precedent for legal decisions.

ADOPTION

Adoption is also an option for those couples who want to raise children. All 50 states have laws regulating adoption. Certain areas of federal law may also affect some aspects of the parent–child relationship established by adoption. For example, the Adoption Assistance and Child Welfare Act of 1980, the Child Abuse Prevention and Treatment and Adoption Reform Act, and the Indian Child Welfare Act all contain provisions that pertain to adoptive parents and their children.

Typically, any adult who shows the desire to be a fit parent may adopt a child. Depending on state law, both married and unmarried couples may adopt, and single people may adopt through a process called single-parent adoption. Some states list special requirements for adoptive parents, such as requiring an adoptive parent to be a specified number of years older than the child. There may also be state requirements concerning residency, or the marital state of the prospective parent. Any adult who wishes to adopt will need to check state law before proceeding, and if potential adoptive parents use an adoption agency, they will also have to meet any agency requirements.

Some single individuals or couples may have a more difficult time qualifying as adoptive parents than others. For example, single men, gay singles, and homosexual couples may not specifically be prevented from adopting by state law, but they may have a more difficult time meeting state and agency requirements than married couples would.

LANDMARK COURT CASE | ## Gestational Surrogacy Contract Held Valid

A married couple was unable to have a child because the wife had undergone a hysterectomy. The wife's ovaries had not been removed, however, and could still produce eggs, so the couple opted for gestational surrogacy. They entered into a surrogacy contract with a woman who agreed to relinquish her parental rights after the child was born in exchange for a $10,000 fee and a paid life insurance policy. The wife's eggs were fertilized in vitro with the husband's sperm, and the resulting embryo was implanted into the surrogate's uterus. While she was still pregnant, the surrogate demanded immediate payment and threatened not to relinquish the child when it was born. The couple who had contracted with the surrogate filed a lawsuit seeking a legal determination that the surrogate had no parental rights to the baby. The surrogate countersued and the court consolidated the two cases.

A trial court found for the married couple. It determined that the couple was the child's "natural parents" and held that the surrogate had no parental rights to the child. An appellate court and the state supreme court upheld this decision.

Johnson v. Calvert, 5 Cal. 4th 84, 851 P.2d 776 (1993).

All states strive to find placements that meet the best interest of the child, so in some cases potential adoptive parents may be asked additional questions about lifestyle and why they want to adopt. (See "Best Interest of the Child Concept" on page 309 for a more thorough explanation of "best interest of the child.")

Generally, couples can adopt a child of a different race. Adoptions of Native American children, however, are governed by the Indian Child Welfare Act, and the act's provisions outline specific rules and procedures that must be followed if the adoption of a Native American child is to be approved.

There are several different types of adoptions, depending on services used and whether or not a blood or marital relationship exists between adoptive parents and children:

- Agency adoptions occur when state-licensed and/or state-regulated public or private adoption agencies place children with adoptive parents. Charities or religious or social service organizations often operate private agencies. Adoption agencies usually place those children who have been orphaned or whose parents have lost or relinquished parental rights through abuse, abandonment, or inability to support.

- Independent or private adoptions are arranged without the involvement of adoption agencies. Potential adoptive parents may hear of a mother who wants to give up her child, or they may advertise in newspapers or on the Internet to find such a mother. At some point in the process, an attorney must be involved to ensure the legality of the adoption. A few states prohibit independent adoptions. In those states where independent adoptions are allowed, they are usually strictly regulated.

- Identified adoptions are those in which adopting parents locate a birth mother, or vice versa, and then ask an agency to take over the adoption process. Prospective parents who find a birth mother willing to give up her child can bypass the long waiting lists that most agencies maintain for adoptions and can perhaps be better assured that the adoption will proceed in an orderly and legal fashion.

- International adoptions occur when couples adopt children who are citizens of foreign countries. In these procedures, adoptive parents must not only meet requirements of the foreign country where the child resides, they must also meet all U.S. state requirements and U.S. Immigration and Naturalization Service rules for international adoptions.

- Relative adoptions are those in which the child is related to the adoptive parent by blood or marriage. Stepparent and grandparent/grandchildren adoptions fall within this category.

LO 11.5

List and discuss those laws affecting health care that pertain especially to children's rights.

parens patriae
A legal doctrine that gives the state the authority to act in a child's best interest.

Rights of Children

Common law has established the rights of parents to make health care decisions for minor children. In some circumstances, under the doctrine of ***parens patriae***, literally "father of the people," the state may act as the parental authority. This doctrine is the legal principle that grants the state the broad authority to act in the child's *best interest,* sometimes overriding parental decisions, and allowing the state to remove abused or neglected children from the custody of offending parents.

BEST INTEREST OF THE CHILD CONCEPT

When alternatives are available for child placement or for determining medical treatment for minor children, the common standard is the "best interest of the child." In other words, which alternative will best safeguard the child's growth, development, and health? This standard is used in child placement situations. It is also used when legal authorities must work with health care practitioners to determine the least harmful and most appropriate treatment for an ailing child.

RIGHTS OF THE NEWBORN

Legally, the legal rights of newborns are the same as those of any other American citizen of any age. For newborns who are severely disabled, however, existing law provides for several treatment options. Under the federal Child Abuse Amendments (U.S. Code, Title 42, Section 5106g), if the parents agree, physicians may legally withhold treatment, including food and water, from infants who:

- Are chronically and irreversibly comatose.
- Will most certainly die and for whom treatment is considered futile.
- Would suffer inhumanely if treatment were provided.

Treatment of newborns who are severely disabled raises many ethical questions. Should the federal government intrude into physicians' and parents' decisions with imposed regulations? Is it ever in an infant's "best interest" to die, or should medical treatment be administered regardless of the probable outcome? Is quality of life an issue that can ethically be considered? Who should decide among treatment options for newborns who are disabled if the parents are unwilling or unable to make such decisions?

ABANDONED INFANTS

Throughout the 1990s, newborn babies abandoned and left to die in dumpsters, public bathrooms, and other locations led to legislation allowing a parent to abandon a newborn at a safe location without legal prosecution or with reduced legal prosecution. By 2010, all 50 states had enacted some form of **safe haven law,** allowing abandonment at certain locations. State laws vary greatly:

safe haven laws
State laws that allow mothers to abandon newborns to designated safe facilities without penalty.

- In some states, the baby can be handed to a doctor or police officer, or left at a fire station or hospital.
- Some states allow either reduction or elimination of prosecution.
- In some states, the parent can remain anonymous, while in others he or she must reveal identity and give a medical history. In some states, medical histories can also be dropped off anonymously.

- Some states place a limit on the age of a baby that can be abandoned. This is to encourage a parent to abandon the baby early, so it can receive adequate nutrition and medical care, rather than hiding the baby and letting it become malnourished or otherwise unhealthy.

- Nebraska is one state that did not specify that its safe haven law, passed in July 2008, applied to infants only, and within a short time 16 children, including teenagers, had been abandoned to the care of the state. Nebraska legislators convened an emergency session to change the word "child" in the state's safe haven law to "infant." (Ironically, in 2010 some states were pushing to up the age for abandonment to 4 or 5, in light of several cases where mothers had murdered their small children.)

See **www.childwelfare.gov/systemwide/laws_policies/statutes/safe haven.cfm** for state-specific information about safe haven laws.

Reports by the National Conference of State Legislatures and the national Evan B. Donaldson Adoption Institute in 2003 indicated that the problem of abandonment of newborns has not been resolved and that, in fact, the laws have caused some undesirable results:

- The "no hassle" provisions discourage mothers from using established adoption and child welfare policies, while encouraging irresponsible and destructive behavior.

- The laws seem to some to be government statements that it's OK to abandon a baby.

- The abandoned children have little hope of learning family medical histories.

- The laws allow one parent to abandon a child, thus stripping the other parent of all rights.

The issue of abandonment also raises many ethical questions for society and for health care practitioners. Is the "safe haven" concept ethical—since prosecution is usually waived for parental abandonment under safe haven laws—or is it a form of child abuse and neglect? Should abandoned infants be eventually returned to the parent(s) who abandoned them, or should such parents be forced to relinquish parental rights? What public health measures might help prevent such events from occurring?

Check Your Progress

13. Define *infertility*.

14. List and define three medical procedures that might be available to infertile couples.

15. Adoptions are regulated primarily by _____.

16. Name four types of adoptions.

17. Under existing child abuse amendments, physicians may, with the consent of parents, withhold treatment for those infants who _____.

18. What are safe haven laws designed to prevent?

19. What are the disadvantages of safe haven laws?

TEENAGERS

While common law has dictated that parents have a right to decide what medical care their young children receive, laws for older children differ from those for newborns. For example, states recognize that some older minors have the capacity to consent to their own medical care. For instance, teenagers considered mature or emancipated minors may give consent for medical treatment.

Mature minors are individuals in their mid- to late teens who are considered mature enough to comprehend a physician's recommendations and give informed consent. Most states allow mature minors to seek medical treatment without the consent of a parent or guardian in certain critical areas, such as mental health, drug and/or alcohol addiction, treatment for sexually transmitted diseases, pregnancy, and contraceptive services.

Emancipated minors legally live outside their parents' or guardians' control. A judge may issue an emancipation order at the request of parents or a minor child after certain important factors have been considered:

- Does the minor live at home with parents or other supervising adults, or is he or she living independently? If living at home, does he or she pay for room and board?

- Does the minor have a job, and does he or she spend his or her earnings without parental supervision?

- Does the minor pay his or her own debts?

- Is the minor claimed as a dependent on the parents' tax return?

The court may declare minors emancipated if one or more of the following criteria are met:

- They are self-supporting.

- They are married, provided the marriage is legal. In most states, persons must be at least 16 to marry and those under the age of 18 must have parental consent. Emancipation is not forfeited if the minor divorces or is separated or widowed.

- They are serving in the armed forces.

Emancipated minors do not usually gain all the rights of adults. Some limits, such as the legal age for purchasing alcohol or tobacco products, voting age, mandatory school attendance age (unless married), and other legal age restrictions, still apply.

Minors have the same constitutional rights as adults, including the right to privacy. This is especially relevant for the increasing numbers of adolescents in the United States who are sexually active. Many hesitate to seek birth control or family planning counseling if they must inform or seek consent from their parents.

No state explicitly requires parental involvement for a minor to obtain any of the services listed above. In some states, however, laws leave the decision about whether or not to inform parents that minor sons and daughters have received or are seeking contraceptives, prenatal care, or STI services to the discretion of the treating physician, based on the best interest of the minor.

mature minors
Individuals in their mid- to late teens who, for health care purposes, are considered mature enough to comprehend a physician's recommendations and give informed consent.

emancipated minors
Individuals in their mid- to late teens who legally live outside parents' or guardians' control.

In addition to the ability to consent to these specific services, laws in some states give minors the right to consent to general medical and surgical care under some circumstances, such as being a parent themselves, being pregnant, or reaching a certain age.

Several states also allow minors who are parents to consent to medical care for their children. In many states, mothers who are minors may also legally place their children up for adoption without the consent or knowledge of the mothers' parents.

In many states, minors seeking an abortion must involve at least one parent in the decision. This means that teenagers who do not tell their parents about a pregnancy must either travel out of state or obtain approval from a judge—a process known as *judicial bypass*—to obtain an abortion. Currently, the trend is toward state and federal legislation making it increasingly difficult for minors to obtain an abortion without parental involvement.

For exact legal restrictions regarding minors, health care practitioners should check statutes in the states where they practice.

In certain cases, the legal right of a minor to decline medical treatment has been upheld.

COURT CASE   Minor Appeals for Judicial Bypass to Obtain an Abortion

A 17-year-old high school senior, called "A.V.P." in her lawsuit, asked the court in her state to issue an order authorizing her to have an abortion without parental approval or notification. Her reasons were that her mother had banished her older sister from their home when she became pregnant, indicating that her mother would also banish her. Furthermore, she had received a college scholarship before her pregnancy that she would probably lose because she would have to forego college to support herself and her child. Additionally, A.V.P. said the father of her child severed their relationship upon learning of her pregnancy, and would not help her support a child. She also told the court that she did not think she was emotionally or financially ready to care for a child, and would not consider adoption because she had heard tales of adopted children being abused.

The court found that A.V.P. "presented herself as a responsible and mature young lady for her age," but denied her petition for an abortion without parental approval or notification, because "[W]e believe that A.V.P. would benefit from consulting with her mother. . .and that this decision is too important to be made without the knowledge and advice of A.V.P.'s mother. . ."

State in Interest of A.V.P., 108 So. 3d. 1204 (La. Ct. App. 2013).

Judge Rules That Minor May Consent to Her Own Medical Treatment

Nancy, a 17-year-old Kansas girl, gave permission for a doctor to transplant some skin from her wrist to her finger. Her mother later sued on Nancy's behalf, on the grounds that Nancy was a minor.

Nancy's mother had been hospitalized for major surgery. After the operation, Nancy accompanied her mother to her hospital room. A nurse asked Nancy to wait in the hallway. She didn't notice that Nancy's hand was resting on the wall near the door jamb, with her right ring finger in the space between the door and the jamb. As the nurse closed the door, Nancy cried out in pain. The door had closed on her finger, severing the tip.

Nancy was taken to the emergency room, where a doctor decided to graft a small piece of skin from Nancy's wrist over the raw tip of her finger. Nancy's mother was still recovering from her surgery, and it would be hours before she could give consent for her daughter's treatment. Nancy's parents were divorced, and her father lived in another city. To spare Nancy a long, uncomfortable wait, the emergency room physician called the girl's family physician and received his agreement that he should treat Nancy.

When Nancy's mother recovered, she sued the hospital, claiming that the nurse had been negligent in causing her daughter's injury and that the doctor had not obtained proper consent to treat her minor daughter.

The nurse was not found negligent. Regarding the question of consent, the Kansas Supreme Court ruled that Nancy "was of sufficient age and maturity to know and understand the nature and consequences of the 'pinch graft' utilized in the repair of her finger."

Younts v. St. Francis Hosp. and School of Nursing, 205 Kan. 292, 469 P.2d 330, 338 (1970).

Check Your Progress

20. Define the term *mature minor.*

21. Name three criteria that may be considered to determine if a minor is to be declared *emancipated.*

22. What effect do the previous designations *mature minor* and *emancipated minor* have on a minor's health care decisions?

23. In what treatment areas are minors most likely to make their own health care decisions?

As we progress into the 21st century, health care practitioners will be constantly challenged to stay current with legal and ethical developments in genetics and reproductive science.

Chapter Summary

Learning Outcome	Summary
LO 11.1 Define *genetics* and *heredity*.	How does the term *genetics* differ from the term *heredity*? • Genetics is the science that accounts for natural differences and resemblances among organisms related by descent. • Heredity is the process by which organisms pass on genetic traits to their offspring. What terms, integral to the study of genetics, are defined in this chapter? • DNA—deoxyribonucleic acid: The combination of proteins, called nucleotides, that is arranged to make up an organism's chromosomes. • Chromosome: A microscopic structure found within the nucleus of all living cells that carries genes responsible for the organism's characteristics. • Gene: A tiny segment of DNA that holds the formula for making a specific enzyme or protein. • Genome: All the DNA in an organism, including its genes. What is the Human Genome Project? • A scientific project funded by the U.S. government, begun in 1990 and successfully completed in 2000, for the purpose of mapping all of a human's genes.
LO 11.2 List several situations in which genetic testing might be appropriate, and explain how it might lead to genetic discrimination.	What is genetic testing? • Testing one's DNA to discover one's genetic makeup. What are the different types of genetic testing explained in this chapter? • Predictive • Carrier • Prenatal • Amniocentesis—testing a sample of amniotic fluid for genetic or other conditions in a developing fetus—is a common prenatal test. • Preimplantation • Forensic • Tracing lineage • Newborn screening • Diagnostic What is a mutation? • A permanent change in DNA. What does a genetic counselor do? • Genetic counselors are qualified to counsel individuals before and after genetic testing. What is genetic discrimination? • Genetic discrimination is different treatment of individuals based on actual or presumed genetic differences. What federal laws are in place to protect Americans against genetic discrimination in health insurance and employment? • Genetic Information Nondiscrimination Act (GINA) of 2008. • Health Insurance Portability and Accountability Act (HIPAA). • Americans with Disabilities Act (ADA). • Patient Protection and Affordable Care Act (ACA) of 2010.

Learning Outcome	Summary

LO 11.3 Define *genetic engineering,* and explain why cloning and stem cell research are controversial issues.	What is genetic engineering?
	
	• Genetic engineering is the manipulation of DNA within an organism's cells through synthesis, alteration, or repair to ensure that certain harmful traits will be eliminated in offspring and that desirable traits will appear and be passed on.
	
	What is a clone?
	
	• An organism produced asexually, usually from a single cell of the parent.
	
	What is xenotransplantation?
	
	• Transplantation of animal tissues and organs into humans.
	
	What are stem cells?
	
	• Cells that can become another type of body cell.
	  • Multipotent: Adult cells that can become a limited number of types of tissues and cells.
	  • Pluripotent: Embryonic cells that can become almost all types of tissues and cells.
	
	What is gene therapy?
	
	• Treatment of harmful genetic diseases or traits by eliminating or modifying the harmful gene.

LO 11.4 Discuss three possible remedies for couples experiencing infertility problems.	What is infertility?
	
	• The failure to conceive for a period of 12 months or longer due to a deviation from or interruption of the normal structure or function of any reproductive part, organ, or system.
	
	What alternatives are available for infertile couples who want to become parents?
	
	• In vitro fertilization (IVF).
	• Artificial insemination
	  • Homologous: partner's sperm/woman's eggs.
	  • Heterologous: donor sperm/woman's eggs.
	• Surrogacy
	• Adoption

LO 11.5 List and discuss those laws affecting health care that pertain especially to children's rights.	Under what doctrine may the state act as a child's parental authority?
	
	• *Parens patriae*
	  • Best Interest of the child concept.
	
	When may physicians, with the parents' consent, legally withhold treatment and nourishment from a newborn who is severely disabled?
	
	• If the child is chronically and irreversibly comatose.
	• If the child will most certainly die, and treatment is considered futile.
	• If the child would suffer inhumanely if treatment were provided.
	
	What are safe haven laws?
	
	• Laws that allow mothers to abandon newborns to designated safe facilities without penalty.
	
	How do mature minors differ from emancipated minors?
	
	• Mature minors: Individuals in mid- to late teens who legally live outside parental or guardian control.
	• Emancipated minors: Individuals in mid- to late teens who legally live outside parental or guardian control, usually through judicial decree, as long as minor
	  • Is self-supporting.
	  • Is legally married.
	  • Is serving in the armed forces.

9. In which of the following situations might DNA testing be indicated?

    a. A man involved in a paternity suit

    b. Parents who suspect they brought the wrong baby home from the hospital

    c. A woman who is a suspect in a murder

    d. All of these

10. *Genetic discrimination* is best described as

    a. A government-sponsored project

    b. A form of favoritism in employment

    c. Differential treatment of individuals based on their actual or presumed genetic differences

    d. None of these

LO 11.3

_____ 11. An experimental treatment for hereditary diseases.

_____ 12. The process that produced Dolly the sheep.

_____ 13. Specialized cells considered most valuable for purposes of genetic manipulation.

_____ 14. Those specialized cells that can become almost any kind of cell.

_____ 15. Those cells that can become only one type of body cell.

a. Multipotent

b. Stem cells

c. Gene therapy

d. Cloning

e. Pluripotent

LO 11.4

16. *Artificial insemination* may be an acceptable remedy for

    a. Pregnancy

    b. Infertility

    c. Surrogacy

    d. Cloning

17. Which of the following best defines *in vitro fertilization?*

    a. The union of egg and sperm

    b. The fusion of egg and cell nucleus

    c. Fertilization taking place outside a woman's body

    d. Cloning

18. Which of the following best defines *surrogacy?*

    a. A woman bears a child for another woman.

    b. A woman is artificially inseminated.

    c. Fertilization takes place outside a woman's body.

    d. None of these

LO 11.5

_____ 19. The government serves as a child's parent.

_____ 20. The common standard when the government makes decisions for minor children.

a. Civil Rights Act

b. *Parens patriae*

c. Safe haven laws

_____ 21. Federal regulations concerning newborns who are severely disabled take their authority from which federal regulation?

_____ 22. State laws that allow a parent to abandon newborns to designated safe locations.

_____ 23. In the past, these laws have dictated that parents have a right to decide what medical care children receive.

d. Best interest of the child

e. Common law

f. Child Abuse Amendments

24. In most states, which of the following age groups can receive some types of medical care without parental permission?

a. Mature minors

b. Minors over age 14

c. Minors under age 18

d. None of these

25. Minors may be declared emancipated only if they

a. Go to court and request emancipation

b. Receive parental permission to request emancipation

c. Are self-supporting

d. None of these

26. Once declared emancipated, a minor can lose that status if he or she

a. Was married but divorces

b. Was in the military but is discharged

c. Was self-supporting but loses a job

d. None of these

27. A physician or other health care practitioner who treats a minor in a nonemergency situation, without parental consent, risks being charged with

a. Kidnapping

b. Assault and/or battery

c. Violating the Civil Rights Act

d. No charges can ever be made

Case Studies

Use your critical thinking skills to answer the questions that follow each case study.

LO 11.1

In March 2012, Nancy K. Rhoden, an Associate Professor of Law, wrote in an issue of _The Hastings Report:_ "The ethical tensions inherent in all Baby Doe treatment decisions are compounded by medical uncertainty. Physicians both here and abroad have adopted various strategies. Swedish doctors tend to withhold treatment from the beginning from infants for whom statistical data suggest a grim prognosis. The British are more likely to initiate treatment but withdraw it if the infant appears likely to die or suffer severe brain damage. The trend in the U.S. is to start treating any baby who is potentially viable and continue until it is virtually certain that the infant will die." Rhoden further states that the "least worst strategy is an individualized one: starting treatment gathering data, and then reassessing the decision."

28. In your opinion, which strategy seems the most ethical?

29. Which strategy seems the least ethical? Explain your answers.

Source: **http://onlinelibrary.wiley.com/doi/10.2307/3563115/abstract.**

LO 11.4

As reproductive technology advanced, headlines announcing "Couple Battles over Frozen Embryos" became more and more commonplace. For example, in the 1980s a man went to court and succeeded in preventing his ex-wife from using their frozen embryos to become pregnant. He maintained that after he and his wife had divorced, he no longer wanted to become a parent, and should not be forced to do so against his will.

In 1998, a divorced woman in New Jersey won a legal battle with her ex-husband over custody of seven frozen embryos the couple had created in vitro while still married. The wife wanted to have the embryos destroyed, while the ex-husband argued his right to adopt his own embryos to be implanted in a future partner or donated to an infertile couple.

30. In your opinion, should frozen embryos be considered property to be awarded during a divorce? Why or why not?

31. Should a man who loses custody of frozen embryos in a lawsuit be responsible for child support if his ex-wife is implanted with the embryos and becomes pregnant at a later date? Explain your answer.

32. Should the husband or wife who wins custody of frozen embryos be allowed to destroy them, against the wishes of the ex-husband or ex-wife? Why or why not?

Internet Activities LO 11.1, LO 11.4, and LO 11.5

Complete the activities and answer the questions that follow.

33. Visit the Web site for the Human Genome Project at **www.ornl.gov/sci/techresources/Human_Genome/home.shtml.** What are three of the medical applications expected to result from the project or presently in use as a result of the project?

34. Visit the fact sheet page for the American Society for Reproductive Medicine at **www.asrm.org/detail.aspx?id=2322.** How does the page define *infertility*? Briefly summarize additional information presented.

35. Visit the Planned Parenthood Federation of America's Web site for teens at **www.plannedparenthood.org/teen-talk/.** Briefly summarize the topics available there. In your opinion, does the site promote valid health care issues? Why or why not? The site is controversial. Comment on why you think this is so.

Resources

Alzheimer's disease gene: **http://ghr.nlm.nih.gov/gene/APOE.**

Cases of genetic discrimination: **www.genome.gov/12513976.**

Cloning humans: **www.ornl.gov/sci/techresources/Human_Genome/elsi/cloning.shtml#humans.**

Disadvantages to safe haven laws: **www.onebyonesafehaven.org/777/the-pros-cons-of-safe-haven-laws/.**

Distinguishing genetic from nongenetic medical tests, Joseph S. Alper and Jon Beckwith: **www.springerlink.com/content/lu7v417x88884185/.**

Dolly dies: **www.newscientist.com/article/dn3393-dolly-the-sheep-dies-young.html.**

Dolly "277 attempts": **www.animalresearch.info/en/medical/timeline/Dolly.**

Evan B. Donaldson Adoption Institute Web site: **http://adoptioninstitute.org/.**

Geller, Lisa N., Joseph S. Alper, Paul R. Billings, Carol I. Barash, Jonathan Beckwith, et al. *Science and Engineering Ethics* 2, no. 1 (1996), 71–88.

Geller study: **www.springerlink.com/content/739823h426q50x51/.**

Genetics articles: **www.mayoclinic.com/health/genetic-testing/MY00370/TAB=expertblog.**

Genetic testing/diseases: **www.nlm.nih.gov/medlineplus/genetictesting.html.**

Genetic testing: **http://ghr.nlm.nih.gov/handbook/testing/uses** and **www.genome.gov/19516567#al-2I.**

How many genetic diseases + types of genetic diseases: **www.genetic-diseases.net/** and **www.aicardisyndrome.org/site/.**

Morrison, Eileen E. and Beth Furlong. *Health Care Ethics: Critical Issues for the 21st Century.* Jones and Bartlett, 2014, p. 125, Boston, MA.

Reproductive ethics ISSUE 1: **www.uic.edu/depts/mcam/ethics/arts.htm.**

Uses of genetic testing (University of Washington): **www.genetests.org/.**

Weise, Elizabeth Weise. "Is It Unfair to Patent Genes?" *USA Today,* April 13, 2010, p. 10B.

Zimmer, Carl. "Voices: What's Next in Science?" *The New York Times,* online ed., November 9, 2010, **www.nytimes.com/interactive/2010/11/09/science/20111109_next_feature.html?nl=todaysheadlines&emc=ab1.**

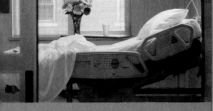

12

Key Terms

Death and Dying

LEARNING OUTCOMES

After studying this chapter, you should be able to:

LO 12.1 Discuss how attitudes toward death have changed over time.

LO 12.2 Discuss accepted criteria for determining death.

LO 12.3 Determine the health care professional's role in caring for the dying.

LO 12.4 Discuss benefits to end-of-life health care derived from the right to die movement.

LO 12.5 Identify the major features of organ donation in the United States.

LO 12.6 Discuss the various stages of grief.

FROM THE PERSPECTIVE OF. . .

ANGELA HAS BEEN A REGISTERED NURSE FOR 22 YEARS. Just as some hospital nurses are drawn to surgery, the emergency room, or the intensive care unit, Angela prefers hospice and palliative care. "Broadly speaking," Angela explains, "medicine is about repairing, extending, and medicating, while end-of-life care is more about the patient as an individual, about basic human needs. In addition, it isn't just the patient you are caring for; you are caring for the entire family group—everybody needs you.

"We live in a time when death has been removed from family and home for the most part," Angela continues, "and people generally have less understanding of the process than a hundred years ago. . . . The family most often feels helpless and confused. The hospice nurse is able to help not just the patient, but the family, too, through a sad and often frightening time."

Sometimes family members are hesitant about approaching a dying loved one. For example, Angela remembers a situation where the mother of two siblings in their thirties was dying. "When I arrived they were practically plastered against the walls of the room, clearly unsure of what they should be doing." Angela encouraged the two family members to come to their mother's bedside and comfort her. "The son pulled a chair to the side of the bed and held his mother's hand. The daughter climbed onto the bed and cradled her mother. . . . I like to think that because I urged them to take a more active part in her passing that they found comfort after their mother was gone."

Angela also recalls a patient in his eighties whose 32 family members joined him in his hospice room. "It was almost a living wake. They talked for hours about his life and the experiences they had each shared with him. They laughed and they cried and it was wonderful. This sharing in their loved one's death was a beautiful experience for those left behind, and I hope it helped him in some way as well."

From Angela's perspective as a hospice nurse, the end of a life is a time when family members can come together to comfort their dying loved one and each other. She sees her job as a facilitator for this natural process.

From the perspective of the individual who is dying, the nearness of family members is comforting, as well as the presence of a nurse who is not uncomfortable with end-of-life issues.

From the perspective of surviving family members, Angela has heard many times that her attitude—don't be afraid to comfort your loved one—gave them the courage to participate in the process, and comforted them after the death occurred.

Attitudes toward Death and Dying

LO 12.1
Discuss how attitudes toward death have changed over time.

Prior to the twentieth century, death was an intimate experience for most families. Antibiotics and chemotherapies had not yet been discovered; genetically engineered drugs, organ transplantation, and life-support machines were still science fiction; and infectious diseases periodically decimated populations. Nearly every husband and wife, mother and father, brother and sister had lost a loved one. Loved ones customarily died at home, surrounded by family members who bade them goodbye and then mourned their passing with funeral rituals and rites, including the following:

- Black has long been worn by undertakers, mourners, and pallbearers to show grief. In ancient times, it was also used as a disguise to protect against malevolent spirits that might be lurking nearby.

- An early custom for mourners was to go barefoot and to wear sackcloth and ashes. This was said to discourage the dead from becoming envious as they might be if mourners appeared at funerals wearing new clothes and shoes.

- Pagan tribes began the custom of covering the face of the deceased with a sheet, since they believed that the spirit of the deceased escaped through the mouth. They often held the mouth and nose of a sick person shut, hoping to retain the spirit and thus delay death.

- In earlier times, traffic was halted for a funeral procession because any delay in transporting a soul might turn it into a restless ghost, reluctant to pass over into the next world.

- Wakes held today come from the ancient custom of keeping watch over the deceased, hoping that life would return. In England, the dead were always carried out of the house feet first; otherwise, their spirits might look back into the house and beckon family members to come with them.

- Pagan beliefs concerning funeral wreaths held that the circle formed by the wreath would keep the dead person's spirit within bounds.

- The firing of a rifle volley over the deceased is similar to the tribal practice of throwing spears into the air to ward off spirits hovering over the deceased.

- In the past, holy water was sprinkled on the body to protect it from demons.

By the late twentieth century, individuals were more likely to die in the hospital, at least in the Western world. Once admitted to hospitals, the dying were isolated from family members and surrounded by machines designed to prolong life as long as possible. Consequently, modern technology has effectively hidden death from view, but in so doing it has also made the end of life a fearful prospect.

Attitudes toward death and dying vary with individuals, of course, but as each of us ages, we will likely begin to think of our own mortality and perhaps to wonder how the end will come. Will I die alone, in an impersonal, clinical hospital environment? Will my health care providers be so committed to preserving life that they delay my dying to an irrational degree? Will I suffer in pain? Will I feel a sense of tasks left unfinished and goals left unrealized, or will I experience a peaceful letting go?

Because the fears associated with death and dying are universal, health care practitioners should evaluate their own attitudes to effectively and compassionately respond to dying patients and their families.

Determination of Death

Modern medical technology and life-support equipment may keep a person's body "alive"—the heart may beat and blood may circulate—long after the brain ceases to function. This makes it difficult in some cases to determine the moment when death actually occurs. For this reason, in 1981 a **Uniform Determination of Death Act** was proposed by the President's Commission for the Study of Ethical Problems in Medicine and Biomedical Research working in cooperation with the American Bar Association, the American Medical Association, and the National Conference of Commissioners on Uniform State Laws. The National Conference of Commissioners on Uniform State Laws has no legislative authority. Acts the commissioners propose must still be approved by state legislatures, and that is sometimes difficult to accomplish. States have their own criteria for determining when death actually occurs, but most have adopted the act's definition of **brain death** as a means of determining when death actually occurs:

- Circulatory and respiratory functions have irreversibly ceased.
- The entire brain, including the brain stem, has irreversibly ceased to function.

When the brain is injured or shuts down due to lack of oxygen, a patient may appear near death when, in fact, he or she is in a **coma,** which is a condition of deep stupor from which a patient cannot be roused by external stimuli. Patients can and do recover from comas, as opposed to a persistent vegetative state. **Persistent vegetative state (PVS)** exists as a result of severe mental impairment, characterized by irreversible cessation of the higher functions of the brain, most often caused by damage to the cerebral cortex. In PVS, only involuntary bodily functions are present, and there exists no reasonable expectation of regaining significant mental function.

Before pronouncing an unresponsive and unconscious patient dead, physicians may perform a series of tests to determine whether death has occurred. Death is indicated if the following signs are present. The patient:

- Cannot breathe without assistance.
- Has no coughing or gagging reflex.
- Has no pupil response to light.
- Has no blinking reflex when the cornea is touched.
- Has no grimace reflex when the head is rotated or ears are flushed with ice water.
- Has no response to pain.

Today the declaration of death occurs only when the last signs of brain and respiratory activity are gone. (An EEG and brain perfusion scan may also be administered to test for brain activity.) Technically, death results from lack of oxygen. When deprived of oxygen, cells cannot maintain metabolic function and soon begin to deteriorate.

AUTOPSIES

After a patient is declared dead, family members (next of kin) may be asked to consent to an autopsy. An autopsy is a postmortem examination

Uniform Determination of Death Act
A proposal that established uniform guidelines for determining when death has occurred.

brain death
Final cessation of bodily activity, used to determine when death actually occurs; circulatory and respiratory functions have irreversibly ceased, and the entire brain (including the brain stem) has irreversibly ceased to function.

coma
A condition of deep stupor from which the patient cannot be roused by external stimuli.

persistent vegetative state (PVS)
Severe mental impairment characterized by irreversible cessation of the higher functions of the brain, most often caused by damage to the cerebral cortex.

1. Briefly explain how attitudes toward death and dying in the United States have changed over the years.

2. The _____, while not a law, was proposed as a universal means of determining when death actually occurs.

3. Distinguish between *comatose* and *persistent vegetative state*.

4. Define *brain death*.

5. Name six signs for which physicians may test that indicate death has occurred.

to determine cause of death and/or to obtain physiological evidence when necessary. Autopsies performed in hospitals may confirm or correct clinical diagnoses, thus providing a measure of quality assurance. Autopsy results can also highlight those cases in which diagnoses tend to be incorrect, or treatments tend to be ineffective, thereby adding to scientific knowledge and revealing areas that need further study. In cases of suspicious deaths, autopsy results can provide information to help law enforcement authorities, such as cause and time of death. (Legal requirements concerning autopsies are discussed in Chapter 9.)

While autopsies must be performed in cases in which the death is suspicious or due to homicide, the number of autopsies performed in all other deaths each year has steadily declined. One reason that fewer autopsies are performed today is cost—insurance companies and government health care programs usually do not pay for autopsies. (However, when patients die in hospitals, often an autopsy can be performed free of charge.) Some clinicians argue that technological advances have made clinical diagnoses more accurate, so that postmortem diagnoses are less essential. Another reason for the decline in autopsies is that in many smaller hospitals, pathologists are not readily available.

Furthermore, even though autopsies can yield information that may clarify causes of death, reveal genetic disease that runs in families, or reassure survivors that their loved ones could not have been saved, when an autopsy is not mandated by law, family members are often reluctant to give consent. They may feel that their loved one has "suffered enough," that the physician already knows the cause of death, or that the procedure would interfere with viewing of the body during funeral rites. Health care practitioners may believe that these perceptions of autopsies are inaccurate, but they must remain sensitive to the beliefs and emotions of surviving family members.

Caring for Dying Patients

When it becomes evident that a patient's disease is incurable and death is imminent, **palliative care** may serve the dying patient better than **curative care.** Curative care consists of treatments and procedures directed toward curing a patient's disease. Palliative care, also called comfort care, is directed toward providing relief to terminally ill patients through symptom and pain management. The goal is not to cure, but to provide comfort and maintain the highest possible quality of life. Going

LO 12.3

Determine the health care professional's role in caring for the dying.

palliative care
Treatment of a terminally ill patient's symptoms to make dying more comfortable; also called comfort care.

curative care
Treatment directed toward curing a patient's disease.

beyond relief of disease symptoms, palliative care includes relief of emotional distress and other problems, so that a patient's last months and days may be as comfortable as possible.

Palliative care is also emerging as a way to help patients with serious illnesses live a more comfortable and fulfilling life, whether their diseases are terminal or not. For example, through palliative care:

- A 90-year-old stroke patient with limited mobility is able to continue living independently in his home.

- An ovarian cancer patient is more comfortable and can actually continue working as she undergoes aggressive chemotherapy treatment.

- A lung cancer patient receives counseling about his disease and help in navigating the complex U.S. health care system.

In many cases, choosing palliative care or curative care is not an either/or proposition. Patients can move in and out of palliative care as treatment needs change, or as a respite from aggressive medical treatment and/or high medical expenses (Figure 12-1).

Palliative care is not the same as hospice care, which is limited to terminally ill patients (see the next section).

The Center to Advance Palliative Care, based in New York, provides information to help patients and their families receive care that addresses all of the patient's needs. (Visit the center's Web site at **www.capc.org** for information about goals and services.)

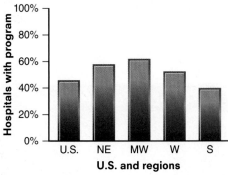

FIGURE 12-1
Numbers of hospitals in the U.S. that have palliative care programs vary with geographic region.

HOSPICE CARE

Terminally ill patients are often referred to facilities or agencies that provide **hospice** care. A hospice in medieval times was a way station for travelers. The first modern hospice facilities were established in England in the 1960s as places where patients could go to die in comfort.

In the United States, hospice care may be provided in facilities built especially for that purpose, in hospitals and nursing homes, or at home. (Angela, in the chapter's opening scenario, practices in a hospital. The floor she supervises is designated a hospice.) Hospice care focuses on relieving pain, controlling symptoms, and meeting emotional needs and personal values of the terminally ill, instead of targeting the underlying disease process. The hospice philosophy also recognizes that family members and other caregivers deserve care and support, continuing after the death of the patient. Hospice programs ease dying; they do not support active euthanasia (a Greek term meaning "good death") or assisted suicide.

Bereavement services are also available through hospice care to help patients discuss such issues as preparing a will and planning a funeral, and to help surviving family members cope with grief and loss after the patient dies. Hospice programs generally provide bereavement services through discussion groups, follow-up visits from hospice personnel, and sometimes referrals to appropriate mental health professionals.

Most in-home hospice programs are independently run in a fashion similar to visiting nurse or home health care agencies. Patients receive coordinated care at home by multidisciplinary teams composed of physicians, nurses, social workers, home health aides, pharmacists, physical

hospice
A facility or program (often carried out in a patient's home) in which teams of health care practitioners and volunteers provide a continuing environment that focuses on the physical, emotional, and psychological needs of the dying patient.

therapists, clergy, volunteers, and family members. Hospice teams meet regularly to work on patients' needs concerning pain and other serious symptoms, depression, family problems, inadequate housing, financial problems, or lack of transportation. The team then expands, amends, or otherwise revises each patient's care plan, as necessary.

For patients to be eligible for hospice care, physicians usually must certify that they are not expected to live beyond six months. Hospice care is generally reimbursed by Medicare, Medicaid, and many private insurance companies and managed care programs.

Check Your Progress

6. Distinguish between *palliative care* and *curative care*.

_____

7. Define *hospice*.

_____

Indicate with a "C" or a "P" whether each of the following actions constitutes a form of curative care or palliative care.

_____ 8. Allowing a patient who is terminally ill with lung and stomach cancer to self-administer morphine patches as needed for pain relief.

_____ 9. Administering radiation treatments after breast cancer surgery.

_____ 10. Surgical severing of certain nerves to relieve suffering for a patient terminally ill with cancer of the spine.

_____ 11. Counseling a terminally ill patient and his or her family concerning funeral arrangements and other end-of-life decisions.

_____ 12. Administering antibiotics to cure an infected tooth.

_____ 13. Cosmetic surgery for a teenaged patient whose face was burned in a fire.

EDUCATING HEALTH CARE PRACTITIONERS ABOUT END-OF-LIFE ISSUES

While modern medicine has effectively delayed the moment of death, in many cases it has dealt less conscientiously with compassionate, comfort care for **terminally ill** patients: those who are not expected to live beyond six months, usually because of a chronic illness that has progressed beyond effective treatment or for which there is no cure.

Studies published within the last decade have shown the need for educating health care practitioners in end-of-life care:

terminally ill
Referring to patients who are expected to die within six months.

- A 2003 Hastings Center Report found that ". . . too many Americans die unnecessarily bad deaths—deaths with inadequate palliative support, inadequate compassion, and inadequate human presence and witness. Deaths preceded by a dying marked by fear, anxiety, loneliness, and isolation. Deaths that efface dignity and deny individual self-control and choice."

- In 2004, the American Medical Students Association (AMSA) formed a death and dying interest group, in response to medical

-
-

Na

en
wh
ne

LI

A l
and
ma
ue
de
siv
no
ple
"he
and
reg
wil
inc

spe
ma
vic

bu
of
age
sio

DL

Th
bu
to
eff
eitl
pla
an
ing
ava

HE

A l
en
att

students' consensus that medical school leaves students inadequately prepared to communicate with terminally ill patients, as
well as poorly equipped emotionally to deal with matters of death
and dying. The AMSA interest group continues to provide guidance, support, and resources for students who wish to supplement
their medical education in the area of death and dying.

- A 2010 study of 12 Washington State hospitals found that programs aimed at improving health care practitioners' ability to
communicate with patients and families in ICUs did not improve
end-of-life care, according to results published online in the
American Journal of Respiratory and Critical Care Medicine. For
example, wrote J. Randall Curtis, MD, one of the study's authors,
"Many patients [in the intensive care unit] die with moderate or
severe pain and physicians are often unaware of patients' preferences regarding end-of-life care." In addition, the study found,
"Family of ICU patients have a high prevalence of symptoms of
anxiety, depression, and post-traumatic stress disorder . . . and
report physician and nurse behaviors that increase their burden."
Study conclusions supported improving education among doctors, patients, family members, nurses, and social workers to
improve end-of-life care and patient/family satisfaction. "This is
an area of care that is especially important in our current time,"
Curtis added.

- A 2010 British study that surveyed 8,500 physicians found that
their religious beliefs often affected the quality of end-of-life care
administered. The more religious the physician, the more likely
he or she is to avoid discussions with very ill patients about comfort care only. Physicians who describe themselves as agnostics
or atheists were more open to patient requests for less aggressive
end-of-life care.

- In 2013, the Association of American Medical Colleges (AAMC)
reported that only five of the nation's 125 medical schools offered
separate courses on death and dying. Instead, most incorporated
medical humanities, ethics, and/or communication into an existing required course.

Source: Jennings B., T. Rundes, C. D'Onofrio, et al. "Access to Hospice Care:
Expanding Boundaries, Overcoming Barriers. The Hastings Center Report." 2003;
33 (2): S3–4.

Fortunately, the need to teach end-of-life care to physicians and other
health care practitioners has been recognized. Increasingly, schools that
train health care providers are offering courses in **thanatology**—the
study of death and of the psychological methods of coping with death.
For instance, the American Board of Internal Medicine (ABIM) requires
that internists seeking certification have training in caring for the dying
during residency. The University of Illinois Chicago College of
Medicine teaches pediatric residents how to communicate with grieving parents. New York Medical College in Valhalla offers a 2-month
course in empathy for first year students. George Washington University medical school teaches students how to deliver bad news to
patients and how to talk to patients about advance directives and other
end-of-life concerns.

thanatology
The study of death and of the
psychological methods of coping
with it.

The message for health care practitioners is to remain flexible in their expectations of other people's grief. That is, to realize that every person grieves in his or her own way, and some are resilient enough to get through grief on their own, while others may benefit from a combination of the helpful measures outlined in this chapter.

FINDING SUPPORT

People who are grieving can find support from a variety of sources. They can read books on the subject, attend a bereavement support group sponsored by a hospital or hospice, visit a counselor, talk with a member of the clergy, or talk with family members and friends.

Health care practitioners can be excellent sources of support for terminally ill patients and their families. Talking and listening are the most helpful activities others can perform, the experts advise. Do not force a conversation, but make yourself available to talk. Do not respond in kind if patients are angry and resentful. Talking about distress helps relieve it, and sensitive listening is effective in itself. The following list of recommendations for talking to a dying patient is adapted from *"I Don't Know What to Say . . . ": How to Help and Support Someone Who Is Dying* (Little, Brown, 1989), by oncologist Dr. Robert Buckman:

- Pay attention to setting. Sit down, relax, do not appear rushed, and act as though you are ready to listen.
- Determine whether or not the patient wants to talk. Ask, "Do you feel like talking?" before plunging into conversation.
- Listen well, and show that you are listening. Pay attention to the patient's words, without the distraction of planning your next remark.
- Encourage the patient to talk by saying, "What do you mean?" or "Tell me more."
- Remember that silence and nonverbal communication, such as grasping a hand or touching a shoulder, are also effective.
- Do not be afraid to describe your own feelings. It is permissible to say, "I find this difficult to talk about" or even, "I don't know what to say."
- Make sure you haven't misunderstood. You can ask, "How did it feel?" or say, "You seem angry."
- Do not change the subject. If you are uncomfortable, admit it. Don't try to distract the patient by changing the subject to something less threatening, such as the weather.
- Do not give advice early. The time may come when the patient asks your advice, but it is usually not prudent to offer unsolicited advice, because it stops the dialogue.
- Encourage reminiscence. Sharing memories can be a wrenching experience, but it can also encourage patients to look positively at the past.
- Respond to humor. Humor allows patients to express fears in a nonthreatening way. Do not try to cheer someone up with your own jokes, but if patients want to tell jokes or funny stories, humor them.

In short, the more you try to understand the feelings of others, the more support you will be able to give.

Chapter Summary

Learning Outcome	Summary
LO 12.1 Discuss how attitudes toward death have changed over time.	**Which Western rituals surrounding death have survived to the present?** • Mourners wearing black. • Halting traffic for a funeral procession. • Wakes • Firing a rifle volley over the deceased. • Funeral wreaths

LO 12.2 Discuss accepted criteria for determining death.	**What is the Uniform Determination of Death Act?**
	• A federal proposal that defines brain death as a means of determining when death actually occurs:
	  • Circulation and respiration have irreversibly ceased.
	  • The entire brain, including the brain stem, has irreversibly ceased to function.
	
	What is the difference between a coma and a persistent vegetative state?
	• Coma: A condition of deep stupor from which the patient cannot be roused by external stimuli.
	• Persistent vegetative state (PVS): Severe mental impairment characterized by irreversible cessation of the higher functions of the brain, most often caused by damage to the cerebral cortex.
	
	What tests may be performed to determine if death has occurred?
	• Cannot breathe without assistance.
	• No coughing or gagging reflex.
	• No pupil response to light.
	• No blinking reflex when cornea is touched.
	• No grimace reflex when head is rotated or ears are flushed with ice water.
	• No response to pain.

LO 12.3 Determine the health care professional's role in caring for the dying.	**What is the difference between palliative care and curative care?** • Palliative care: Treatment of a patient's symptoms to make him or her more comfortable—also called comfort care. • Curative care: Treatment directed toward curing a patient's disease. **What is a hospice?** • A facility or program in which health care practitioners and volunteers provide a continuous environment that focuses on the physical, emotional, and psychological needs of the dying patient. **What is meant by the phrase *terminally* ill?** • A patient has six months or less to live. **What is *thanatology*?** • The study of death and psychological coping methods.

LO 12.4 Discuss benefits to end-of-life health care derived from the right to die movement.	**What is the Uniform Rights of the Terminally Ill Act?**
	• A 1989 federal proposal to guide state legislatures in constructing laws concerned with advance directives.
	
	What is euthanasia?
	• Mercy killing of the hopelessly ill.
	  • Active euthanasia: A conscious medical act that results in the death of a dying person.
	  • Passive euthanasia: Allowing a dying patient to die without medical interference.
	  • Voluntary euthanasia: Requires the patient's consent or the consent of the patient's legal representative to implement.

Learning Outcome	Summary
	• Involuntary euthanasia: The use of medical means to end a dying patient's life without his or her consent.
	• Physician-assisted suicide: Any of the previously listed methods in which a physician takes part in the patient's suicide.
	What is the Patient Self-Determination Act?
	• A federal act that requires hospitals and other health care providers to give written information to patients regarding their rights under state law to make medical decisions and to execute advance directives.
	• Living will: An advance directive that specifies a patient's end-of-life wishes.
	• Durable power of attorney: An advance directive that gives a designee authority to make a variety of legal decisions for a patient, including health care decisions.
	• Health care proxy: A durable power of attorney for health care decisions only.
	• Do-not-resuscitate order (DNR): The patient specifies in writing that he or she does not wish to be resuscitated if his or her heart stops.
LO 12.5 Identify the major features of organ donation in the United States.	**What is the National Organ Transplant Act?**
	• A 1984 federal law that provides grants to qualified organ procurement organizations and that established an Organ Procurement and Transplantation Network (OPTN).
	• Established the United Network of Organ Sharing (UNOS) to administer the OPTN. The UNOS
	• Increases the effectiveness and efficiency of organ sharing and equity in the national system of organ allocation.
	• Increases the supply of donated organs available for transplant.
	What is the Uniform Anatomical Gift Act?
	• A federal proposal that states enact laws allowing anyone 18 or older, of sound mind, to make a gift of his or her body or certain organs for use in medical research, transplantation, or storage in a tissue bank. The act recommends that:
	• Donations made through a legal will are not to be held up by probate.
	• Except in autopsies, the donor's rights override those of others.
	• Survivors may speak for the deceased if no arrangements for donation were made prior to death, provided the deceased did not express an objection to donation before death.
	• Physicians who rely on donation documents for the acceptance of bodies or organs are immune from civil or criminal prosecution.
	• Hospitals, surgeons, physicians, accredited medical or dental schools, colleges and universities, and tissue banks or storage facilities may accept anatomical gifts for research, advancement of medical or dental science, therapy, or transplantation.
	• Time of death of the donor must be established by a physician who is not involved in transplanting the donor's designated organs, and the donor's attending physician cannot be a member of the transplant team.
	• Donors may revoke the gift, and gifts may be rejected.
	What is grief?
	• The human reaction to loss.
LO 12.6 Discuss the various stages of grief.	**What are Elizabeth Kübler-Ross's stages of grief?**
	• Denial
	• Anger
	• Bargaining
	• Depression
	• Acceptance
	What are Roberta Temes's stages of grief?
	• Numbness
	• Disorganization
	• Reorganization

Ethics Issues Death and Dying

Ethics ISSUE 1:

An understanding of the principles that underlie biomedical ethics is important in addressing the issues that confront health care practitioners and their patients at the end of life. The ethical principles include autonomy (the patient's right to self-determination), beneficence (acting in the patient's best interest), nonmaleficence (do no harm), justice (determine what is fair and just), and fidelity (truthfulness and faithfulness).

Discussion Questions

1. Assume you are an emergency medical technician (EMT) responding to a 911 call at a grocery store. An elderly shopper has collapsed, and she is unconscious on the floor when you arrive. Her vital signs are weak. The woman is placed in the ambulance, where she arrests. You notice that the woman is wearing a bracelet that says "DNR," and a quick check of her purse reveals a signed and witnessed DNR order. What do you do?

_____

_____

2. An 80-year-old woman has suffered a massive heart attack and is on a ventilator in the hospital's ICU. She apparently has no advance directive. Her three daughters arrive from different areas of the United States and express their opinions about their mother's medical care. One daughter says her mother would "not want to be kept alive" in her present state, while a second, more aggressive daughter demands that "everything" be done to keep her mother alive. The third daughter expresses no opinion. In your opinion, what should be done?

_____

_____

Ethics ISSUE 2:

In some states, state law allows EMTs to do what is right for the patient when transporting them for care. In other states, the law may say you must obey the patient's instructions, regardless of what those instructions are.

Discussion Questions

1. As an EMT in a state where the law says you must do what is right for the patient, you are transporting a patient with chest pain, and you decide to transport her to a hospital with heart catheterization capabilities, even though the patient has expressed a desire to go to a less well-equipped hospital in the area. Legally and ethically, how will you respond?

_____

_____

2. You are an EMT in a state where state law says the patient has the last word. The patient has been injured in a car accident, and you want to take him to a hospital with a level 1 trauma center, but he says no, take him to a different hospital, without a level 1 trauma center. Legally and ethically, what will you do?

_____

_____

Ethics ISSUE 3:

As a health care practitioner, you are committed to acting in the patient's best interest, and you believe that the wishes of patients in end-of-life situations should be followed. Furthermore, professional codes of ethics generally state that the social commitment of health care practitioners is to sustain life and relieve suffering, and that when the performance of one duty conflicts with the other, the preferences of the patient should prevail.

Discussion Questions

1. As a nurse, you are assigned to help care for a middle-aged patient with a terminal, end-stage disease. He is in pain, but has asked that pain medication not be prescribed, so he can keep his mind clear. He has also expressed a fear of addiction. You know that the patient could be relieved of his pain if he would only agree to be medicated. What will you do?

   _____

   _____

2. A young mother who was severely injured in a car accident is brought into the hospital trauma center where you work. She belongs to the Jehovah's Witnesses church, and emphatically states that she refuses to have a blood transfusion. You know she risks death without a transfusion, but she believes her decision is a matter of her salvation. As a member of the patient's health care team, what will you do?

   _____

   _____

3. The female patient in the car accident scenario is unconscious, but her husband makes her wishes known regarding blood transfusions. Can you accept the husband's decision on the patient's behalf? Explain your answer.

   _____

   _____

Ethics ISSUE 4:

Health care practitioners are ethically bound to respond to the needs of the patient at the end of life, but they are also ethically bound to practice fidelity.

Discussion Question

1. When asked in a survey if they would ever withhold the truth about a terminal or pre-terminal diagnosis from a patient in order to keep his or her spirits up, physicians' responses were:

   "Most of the time, I tell them exactly as it is; they need to know the truth, and who am I to judge what they should or shouldn't know? However, if the patient is very frail emotionally and physically and has a very supportive family, I may not."

   "It's not about hiding information. It's learning how to talk to patients and giving bad news in the best way possible. All the information should be given, but any positive that exists should be also talked about."

   "The truth, delivered with compassion, is a gift."

   "I think patients deserve total honesty from their physician. They want to know."

   "An elderly patient who is senile will not understand, benefit, or prepare, so it is senseless to inform them. However, a family member, next of kin, or whoever is the health proxy will be notified."

   Which of the preceding statements most closely matches your opinion? Explain your answer.

   _____

   _____

Ethics ISSUE 5:

Your elderly aunt has asked you to take on her health care power of attorney. She makes the request while she is healthy and able to make her own decisions. You agree and sign the appropriate legal papers. She tells you at this time that she never wants "heroic measures" to be undertaken to save her life, if her quality of life would suffer.

Discussion Questions

1. Five years later, your aunt is 86 and suffering from diabetes, coronary problems, and dementia. While in a long-term care facility, your aunt suffers a severe heart attack and is transported to the local hospital's

emergency room. She is conscious when she reaches the emergency room, and when the attending physician asks her if she wants "all measures taken to preserve her life," she says yes. When you arrive at the hospital, your aunt is comatose and has been placed in the intensive care unit. Her physician says she cannot recover, but he could transport her to a larger hospital where physicians could "try" a pacemaker. How will you respond?

_____

_____

2. What ethical issues will influence your decision?

_____

_____

Chapter 12 Review

Enhance your learning by completing these exercises and more at
http://connect.mheducation.com!

Mc Graw Hill Education **connect**®

Applying Knowledge

LO 12.1

1. Before the twentieth century, death most likely occurred

   a. In a hospital

   b. In a hospice

   c. At home

   d. At work

2. Which of the following is a modern-day custom regarding death?

   a. Holding a funeral

   b. As a survivor, wearing sackcloth and ashes for several days

   c. As a survivor, wailing loudly at certain times in public places

   d. None of these

3. Which of the following is true of death in the United States in the twenty-first century?

   a. Most deaths are occurring among teenagers.

   b. Most deaths occur in hospitals.

   c. All deaths result in autopsies.

   d. Infants seldom die.

LO 12.2

4. The purpose of the Uniform Determination of Death Act was to

   a. Define guidelines for determining when death actually occurs

   b. Teach caregivers how to prepare patients for death

   c. Teach caregivers how to use technology to prolong life

   d. None of these

5. The Uniform Determination of Death Act defines _____ as a means of determining when death actually occurs.

   a. Cessation of breathing

   b. Brain death

   c. Blood pressure reading

   d. Cessation of ability to speak

6. *Coma* is best defined as

   a. A deep sleep

   b. Severe mental impairment

   c. Deep stupor from which the person cannot be roused by external stimuli

   d. Cessation of all brain function

7. Persons said to be in a *persistent vegetative state*

   a. Cannot breathe on their own

   b. Can be aroused by external stimuli

   c. Have severe brain damage

   d. Are in a deep coma

8. Technically, death results from

   a. Loss of oxygen

   b. Circulatory system collapse

   c. Coma

   d. None of these

9. Before pronouncing a nonresponsive and unconscious patient dead, physicians may perform certain tests. Which of the following is *not* a condition denoting death has occurred?

   a. Cannot breathe without assistance

   b. Cannot stand unaided

   c. Has no coughing or gagging reflex

   d. Pupils' lack of response to light

10. Recent reports indicate a decline in the number of nonmandatory autopsies performed in hospitals. Which of the following is a probable reason for the decline?

    a. Fewer patients are dying.

    b. Family members of deceased patients are often reluctant to give permission for an autopsy.

    c. No one wants to perform them.

    d. The law does not allow hospitals to perform autopsies.

11. Recent reports also indicate a continuing decline in the number of all autopsies performed in the United States. Of what value is a nonmandatory autopsy performed after a hospital patient dies?

    a. Helps determine cause of death

    b. Helps advance medical knowledge about disease

    c. Helps reassure family members of the deceased that everything possible had been done for their loved one

    d. All of these

12. Care provided to relieve pain and make a patient's last days as comfortable as possible is referred to as

    a. ICU care

    b. Palliative care

    c. Curative care

    d. Hospital care

13. The Greek term for "good death" is

    a. Palliative

    b. Thanatology

    c. Euthanasia

    d. DNR

14. If one has six months or less to live, he or she is said to be

    a. Under palliative care

    b. Eligible for curative care

    c. Terminally ill

    d. Not eligible for hospice care

15. The right to die movement is largely responsible for educating people about

    a. Advance directives

    b. Hospice care

    c. Palliative and curative care

    d. Wills

16. A document serving to appoint an individual, chosen by the patient, to represent the patient's interests is a(n)

    a. Advance directive

    b. Living will

    c. Durable power of attorney

    d. Guardian *ad litem*

17. An authorization in advance to withdraw artificial life support is

    a. Assault

    b. Battery

    c. An advance directive

    d. Uniform Anatomical Gift

18. Landmark events in the right to die movement include

    a. The *Karen Ann Quinlan* case

    b. The *Nancy Cruzan* case

    c. The *Terry Schiavo* case

    d. All of these

19. Which of the following is *not* true of the Uniform Rights of the Terminally Ill Act?

    a. Recommended by the National Conference of Commissioners on Uniform State Laws

    b. Intended to guide state legislatures in constructing laws to address advance directives

    c. Was repealed in 1994

    d. None of these

20. The Uniform Anatomical Gift Act does *not* include the provision(s) that

    a. Persons 18 and older and of sound mind may donate organs and tissues for transplantation.

    b. Donations made through a will are not to be held up in probate.

    c. Organs are not accepted from patients over 60 years of age.

    d. Except in autopsies, the donor's rights override the rights of others.

21. The Patient Self-Determination Act does *not* provide for

    a. Documenting the existence of an advance directive in the patient's medical record

    b. Nondiscrimination regarding whether or not a patient has an advance directive

    c. Compliance with state laws respecting advance directives

    d. Legal prosecution of health care practitioners who influence a patient's decision in preparing an advance directive

22. Physician-assisted suicide is legal

    a. In all 50 states

    b. Presently, only in 4 states

    c. Only when the patient agrees to be euthanized

    d. Never

23. A form of advance directive that allows hospital patients to tell health care practitioners not to revive them if breathing stops is called a

    a. Durable power of attorney

    b. Will

    c. Do-not-resuscitate order (DNR)

    d. Summons

LO 12.5

24. Which legislation paved the way for organ transplantation in the United States?

    a. Patient Self-Determination Act

    b. Uniform Rights of the Terminally Ill Act

    c. Uniform Anatomical Gift Act

    d. Death with Dignity Acts

25. Which legislation established organ procurement and transplantation networks in the United States?

    a. Uniform Rights of the Terminally Ill Act

    b. Death with Dignity Acts

    c. DNR order

    d. National Organ Transplant Act

26. Which of the following is true of organ transplants?

    a. Organ donors or their families must pay if a transplant occurs.

    b. Only individuals under the age of 55 can serve as organ or tissue donors.

    c. Prospective donors should inform family members of their wishes.

    d. Only family members can donate certain organs for transplantation.

LO 12.6

27. Which of the following best describes grief?

    a. An emotion one feels when loss has occurred

    b. The wish to die

    c. An emotion that should be denied

    d. None of these

28. Dr. Elisabeth Kübler-Ross's five stages of coping with a death or with a terminal illness do *not* include which of the following?

    a. Acceptance

    b. Bargaining

    c. Depression

    d. All of these are included

29. Which of the following is *not* true of the stages of grief?

    a. All grieving people progress through the stages in order.

    b. Grieving people may not experience one or more of the stages of grief.

    c. A person may experience the second stage of grief before the first, or the third stage before the second.

    d. A person may go back and forth among the stages until resolution is accomplished.

30. Which of the following behaviors is probably most helpful to a dying person?

    a. Ignoring the fact that the person is dying

    b. Avoiding any discussion of future events

    c. Giving the person your attention and listening well

    d. Telling jokes

Case Studies

Use your critical thinking skills to answer the questions that follow each case study.

LO 12.3

31. You are the health care practitioner assigned to speak with a deceased patient's family about permission to do an autopsy, and you find yourself feeling reluctant to do so. What reasons can you think of that might make one feel reluctant in such a situation?

_____

_____

32. How might you phrase a request to surviving family members to allow their deceased loved one's organs/tissues to be donated?

_____

_____

LO 12.3

You are a member of a hospital resource allocation committee that must decide which three out of seven critical patients will receive immediate live-saving surgery. The hospital has resources to save just three of the seven, but without surgery, all seven patients will die. The situation is further complicated by the fact that a blizzard is raging outside, and none of the patients can be transferred to another hospital. All seven are too critically ill to be moved by snowmobile.

33. Working alone or in a group, decide what criteria will be used to make the decisions (consider age, social standing, benefit to society, lifestyle, degree of physical deterioration, etc.).

_____

_____

34. Obtain a list of the seven patients from your instructor, and choose three patients to receive immediate life-saving surgery. Write your decisions, and/or discuss the rationale for your choices with the class.

_____

_____

Internet Activities LO 12.4 and LO 12.6

Complete the activities and answer the questions that follow.

35. Visit the Web site for Caring Connections at **www.caringinfo.org.** Download a living will and a health care power of attorney form, and compare the forms with those of a classmate from another state. Overall, how do the forms from another state differ from those for your state?

_____

_____

36. Visit the Hospice Patients Alliance at **www.hospicepatients.org/hospic4.html.** List three recommendations offered at the site for choosing the right hospice for a dying family member.

_____

_____

37. Visit the Web site for Healing Resources at **www.webhealing.com.** List three grief links found at the site that might help the bereaved. Why might these resources prove helpful?

_____

_____

Resources

"Before I Die"—WNET, New York: **www.wnet.org/bid/sb-medschool.html.**

Donate the Gift of Life—U.S. Department of Health and Human Services: **www.organdonor.gov/index .html.**

Intervention and end-of-life care in ICU: **www.medscape.com/viewarticle/728356.**

Konigsberg, Ruth Davis. *The Truth about Grief.* New York: Simon & Schuster, 2011.

Konigsberg's book synopsized in *Time,* January 24, 2011, pp. 42–46.

Kübler-Ross, Elisabeth. *On Death and Dying.* New York: Scribner, 1969.

Medscape 2010 Physician Ethics Study: **www.medscape.com/features/slideshow/public/ethical-dilemmas.**

National organ transplant data: **http://optn.transplant.hrsa.gov/latestData/step2.asp**

Rafinski, Karen. "Easing Pain: Palliative Care Is Not What You Think." *AARP Bulletin* (June 2011), p. 14.

States with laws preventing/accepting assisted suicide: **www.euthanasia.com/bystate.html.**

Study on end-of-life care—physicians' religion: **http://religion.blogs.cnn.com/2010/08/26/study-doctors -religious-beliefs-affect-end-of-life-care/.**

Telephone interview November 10, 2007, with Don Lundy, EMS director for Charleston County, South Carolina.

Temes, Roberta. *Solace: Finding Your Way through Grief and Learning to Live Again.* New York: Amacon Books, 2009.

U.S. Supreme Court upholds Oregon's right to die law: **http://abcnews.go.com/Politics/SupremeCourt/ story?id=1514546.**

Washington's assisted-suicide law: **www.nytimes.com/2010/03/05/us/05suicide.html.**

Worden, W. *Grief Counseling and Grief Therapy.* New York: Springer, 1982.

13

Key Terms

access
Agency for Healthcare Research and Quality (AHRQ)
cost
epigenetics
genometrics
gross domestic product (GDP)
life expectancy
life span
personalized medicine
pharmacogenomics
proteomics
quality
stakeholders

Health Care Trends and Forecasts

LEARNING OUTCOMES

After studying this chapter, you should be able to:

LO 13.1   Identify the major stakeholders in the U.S. health care system.

LO 13.2   Describe the major areas of concern to those stakeholders.

LO 13.3   Describe those trends that are likely to continue to affect patient care in the future.

LO 13.4   Discuss those broader movements that forecast the future of health care.

FROM THE PERSPECTIVE OF. . .

WHEN STEVE, a speech pathologist and gerontologist, meets with his group, they sometimes build a swimming pool—virtually, not literally. They discuss such steps in the process as: What are the pool's dimensions? How much dirt, in cubic feet, will we have to move? How much cement will we need? How many gallons of water will the pool hold? On days when they aren't building swimming pools Steve's group may be reviewing little-known countries and areas in the world, such as Uruguay, or the Ivory Coast.

Steve helps rehabilitate people recovering from head injuries who come to him as a result of on-the-job accidents, car crashes, adverse drug reactions, strokes, West Nile Virus and Legionnaire's Disease, rodeo/sports mishaps, and other occurrences that result in brain injury. A neuropsychologist evaluates the individuals and draws up individual therapy plans and goals. The therapy is intense, Steve says, and repetitive. Because the brain is "an intricate little piece of equipment, no two cases of brain injury are alike in more than one or two functional aspects." But "we generally work on cognitive skills, such as listening, learning, and memory." For example, one of Steve's people had trouble remembering the names for everyday items. When asked to name a "door," she could recall "hinge," and "knob," but not the more common "door." Until Steve asked her for directions to an office in the building and she said, "You go through this door . . . "

Steve celebrates successes with his people—no matter how small—but many times wishes doctors had referred brain-injured individuals earlier. "For too long, the general consensus has been based on a false assumption that injuries to the brain are incurable and the consequences permanent." While it is true that the site of the damaged tissue remains permanently in place, "the brain has the remarkable ability to find neural pathways around the damaged tissue and recover lost functioning." Refer brain-injured people as early as possible, Steve advises physicians, and know that "it's never too late to start therapy."

From Steve's perspective, brain-injured people should begin therapy as quickly as possible, and it's never too late to start therapy.

Too often from a physician's perspective, brain injuries cause permanent loss of function.

From an injured person's perspective, therapy may be tedious, but regaining lost function is often possible and always worth the struggle.

As you have progressed through *Law & Ethics for the Health Professions*, you have gained knowledge about legal issues affecting every health care practitioner. You have also learned that in addition to the law, ethics play a crucial role in health care decisions. This final chapter outlines major concerns all Americans have with the country's health care system, and offers a glimpse of possibilities for the future.

LO 13.1

Identify the major stakeholders in the U.S. health care system.

stakeholders

Those who have a vested interest in the health care industry in the United States, and in any efforts to reform the industry.

Whom Does the Health Care System Serve?

Those who have a vested interest in the health care industry in the United States, and in any efforts to reform the industry, are called **stakeholders.** They include, but are not limited to, the following:

1. **The public.**

   The patients who use health care services will always be at the head of the list of stakeholders. When health problems arise, everyone wants the best medical care available, conveniently delivered, at an affordable cost.

2. **Employers.**

   Since employers often provide health care benefits for employees, they hope to contract with health care providers who can deliver quality services at reasonable cost.

3. **Health care facilities and practitioners.**

   As the providers of health care services, facilities such as hospitals, skilled nursing care organizations, physicians' practices, medical and dental clinics, laboratory and radiology services, rehabilitation hospitals, and many others influence the health care system in the quality, range, and cost of services provided.

4. **Federal, state, and local governments.**

   Governments help pay the cost of health care services through Medicare, Medicaid, Federal Employees Health Benefits Program, Military Health System, Veterans Health Administration, Indian Health Service, State Children's Health Insurance Program, and other state and federal government-financed programs. For that reason, governments are near the top of the list of health care stakeholders.

5. **Managed care organizations.**

   Managed care organizations provide funds to help cover the costs of health care services for all the employees of a certain business or for other groups who have come together to buy coverage for health care at lower cost than each member of the group could get individually. As for-profit organizations, their focus is on the bottom line—helping reimburse health care providers while at the same time earning a profit.

6. **Private insurers.**

   Private insurance companies sell health care policies to individuals, agreeing to pay certain health care costs for policyholders for a fee. Fees are based on age, general state of health, preexisting medical conditions, and other factors that result in lower or higher rates, depending on each client's profile.

7. **Voluntary facilities and agencies that provide health care or influence health care policies.**

   Disaster relief agencies and nongovernmental volunteer organizations that provide health care or funds for health care are also important stakeholders in the national health care system.

8. **Health care practitioner training institutions.**

   Any training institution that prepares health care practitioners to administer health care has a huge stake in the health care system, and also influences the system proportionately according to the quality and quantity of practitioners they prepare.

9. **Professional associations and other health care industry organizations.**

   While each state's medical practice acts mandate licensing and/or certification for certain health care practitioners, professional associations and other industry organizations also establish and monitor health care practitioner ethics, and offer advice and support for members of their diverse groups.

10. **Medical, biotechnological, pharmaceutical, and other health care companies.**

    For-profit companies that develop treatments and cures for diseases and other medical conditions, which look at the business of health care to make a profit while serving the consumer, also have a vested interest in the health care system.

Cost, Access, and Quality

Key issues of concern to *stakeholders* within the American health care system are *cost, access,* and *quality.*

Cost refers to the amount individuals, employers, state and federal governments, managed care organizations, private insurers, and other stakeholders spend on health care in the United States. As explained in the section entitled "Access," the number of people who have **access** to health care services—that is, the number of people for whom the services are available and for which they as consumers can pay—also helps determine cost. In addition, the cost of health care services also directly affects the **quality,** or degree of excellence, of health care services offered.

COST

Just as preparing a budget shows you how much of your income is spent on food, housing, clothing, insurance, and so on, the total cost of health care in the United States is often expressed as a percentage of the country's gross domestic product. The **gross domestic product (GDP)** represents the total value of all goods produced and services provided in a country in one year. The percentage of the GDP represented by *total* health care spending (both government and private) was first determined in 1960, and it has been steadily increasing ever since. In 1960, health care spending accounted for slightly more than 5 percent of the GDP. In early 2014, according to figures compiled by the Organization for Economic Cooperation and Development (OECD), health care spending in the United States had risen to 17.7 percent of GDP, and health care spending per each American was still the highest of any OECD member nation, at $8,508. Figure 13-1 shows the government health care spending as a percentage of the GDP of the United States, as compared with other member nations of the Organization for Economic Cooperation and Development (OECD).

LO 13.2

Describe the major areas of concern to those stakeholders.

cost
The amount individuals, employers, state and federal governments, HMOs, and insurers spend on health care in the United States.

access
The availability of health care and the means to purchase health care services.

quality
The degree of excellence of health care services offered.

gross domestic product (GDP)
The total value of goods produced and services provided in a country during one year.

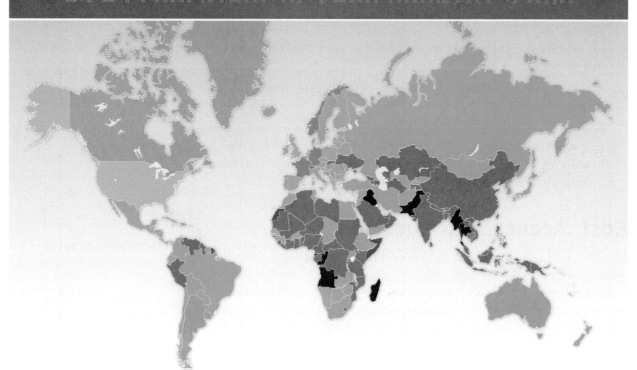

HEALTH CARE SPENDING WORLDWIDE, AS A PERCENTAGE OF EACH COUNTRY'S GDP

International Health Spending as Percentage of GDP

- Less than or equal to 3
- 3.1–5.0
- 5.1–8.0
- 8.1–10.0
- 10.1–13.0
- More than 13
- No data

In most countries, government health care spending is financed from taxes and/or Social Security contributions, with private insurance or out-of-pocket payments playing a secondary role. The government share of health care expenditure in the United States was 47.8 percent in 2012, lower than the OECD average of 72.2 percent.

Source: www.bcbs.com/blueresources/mcrg/chapter1/ch1_slide_1.html.

As shown in Figure 13-2, most federal spending goes toward defense, Social Security and health programs.

Based on past increases in health care spending—approximately 8 percent per year from 1960 to 1990—the Congressional Budget Office projected in September 2013 that health care spending as a percentage of the GDP in the U.S. could be 22 percent by 2038.

One of the major purposes of the Patient Protection and Affordable Care Act, passed in 2010, was to stem the rapidly rising cost of health

FIGURE 13-2 Where Does the Money Go?

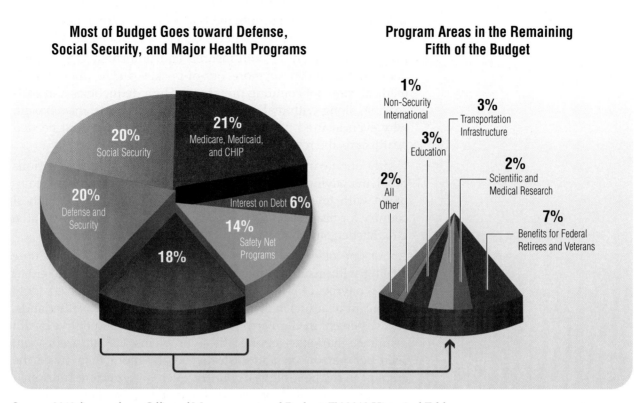

Most of Budget Goes toward Defense, Social Security, and Major Health Programs

- 21% Medicare, Medicaid, and CHIP
- 20% Social Security
- 20% Defense and Security
- 18%
- 14% Safety Net Programs
- Interest on Debt 6%

Program Areas in the Remaining Fifth of the Budget

- 1% Non-Security International
- 3% Transportation Infrastructure
- 3% Education
- 2% All Other
- 2% Scientific and Medical Research
- 7% Benefits for Federal Retirees and Veterans

Source: 2012 figures from Office of Management and Budget, FY 2012 Historical Tables.

Note: Percentages may not total 100 due to rounding.

care in the United States, and first indications were that it was helping, since reports at the end of 2013 indicated that total health care spending had increased just 4 percent during that year.

However, a 2013 study by the Pew Charitable Trusts showed that the reduction in spending for federal, state, and local governments had still not occurred at the end of 2013, due to the Affordable Care Act mandates that placed more individuals on Medicaid, Medicare, and other forms of government-subsidized health care. In 2013, in fact, state and local governments spent 31.5 percent of their budgets on health care costs, according to the Centers for Medicare and Medicaid Services and the U.S. Bureau of Economic Analysis. Since the PPACA won't be fully implemented until at least 2018, reports on its effectiveness regarding a reduction in total health care spending are not yet available.

Why should health care stakeholders be concerned about the rising share of the GDP that health care expenditures consume? Because state and federal governments bear about 50 percent of the nation's health care costs, and higher health care spending means that money remaining in the allocation pot, therefore, *can't* be spent on roads, schools, parks, defense, scientific and medical research, the environment, or other concerns.

Furthermore, aside from concerns about the high cost of health care for federal, state, and local governments, high costs mean that individual Americans can't always afford the price of health care.

According to a 2013 study by the Commonwealth Fund:

- In 2013, more than one-third (37 percent) of U.S. adults went without recommended health care, did not see a doctor when they were sick, or failed to fill prescriptions because of costs, compared with as few as 4 percent to 6 percent in the United Kingdom and Sweden.

- Roughly 40 percent of both insured and uninsured U.S. respondents spent $1,000 or more out-of-pocket during the year on medical care, not counting premiums. High deductibles and cost-sharing, along with no limits on out-of-pocket costs, may explain why even insured people in the U.S. struggled to afford needed health care, the researchers said.

- Nearly one-quarter (23 percent) of U.S. adults either had serious problems paying medical bills or were unable to pay them, compared with fewer than 13 percent of adults in the next-highest country for health care costs, France; and 6 percent or fewer in the UK, Sweden, and Norway.

- About one of three (32 percent) U.S. adults spent a lot of time dealing with insurance paperwork and disputes and were either denied payment for a claim or were paid less than expected. Only 25 percent of adults in Switzerland, 19 percent in the Netherlands, and 17 percent in Germany—all countries with competitive health insurance markets—reported these problems. U.S. insurers spent $606 per person on administrative costs, more than twice the amount in the next-highest country. Such high costs result from a complex, fragmented insurance system, the researchers write.

- The vast majority (75 percent) of U.S. adults surveyed said their health system needs to undergo fundamental changes or be rebuilt completely.

- The U.S. spends $8,508 per person on health care, nearly $3,000 more per person than Norway, the second-highest spender.

According to the Health Care Cost Institute, a research organization formed in 2011 to provide comprehensive information on health care activity and spending, increases in health care costs can be attributed to the following:

- **Medical technology.** New medical technology accounts for between 38 and 64 percent of increasing health care costs. New computer-aided diagnostic and therapeutic equipment and techniques generally cost more to acquire and use than older methods and equipment. Duplication of expensive medical equipment instead of shared use, as when nuclear imaging equipment is found in every hospital, has also been listed as adding to health care costs.

- **Administrative costs.** Health care providers must hire personnel to handle filing insurance forms and other forms of payment for service, chart patients' treatment, and otherwise keep records required to run a health care business. This expense is then passed on to consumers.

- **Widespread adoption of health information technology (HIT)** also adds to rising health care costs, since hardware, software, and personnel trained in HIT are costly.

- **Wasteful spending and fraud.** As discussed in Chapter 8, fraud and waste contribute significantly to health care costs.

U.S. Census Projection for Population Growth by Age

Growth of the Population by Age, 1900–2030

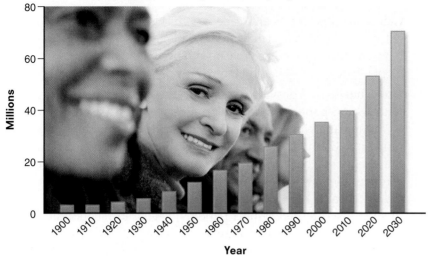

FIGURE 13-3
U.S. Census Projection for Population Growth by Age

Source: U.S. Bureau of the Census, **www.census.gov/.**

- **Unhealthy lifestyles.** Chronic diseases caused by smoking, alcoholism, drug addiction, obesity, unhealthy diets, lack of exercise, and other bad habits also add to health care costs. Researchers predict a 42 percent increase in chronic disease cases by 2023, adding $4.2 trillion in treatment costs and lost economic productivity.

- **Aging population.** Individuals age 65 and older, who use more health care services than younger individuals, will make up one-fifth of the population by 2050. Both older and younger health care consumers spend most of their health care dollars on hospital care and physician services, but health care expenses are greater for older Americans: $12,271 per person on average for people age 65 and older, versus $2,761 per person for people under age 65 (see Figure 13-3).

Other health care industry reports also list increasing hospital charges due to consolidation of hospitals, higher health care provider costs, increasing use of medical specialists, higher costs for prescription drugs, and increasing insurance provider taxes, which in turn cause increases in insurance premiums and co-pays, as contributors to increasing health care costs.

Check Your Progress

1. Who are the major stakeholders in the American health care system?
2. What three issues are of primary concern to stakeholders within the American health care system?
3. Discuss how the three factors identified in question 2 are interrelated.
4. Identify five factors that have added to health care costs.
5. Of what significance is the percentage of the gross domestic product represented by health care spending?
6. How do waste and fraud add to health care costs?

ACCESS

Access to health care means having the timely use of personal health services to achieve the best health outcomes (Institute of Medicine, 1993). There are three steps vital to attaining access to care:

1. Gain entry into the health care system. Health insurance facilitates entry into the system. Uninsured people, therefore, are less likely to have an entry into the health care system, where they can seek treatment when it is most helpful for treating or preventing major illnesses.

2. Find a health care provider who meets the needs of each patient and with whom patients can develop a relationship based on mutual communication and trust. Seeing primary care providers—doctors, nurse practitioners, physician assistants—regularly helps increase the likelihood that patients will receive appropriate care. Primary care providers who see patients over time learn about their patients' diverse health care needs, and can coordinate care (e.g., visits to specialists) to better meet patients' needs. In fact, studies have shown that patients with regular primary care providers receive higher-quality care, have better health outcomes, and maintain better health than those without such a health care provider.

3. Access health care service sites offering ongoing care. "On-going" means that patients can continue to see their chosen providers over time. It also means that patients with conditions that require more than one source of care will be able to see other providers as necessary. For example, women of childbearing age and older people tend to have more than one doctor. Specific facilities providing ongoing care include urgent care/walk-in clinics, doctor's offices, medical clinics, health center facilities, hospital outpatient clinics, health maintenance organizations/preferred provider organizations, military or other Veterans Affairs health care facilities, or some other similar source of care. (Hospital emergency rooms are excluded as sources of ongoing care.)

QUALITY

Agency for Healthcare Research and Quality (AHRQ)
The lead federal agency responsible for tracking and improving the quality, safety, efficiency, and effectiveness of health care for Americans.

The **Agency for Healthcare Research and Quality (AHRQ)** is the lead federal agency responsible for tracking and improving the quality, safety, efficiency, and effectiveness of health care for Americans.

Since 2003, the AHRQ has studied the health care industry and tracked quality of health care. The agency's findings are published in an annual report, the National Healthcare Quality Report (NHQR). The first NHQR, issued in 2003, found certain key issues to be problematic, as listed in the following text. Findings from the most recent (2012) NHQR followed three themes that emphasize the need to accelerate progress if the United States is to achieve higher quality and more equitable health care in the future.

One of the primary purposes of the Affordable Care Act, in addition to lowering costs, was to make health care more accessible to those individuals denied access due to the inability to pay. To that end, in 2013 and 2014 people who were either uninsured or underinsured gained access to either Medicaid or government-subsidized insurance policies, depending on income. Young people up to the age of 26 could remain on their parents' policies. Others gained access to insurers if they had been shut out due to preexisting conditions, since the ACA prohibited insurance companies from refusing to cover such individuals.

With more people gaining entry into the health care system, a projected shortage of primary care providers became a concern. To address this concern, another provision of the ACA, effective in 2010, offered incentives to primary care physicians, nurses, physician assistants, and nurse practitioners that included scholarship funding and education loan forgiveness for practicing in underserved areas.

Time will tell if the sweeping changes mandated in the ACA will be sufficient to lower health care costs and increase access to health care for all Americans.

The AHRQ receives reports from certain health care providers and facilities throughout the United States to determine how cost, access, and quality are faring. The latest (2012) report found that:

1. Health care quality and access are often suboptimal, especially for minority and low-income groups.

2. Overall quality is improving, access is getting worse, and disparities are not changing.

3. Urgent attention is warranted to ensure continued improvements in:

    -   Quality of diabetes care, maternal and child health care, and adverse events.

    -   Disparities in cancer care.

    -   Quality of care among states in the South.

Table 13-1, published in the AHRQ report for 2012, shows some of the important quality measures used to analyze access and quality for adult health care consumers. All quality and access measurements are also analyzed for children and for race, ethnicity, and socioeconomic status.

In Table 13-1, of the 10 quality measures that are improving at the fastest pace, 9 are CMS publicly reported measures (blue). Of the 10 quality measures that are getting worse at the fastest pace, 3 relate to diabetes (light green), 2 relate to maternal and child health (gray), and 2 relate to adverse events in health care facilities (dark green).

The AHRQR also found that quality of care within the United States differs across geographic regions:

> For overall quality of care, states in the New England (CT, MA, ME, NH, RI, VT) and West North Central (IA, KS, MN, MO, ND, NE, SD) census divisions were most often in the top quartile for quality.

> States in the South Atlantic (DC, DE, FL, GA, MD, NC, SC, VA, WV), East South Central (AL, KY, MS, TN), and West South Central (AR, LA, OK, TX) census divisions were most often in the bottom quartile.

The report emphasizes that access to health care and receiving quality health care are vital components of any health care system: "It makes a difference in people's lives when breast cancer is diagnosed early; when a patient having a heart attack gets the correct lifesaving treatment in a timely fashion; when medications are correctly administered; and when doctors listen to their patients and their families, show them respect, and answer their questions in a culturally and linguistically skilled manner. All Americans should have access to

Table 13-1 Quality Measures with the Most Rapid Pace of Improvement or Deterioration

Quality Improving	Quality Worsening
Adult surgery patients who had prophylactic antibiotics discontinued within 24 hours after surgery end time	Children ages 19–35 months who received 3 or more doses of *Haemophilus influenzae* type B vaccine
Adult surgery patients who received prophylactic antibiotics within 1 hour prior to surgical incision	Maternal deaths per 100,000 live births
Hospital patients with heart attack who received percutaneous coronary intervention within 90 minutes of arrival	Adults age 40+ with diagnosed diabetes who had their feet checked for sores or irritation in the calendar year
Hospital patients age 65+ with pneumonia who received a pneumococcal screening or vaccination	Postoperative pulmonary embolism or deep vein thrombosis per 1,000 surgical admissions, age 18+
Hospital patients age 50+ with pneumonia who received an influenza screening or vaccination	Admissions for asthma per 100,000 population, age 65+
Hospital patients with pneumonia who had blood cultures collected before antibiotics were administered	Adults age 40+ with diagnosed diabetes who received 2+ hemoglobin A1c measurements in the calendar year
Hospital patients with heart failure who were given complete written discharge instructions	Suicide deaths per 100,000 population
Hospital patients with heart failure and left ventricular systolic dysfunction who were prescribed an ACE inhibitor or ARB at discharge	Women ages 21–65 who received a Pap smear in the last 3 years
Long-stay nursing home residents who were assessed and given pneumococcal vaccination	Admissions with stage III or IV pressure ulcer per 1,000 medical and surgical admissions of length 5+ days
Patients with colon cancer who received recommended treatment: surgical resection of colon specimen that had 12+ regional lymph nodes pathologically examined	Admissions with diabetes with short-term complications per 100,000 population, age 18+

Source: National Healthcare Disparities Report, 2012, **www.ahrq.gov/research/findings/nhqrdr/nhqr12/2012nhqr.pdf.**

Note: In the above table, of the 10 quality measures that are improving at the fastest pace, 9 are CMS publicly reported measures (blue). Of the 10 quality measures that are getting worse at the fastest pace, 3 relate to diabetes (light green), 2 relate to maternal and child health (gray), and 2 relate to adverse events in health care facilities (dark green).

quality care that helps them achieve the best possible health." Read the entire report at **www.ahrq.gov.**

Life Expectancy and Life Span

Since the United States is one of the wealthiest countries in the world, and the country that spends the most per capita on health care, observers might assume that Americans also live longer and enjoy a healthier life span than citizens of other countries (see Figure 13-4). Not so. In 2013–early-2014, OECD statistics noted that Americans, with a life expectancy of 78.64 years, are 26th when compared with 33 other countries. Canadians, for example, are expected to live 80.93 years, the British 80.75 years, and the Japanese and Italians for 83 years. (**Life expectancy** refers to the number of years one can expect to live at birth, and **life span** is the number of years one actually lives.)

When compared with citizens in other developed countries, Americans weigh more, don't always see doctors when they need to, are too inactive, don't get the recommended nutrients in their diets, and, except for strokes and cancer, don't always get good treatment for many diseases. Researchers have also found that we take more legal and illegal drugs and are more likely to die in car accidents or to be murdered.

In one major measure of a country's health system—infant mortality—the U.S. ranks near the bottom, with an infant mortality

life expectancy
The number of years an individual can expect to live, calculated from his or her birth.

life span
The number of years an individual actually lives.

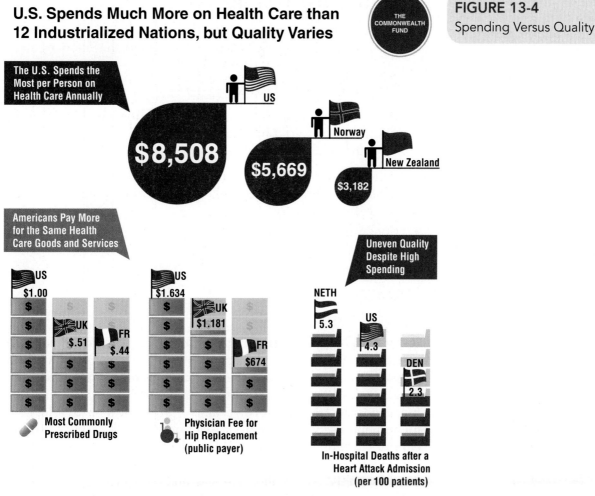

U.S. Spends Much More on Health Care than 12 Industrialized Nations, but Quality Varies

THE COMMONWEALTH FUND

FIGURE 13-4
Spending Versus Quality

The U.S. Spends the Most per Person on Health Care Annually

US
$8,508

Norway
$5,669

New Zealand
$3,182

Americans Pay More for the Same Health Care Goods and Services

US
$1.00

UK
$.51

FR
$.44

Most Commonly Prescribed Drugs

US
$1.634

UK
$1.181

FR
$674

Physician Fee for Hip Replacement (public payer)

Uneven Quality Despite High Spending

NETH
5.3

US
4.3

DEN
2.3

In-Hospital Deaths after a Heart Attack Admission (per 100 patients)

Explaining High Health Care Spending in the United States: An International Comparison of Supply, Utilization, Prices, and Quality, The Commonwealth Fund, **May 2012. http://www.commonwealthfund.org/Publications/Issue-Briefs/2012/May/ High-Health-Care-Spending.aspx.**

Note: Per capita spending figures are from the OECD.

rate of 6.1 deaths for every 1,000 live births, which is well below the OECD average of 4 deaths per 1,000. In Iceland, 1.6 babies out of every 1,000 die; and in Sweden, Japan, and Finland, the number is about 2 per 1,000.

Cost and access are most often listed as the reasons for America's too-high infant mortality rate, as well as too few resources devoted to public health and primary care, and its large percentage of uninsured individuals.

Check Your Progress

7. Check the 10 amendments to the U.S. Constitution called the Bill of Rights at **www.archives.gov/ exhibits/charters/bill_of_rights.html**. Is health care listed as a right for all Americans?

8. What are two areas of continuing concern revealed in the most current National Healthcare Quality Report (NHQR)?

9. What is the difference between life expectancy and life span?

10. In your opinion, why is the United States 26th on a list of life expectancies in various countries?

LO 13.3

Describe those trends that are likely to continue to affect patient care in the future.

Health Care Trends

Trends in health care that are emerging as medicine moves into the twenty-first century include, but are not limited to, the following areas:

MEDICAL TECHNOLOGIES

New medical technologies are a major driving force within the health care industry. Advanced medical technologies that will affect patient care over the next decade include:

- Rational drug design—use of computers to create drugs designed to attack specific diseased cells or to otherwise pinpoint delivery and enhance efficacy.
- Continuing advancement in imaging equipment and techniques.
- Genetic mapping and testing.
- Gene therapy
- Use of stem cells.
- Personalized medicine

Rational Drug Design   Rational drug design refers to the use of increasingly powerful computers to develop new drugs by looking at the molecular structure and chemical composition of target cells and creating substances that will bind to certain molecules, affecting their function inside the body. For example, drugs now in development for antiviral use will prevent viruses from using the body's protease enzymes to chop up amino acids for viruses to use as building blocks for replicating. These new antiviral drugs may be used to combat such diseases as HIV, encephalitis, measles, and influenza.

Drugs are also in development that can bind with receptors for various neurotransmitters in the nervous system, helping to reduce symptoms in patients suffering from neurological and mental diseases.

Similarly, drugs in development to combat cancer will target cancer cells for destruction, but will not destroy normal cells in the body, thus eliminating many of the noxious side effects cancer patients often suffer during chemotherapy.

Advances in Imaging   The improvement of computers is also leading to advances in imaging equipment and techniques.

Energy sources currently used for imaging include X-rays, ultrasound, electron beams, positrons, magnets, and radio frequencies. By precisely pinpointing areas of the body to be imaged and closely focusing the energy source, new imaging devices will be better able to avoid damaging normal tissue. The use of concentrated ultrasound energy to destroy kidney stones is one example of a relatively new technique now in use.

Future imaging equipment will also take advantage of the trend toward smaller, yet more powerful, computerized devices. Smaller magnetic resonance imaging (MRI) machines, for example, will soon be available for use in orthopedics, neurology, and mammography, which developers predict will not only provide clearer, more detailed images, but also lower purchasing and operating costs.

Genetic Mapping and Testing   The Human Genome Project, discussed in Chapter 11, launched an era of unprecedented interest in mapping the human genome. The project was begun in 1990 and progressed so quickly that it was ended ahead of schedule, in mid-2000. During that time, scientists identified approximately 20,000 to 25,000 genes present in human DNA. They also developed protocols for researching DNA, and passed on their acquired knowledge to other scientists.

The project's results have led to applications in **pharmacogenomics,** the science that defines how individuals are genetically programmed to respond to drugs. The results have also speeded the development of specific tests for genes causing cancers of the breast, colon, and prostate, and have added to scientists' knowledge of how genes cause the expression of certain traits in individuals—a science called **genometrics.**

Also associated with advances in genometrics is a new field of research called **epigenetics,** or the study of changes in gene activity that do not involve alterations to the genetic code, but are still passed down to at least one successive generation. The process works like this: Certain cellular materials sit above the DNA in one's genome—hence the prefix *epi-,* which means "above"—and are responsible for telling genes when to switch completely or partially on and off. Through these epigenetic markers, a parent's bad habits, such as smoking, overeating, or not following a nutritious diet, can imprint genes so that undesirable characteristics are passed on to at least one generation. That means that the genes for obesity, for example, can express themselves too strongly in your offspring, or the genes for longevity to express themselves too weakly, thus causing your bad habits to affect your children through your DNA.

Pharmacogenomic research has led to genometric drug design—the process of using a person's DNA profile to design a drug specifically for that person. This procedure is showing promise for extending the lives of cancer patients. For example, Dendreon Corporation's drug Provenge was approved for use in April 2010 for patients suffering from incurable prostate tumors. The drug is not a "one-size-fits-all" treatment but is similar to a vaccine, designed to train the immune system to fight prostate cancer cells. The drug is individually prepared using each patient's DNA profile and a protein found on most prostate cancer cells. Unfortunately, the price tag for a year's treatment with Provenge in 2010 was an astounding $93,000, and the drug does not cure the disease but may extend the life of patients an additional few months. Other cancer drugs designed for specific patients can run as much as $10,000 a month.

The future of such drugs seems promising, but cost then becomes an issue. If Medicare and private insurance plans pay for such drugs, will all enrollees share the cost in the form of higher premiums and fees? Since 85 percent of Americans earn less than $100,000 a year, will the price of such drugs limit their use and lead to rationing based on resources?

The Human Genome Project also revealed future ramifications of genetic testing, including social and ethical implications. If a health insurance company obtains a client's genetic testing results, for example, and learns that he or she is at risk to develop a genetic disease, can the company drop coverage for the client? Will reproductive rights of certain individuals be restricted if genetic testing reveals that their

pharmacogenomics
The science that defines how individuals are genetically programmed to respond to drugs.

genometrics
The science of determining how genes cause the expression of certain traits in individuals.

epigenetics
The study of changes in gene activity that do not involve alterations to the genetic code, but are still passed down to at least one successive generation.

offspring are at risk for inherited disabilities or diseases? Will prenatal genetic testing result in "designer" children for many couples? Will self-administered genetic testing kits eventually become available, bypassing valuable genetic counseling for consumers?

Gene Therapy Gene therapy, which involves correcting defective genes responsible for disease, is also on the horizon for the future. Researchers may use one of several approaches for correcting faulty genes:

- A normal gene may be inserted into a nonspecific location within the genome to replace a nonfunctional gene. This approach is most common.

- A normal gene could be substituted for an abnormal gene through an exchange of sections of chromosomes during meiosis.

- The abnormal gene could be repaired through selective reverse mutation, which returns the gene to its normal function.

- The regulation (the degree to which a gene is turned on or off) of a particular gene could be altered.

Both genetic testing and gene therapy are in evolving stages of development. Widespread utilization of the science will require practicing health care practitioners to acquire the knowledge and techniques necessary to practice genomic medicine—a field in which specialists are currently limited in number.

Utilizing gene therapy will undoubtedly also require testing in court.

Use of Stem Cells The largest barrier to using stem cells to treat disease has been political objection, on religious and ethical grounds, to the destruction of human embryos that are most useful in stem cell research.

In 2007, researchers announced that human skin and bone cells had been used to produce the stem cells that might someday be useful to patients with spinal cord injuries, Parkinson's disease, diabetes, damaged hearts, and other diseases or conditions.

LANDMARK COURT CASE *Mayo Collaborative v. Prometheus Labs*

The Mayo Clinic had been using a Prometheus Labs thiopurine drug to treat certain autoimmune diseases, such as Crohn's disease and ulcerative colitis. The method of determining dosages was patented by Prometheus Labs. When a patient ingested the compound, his body metabolized the drug, causing metabolites to form in his bloodstream which could be useful in treatment. Because the way in which people metabolize thiopurine compounds varies genetically, the same dose of a thiopurine drug affects different people differently, making it complicated for doctors to determine dosages. Mayo doctors developed their own thiopurine drug protocol, and

Prometheus Labs protested that they held the patent for administering the drug, so Mayo Clinic was in copyright violation.

The case reached the U.S. Supreme Court, where justices decided: "simply appending conventional steps, specified at a high level of generality, to laws of nature, natural phenomena, and abstract ideas cannot make those laws, phenomena, and ideas patentable." Therefore, "the patent claims at issue here effectively claim the underlying laws of nature themselves. The claims are consequently invalid."

Mayo Collaborative v. Prometheus Labs, 132 S. Ct. 1289, 566 U.S. 10, 182 L. Ed. 2d 321 (2012).

Progress in growing stem cells from tissues other than embryos has continued, and as of 2014, through a process called tissue engineering, scientists have been able to grow functioning bladders, urethras, and even heart and lung tissue from a person's own cells. Using cells taken from an individual, an organ such as a bladder is grown over a scaffold. The bladder can be transplanted into that same individual without the fear of rejection, since the recipient's own cells were used to grow the bladder. Once transplanted, the scaffold disintegrates, and the bladder adapts to its new location. To date, several individuals have received such transplants, and the laboratory-grown bladders have functioned successfully. So far, tissue-engineered hearts and lungs are still in the experimental stage.

Wake Forest University Medical Center in Winston-Salem, North Carolina, pioneered the world's first lab-grown bladder, and it remains at the forefront of the organ-growing field. Wake Forest is the world's largest regenerative medicine research center, and its current research is in growing 22 different types of tissue: heart valves, muscle cells, arteries, and even fingers. As the technique improves, it will bring new meaning to the term "personalized medicine."

Personalized Medicine   Imagine that sometime in the near future you visit your doctor for your annual physical. On your first visit, the medical facility's lab analyzed your genome, so your physician is aware that you carry genes for certain gastrointestinal disorders and for late-onset breast cancer. You have not yet developed symptoms of any disorder, but your physician orders all appropriate tests. You have lost 10 pounds since your last visit, making your weight now appropriate for your height and age, so your physician recommends that you continue with the wellness activities outlined during your first visit. Since scientists estimate that one gene can trigger the manufacture of as many as 1,000 proteins responsible for various bodily functions—both normal and abnormal—your physician also orders a protein panel. (The study of the proteins associated with one's genome is called **proteomics**.) After she completes her physical examination and all laboratory results are in, your physician prescribes a regimen of care that includes wellness recommendations and perhaps a medication tailored especially for you. This is **personalized medicine,** and it's coming to a medical facility near you.

Although still in its infancy, the concept of personalized medicine continues to grow as a trend in the United States. PricewaterhouseCoopers, a global accounting and business consulting firm, defines it as "the products and services that leverage the science of genomics and proteomics (directly or indirectly) and capitalize on the trends towards wellness and consumerism to enable tailored approaches to prevention and care."

The personalized medicine industry includes nutrition and wellness components—made up of complementary and alternative medicine, health clubs, organic care, and the medical retail establishment—and unique-to-each-patient aspects that include telemedicine, electronic and personal health records, tests to analyze DNA, and target therapeutics to help providers find the right therapy at the right time. PricewaterhouseCoopers estimates that this was a $225 billion industry in 2009.

proteomics
The study of the proteins that genes create or "express."

personalized medicine
The products and services that leverage the science of genomics and proteomics and capitalize on the trends toward wellness and consumerism to enable tailored approaches to prevention and care.

The hope with personalized medicine is that there will be better patient outcomes, not just in disease management, but in maintaining wellness and improving each patient's participation in his or her own care. Most experts believe that personalized medicine can only become reality with coordination of services and long-term business strategies consistent among all of the players.

Diabetes, Obesity, and the Future   In October 2010, the Centers for Disease Control and Prevention issued a report predicting that one in three people may develop diabetes in the next 40 years. According to the CDC, diabetes is presently the number one cause of adult blindness, kidney failure, and limb amputation and is seventh on the list of diseases that cause death in the United States. The 2012 costs for diabetes and related problems were $245 billion.

The predicted increase in diabetics is partially because people are living longer with the disease. However, there is some evidence to suggest that obesity and diabetes are related, and obesity has become epidemic in the United States. (See Figure 13-5 for trends in obesity

FIGURE 13-5 Trends in Overweight, Obesity, and Extreme Obesity

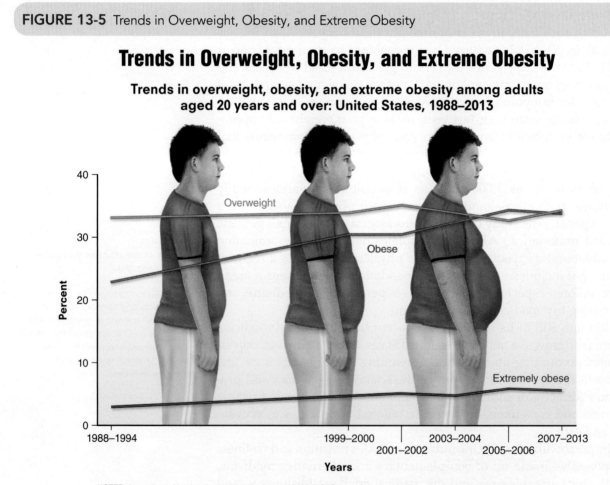

Trends in Overweight, Obesity, and Extreme Obesity

Trends in overweight, obesity, and extreme obesity among adults aged 20 years and over: United States, 1988–2013

NOTES: Age-adjusted by the direct method to the year 2000 U.S. Census Bureau estimates, using the age groups 20–39, 40–59, and 60 years and over. Pregnant females were excluded. Overweight is defined as a body mass index (BMI) of 25 or greater but less than 30; obesity is a BMI greater than or equal to 30; extreme obesity is a BMI greater than or equal to 40.

Source: CDC/NCHS, National Health and Nutrition Examination Survey III 1988–1994, 1999–2000, 2001–2002, 2003–2004, 2005–2006, and 2007–2008.

Source: Centers for Disease Control and Prevention, **www.cdc.gov/NCHS/data/hestat/obesity_adult_07_08/obesity_adult_07_08.pdf.**

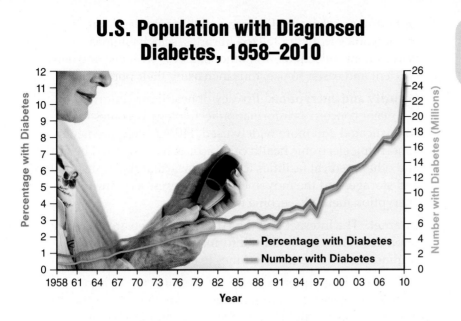

U.S. Population with Diagnosed Diabetes, 1958–2010

FIGURE 13-6
U.S. Population with Diagnosed Diabetes, 1958–2010

and Figure 13-6 for expected increase in diabetes cases.) According to a report released by the CDC in 2013, approximately 35.7 percent of adults 20-years-old and over are obese—that is, these individuals are at least 20 percent over their ideal body weight. Additionally, in 2013 approximately one-third of children and adolescents were overweight or obese. Obesity is a medical condition in which excess body fat has accumulated to the point that it has an adverse effect on health, and may shorten one's life expectancy.

HEALTH INFORMATION TECHNOLOGIES

Polls indicate that most Americans believe that their health care providers routinely use computer technology for storing and managing their medical records. Unfortunately, too often this is not the case. The health care industry has lagged behind other industries in adopting technology for performing daily business chores. For instance, many physician offices still keep reams of paper patient files, filled with hastily scrawled notes, test results, X-rays, illegible copies of prescriptions written, and other materials that are subject to fire, flood, rot, and other natural forces.

Over the next decade, advances in the following areas of communications and information technology will significantly affect the health care industry:

Computer hardware. Faster microprocessors and larger memory capabilities will make managing health care information faster and easier for HCI specialists.

Data storage. Nearly unlimited digital storage capabilities will make it possible to store a population's health care data in smaller and smaller spaces.

Wireless technology. Health care practitioners currently use handheld computers as study aids and to access digitalized patient records, and such use will increase in the future.

Networking bandwidths and data compression. Faster networking systems with larger information transmission capabilities will be the rule, increasing the use of these technologies.

Data storage retrieval. Programs that can find and retrieve information—from digitalized libraries, search engines, government collections, and other sources—will become more efficient and easier to use, thus increasing their popularity.

Security and encryption. Privacy of health care information is a major concern as information technology becomes more sophisticated and more widely used. HIPAA's requirements concerning electronic health care records have spurred hospitals and other medical facilities to move toward digital transmission and storage, and the movement will progress as security and encryption methods become more reliable.

Internet. The Internet and the World Wide Web are currently popular sources for medical information, and the trend will continue as the Internet continues to evolve.

3-D computing. Interior designers, architects, car and equipment designers, animated movie makers, and others in various design fields have access to computer programs, called computer-aided design (CAD) programs, that let them work in 3-D. In the future, CAD programs will become more readily available to health care practitioners, as a means both of visualizing medical procedures and of displaying large amounts of information at one time.

Database software. Already used extensively in business, database software will evolve into new classes that will increase the capacity to store, present, sort, and analyze data.

Sensors. Just as implanted pacemakers and insulin pumps sense when a patient's heart rate or insulin levels must be adjusted, future devices will allow health care practitioners to monitor and adjust a wider range of patient symptoms and events.

Social media. Research for the 2014 report by the IMS Institute for Healthcare Informatics showed that "the Internet is increasingly becoming the first source for general and specific health information." Seventy to 75 percent of people online regularly reported using the Internet for health information. Younger people, however, were using social media for health information more frequently and consistently than older people. (Eighty-nine percent of 18- to 29-year-olds, compared to just 43 percent of people 65 and over.) Since consumers are looking to the Internet for health care information, providers and health care product producers are also using the broader Internet and such platforms as Facebook, Twitter, and YouTube to communicate. The IMS Institute report found that physicians, on average, spend three hours per week watching online videos for professional purposes and cite Medscape and YouTube followed by pharmaceutical company Web sites as the most important sources of video.

As all of these devices and systems become less expensive, larger numbers of health care practitioners and facilities will adopt them for routine use.

Choose three of the medical technologies listed previously that are forecast to improve or otherwise change in the future, and give one specific example of how each might be applied in medical situations.

11. _____

12. _____

13. _____

Choose three of the health information technologies listed previously that are forecast to improve in the future, and give one specific example of how each might be applied in medical situations.

14. _____

15. _____

16. _____

Implications for the Future of Health Care

LO 13.4
Discuss those broader movements that forecast the future of health care.

Experts predict that the key health care issues of cost, access, and quality will continue to be of concern for Americans, and as legislation is implemented changing the health insurance industry, a new group of issues will probably emerge. The Institute for the Future, an independent, nonprofit research group based in California, studies and issues forecasts concerning certain aspects of life in the United States, including health and health care.

In 2014, the group's concerns about health and well-being were accessible online in several publications. In *Healthcare 2020* (**www .iftf.org/our-work/health-self/health-horizons/healthcare-2020/**), the following statement outlined the American health care dilemma and possibilities for the future: "One thing we all agree on, the challenges we face are daunting. At a glance, the United States seems to be the healthiest nation in the world, yet we rank low on longevity and other indicators of health. We spend more of our disposable income on medical care than food or housing, yet more than 130 million people suffer from chronic illness. And despite recent efforts by educators, public health officials, and the media to focus attention on the problem, one in five American 4-year-olds is now obese."

Responses to the nation's health care problems, the report states, should be focused on the following areas:

- **Common interests.** That is, when individuals and communities recognize that cooperation can help solve the problems of chronic disease, obesity, depression, and unhealthy nutrition, results are optimized. For example, this is happening in many communities, in the form of city-sponsored exercise and nutrition classes and wellness clinics where citizens can get blood pressure, cholesterol, and blood sugar readings at no cost.

- **Markets.** Products are tailored to help consumers make healthier choices, with lower fat and salt content and a reduction in other additives with dubious health benefits. Food labels could become easier to read and offer more helpful information, such as more realistic guides concerning calories and serving sizes.

- **Policy.** Governments respond to the nation's health problems and health care burden and address issues of equity, funding, and oversight through programs designed to improve the health of entire populations.

- **Science and technology.** Science and technology resources are used to address health and health care challenges. For example, technology allows individuals to monitor their own exercise and weight goals, and cutting-edge research leads to more effective diagnoses and treatment.

More than ever, stakeholders in the health care system need to know what to expect in the future. Reports from the experts stress the following as necessary for a health care system that works well for patients and their families, health care practitioners, health care facilities, payers, administrators, and every stakeholder named earlier in this chapter:

DATA AND CONNECTIVITY

Within the health care system, we are building electronic systems to connect health care practitioners to each other, laboratories to health care team members, suppliers to hospitals and other medical facilities, and patients to their care givers, and these systems will need to expand exponentially as health care moves into the future.

Patients in most communities are now have access to providers through patient portals to e-schedule appointments, request prescription refills, learn the results of blood tests, X-rays, and other procedures, and discuss concerns. But the vision for the future of health care is that patients will not always need to make a trip to a health care facility—sometimes over great distances or at great inconvenience—to visit a physical facility.

In fact, the day-to-day business of health care may eventually be so electronic that the inconveniences providers and patients have long wrestled with will become obsolete. No more paper records stored in boxes anywhere; no more sniffling, coughing crowds in waiting rooms during flu season; no more physically carrying reams of paper between doctors for patients seeing specialists.

This is the vision for the electronic future of health care, and further predictions can be read in the Kaiser Permanente report, "Our Vision For the Future of Health Care," at **https://xnet.kp.org/future/.**

Awareness of biological and physiological traits is driving people to forge new connections and networks through social media platforms. Sometimes the self-constructed health records posted through social media are more thorough and informative than those stored in hospitals and clinics. Furthermore, networking has allowed people with rare conditions, such as ALS, and with uncommon genetic mutations to form self-organized epidemiological and clinical trials. These individuals hope to find treatment options for their own conditions, as well as aid research in finding new treatments and cures.

PREVENTION AND POPULATION HEALTH

When health data, accessibility to the data, and connectivity are in place, tracking the health of the general population should lead to better health care results, as well as a more advanced way of practicing medicine. Instead of individual physicians relying on personal knowledge and experience to treat one patient at a time, groups of health care providers can be responsible for the care of patients with certain attributes in common, such as symptoms, genetic history for propensity for developing a disease or condition, and so on. With health care costs spiraling ever upward, patients will need to assume more responsibility for their own health, such as maintaining a healthy weight and exercise level, following healthy nutrition plans, and monitoring blood pressure or blood sugar levels.

As the Institute for the Future forecasts, "Medical care is moving from its model as a healing art provided by independent practitioners to one in which care is delivered by coordinated groups of physicians and other professionals; and is being designed, tracked, and refined through the systematic application of processes aimed at delivering consistent, efficient, and accountable results based on current scientific knowledge. Periodic encounters between patients and providers will be replaced by an ongoing relationship that includes remote monitoring of health status and virtual consultations. Rather than focus on caring for isolated individuals, providers will be responsible for optimizing the health of defined populations of patients."

PERSONALIZATION AND PARTICIPATION

Hand-in-hand with the promotion of population health is the development of personalized medicine. While the concept is not new, it is ever more in the spotlight with the availability of DNA analyses. Since each person is genetically unique, statistical averages are not always helpful in determining medical treatment. A person's genome will determine the effectiveness of medications, as well as what side effects are likely, and what drug regimens are appropriate. Regular diagnostic tests will need revision as genetic markers are considered. Since DNA analysis is presently expensive, the methods of pricing and payment will also need revision.

The personalization of health care includes, again, the participation of each individual in maintaining a healthy lifestyle and learning enough about family history and his or her unique bodily responses and characteristics to make healthy choices. As a sign in one medical clinic proclaims, "Good health is not a spectator sport."

Achieving the forementioned improvements in the health care system will also require changes in the way insurances and other payers determine payment. Instead of paying for each test, examination, or treatment performed, as is the current policy, payment will undoubtedly be based on treatment outcome. Readmission to hospitals is already a measurement of efficacy of medical treatment and a basis for payment penalties, and outcome will continue to be the determining factor for payment.

As a health care practitioner, not only is it your responsibility to offer patient-centered, thoughtful, professionally competent care, it is also your duty to stay abreast of current trends in the health care industry and to know what is forecast for the future.

Chapter Summary

Learning Outcome	Summary
LO 13.1 Identify the major stakeholders in the U.S. health care system.	Who are health care *stakeholders*?

Who are health care *stakeholders*?

- Anyone with a vested interest in the health care industry.

Who are the major stakeholders in the United States health care industry?

- The public
- Employers
- Health care facilities and practitioners.
- Federal, state, and local governments.
- Managed care organizations.
- Private insurers
- Volunteer facilities and agencies.
- Health care practitioner training institutions.
- Professional associations and other health care industry organizations.
- Medical and pharmaceutical research groups.

LO 13.2 Describe the major areas of concern to those stakeholders.

What are the key issues of concern to health care industry stakeholders?

- Cost: The amount individuals, employers, state and federal governments, HMOs, and insurers spend on health care in the United States.
  - Health care costs as a percentage of gross national product (GDP) rise yearly.
  - GDP: Total value of all goods produced and services provided in America for one year.
  - Factors adding to health care costs annually include:
    - Medical technology
    - Administrative costs
    - Widespread adoption of health information technology (HIT).
    - Wasteful spending and fraud.
    - Unhealthy lifestyles
    - Aging population
- Access: The availability of health care and the means to purchase health care services.
  - Three steps for attaining access:
    1. Gain entry into the health care system.
    2. Find a health care provider who meets the needs of each patient and with whom patients can develop a relationship based on mutual communication and trust.
    3. Access health care service sites offering ongoing care.
- Quality: The degree of excellence of health care services offered.
  - What is the Agency for Healthcare Research and Quality (AHRQ)?
    - The lead federal agency responsible for tracking and improving the quality, safety, efficiency, and effectiveness of health care for Americans.
  - Latest AHRQ report shows
    - Health care quality and access are often suboptimal, especially for minority and low-income groups.
    - Overall quality is improving, access is getting worse, and disparities are not changing.
    - Urgent attention is warranted to ensure continued improvements in:
      - Quality of diabetes care, maternal and child health care, and adverse events.
      - Disparities in cancer care.
      - Quality of care among states in the South.

Learning Outcome	Summary
LO 13.3 Describe those trends that are likely to continue to affect patient care in the future.	What health care advances have been forecast for the near future? • Rational drug design—use of computers to create drugs designed to attack specific diseased cells or to otherwise pinpoint delivery and enhance efficacy. • Continuing advancement in imaging equipment and techniques. • Genetic mapping and testing. • Gene therapy • Use of stem cells. • Personalized medicine What are three additional areas where we should see improvement/advancement in the near future? • Use of stem cells. • Tissue engineering • Health information technologies (HITs).

LO 13.4 Discuss those broader movements that forecast the future of health care.	What are those broader movements that forecast the future of health care?
	
	• Responses should be focused on:
	  • Common Interests
	  • Markets
	  • Policy
	  • Science and technology.
	• Areas for change in the future:
	  • Data and connectivity.
	  • Prevention and population health.
	  • Personalization and participation.

Ethics Issues Health Care Trends and Forecasts

As the world progresses into the twenty-first century, one aspect of health care—disaster planning—requires urgent attention. Not only does each year bring killer tornadoes, hurricanes, blizzards, floods and wildfires, the threat of spreading diseases and terrorist attacks continues to loom. Health care practitioners are on the front lines during any disaster, and the logistical and ethical concerns associated with caring for populations during these events fall heavily on their shoulders. If all assigned health care practitioners can't report for duty, who will take charge? Should triage (an assessment of which of the injured should receive treatment first) proceed as in normal times, and who will be responsible for deciding? Will nurses be expected to perform as surgeons, technicians as pharmacists, or aides as nurses?

In "Adapting Standards of Care under Extreme Conditions: Guidance for Professionals during Disasters, Pandemics, and Other Extreme Emergencies," the American Nurses Association addresses the ethics-wrought issue of planning for maintaining medical services during widespread emergencies. FEMA's National Incident Management System (NIMS) and Homeland Security's all-hazards National Response Plan provide guidelines for communities and individuals during a disaster, but the ANA's publication specifically addresses the issues health care practitioners will face during extreme emergencies. In addition, The Joint Commission offers "Revisions to Emergency Management Standards for Critical Access Hospitals, Hospitals, and Long Term Care," defining an "all-hazards" approach that will allow some flexibility in responses to disasters.

Ethics ISSUE 1:

Every health care facility should have a disaster plan and should practice implementation of the plan periodically.

Discussion Questions

1. Without having read the fore-mentioned publication, in your opinion would it be ethical, in case of a disaster, for triage personnel to recommend treating only those injured individuals who could recover?

2. If materials were sorely lacking and some health care team members had been unable to report in during a disaster, in your opinion should ethics be suspended and volunteers used to perform patient care duties?

---

3. Which patient care duties could reasonably be suspended during an extreme emergency, if materials, personnel, and perhaps even the usual medical facility were not available?

Source: For a thorough accounting of health care practitioners under stress during a disaster (Katrina), read *Five Days at Memorial: Life and Death in a Storm-Ravaged Hospital*, by Sheri Fink, Crown Publishers, New York, 2013.

Chapter 13 Review

Enhance your learning by completing these exercises and more at
http://connect.mheducation.com!

McGraw Hill Education **connect**

Applying Knowledge

LO 13.1

1. Those who have a vested interest in the American health care industry are called

   a. Employers

   b. The public

   c. Stakeholders

   d. Insurers

2. What is the term for the total value of all goods produced and services provided in America for one year?

   a. Stakeholders

   b. Gross domestic product

   c. Net income

   d. Gross income

LO 13.2

3. Three key issues of concern to everyone within the American health care industry are

   a. Cost, access, quality

   b. Cost, availability, insurance

   c. Competition, education, quality

   d. Cost, access, hospitalization

4. What is the main force expanding the federal budget?

   a. Price of oil

   b. Health care costs

   c. Foreign aid

   d. Construction industry

5.–7. List three steps vital to attaining *access* to health care.

_____

_____

_____

8. What is most often cited as the reason for being uninsured or underinsured?

a. Physicians won't accept Medicare

b. Costs

c. Advanced technology

d. Refused insurance

9. The largest purchasers of health care for most working adults are

a. Parents

b. Single individuals

c. Government and employers

d. Insurance companies

10. Which of the following is *not* a reason for the relatively high rate of infant mortality in the United States?

a. High cost

b. Restricted access to health care

c. Fewer births than other nations

d. High rate of uninsured

11. What is the name of the lead federal agency responsible for tracking and improving the quality, safety, efficiency, and effectiveness of health care for Americans?

a. AHRQ

b. HIPAA

c. PPACA

d. NHQR

12. High-quality health care in the U.S. is *not*

a. Possible

b. Expensive

c. Universal

d. Practical

LO 13.3

13. What is the term for the statistically probable number of years a newborn ought to live, based on environment, heredity, lifestyle and health practices, risk factors, and so on?

a. Lifetime

b. Life expectancy

c. Life span

d. Adulthood

14. What is the number of years an individual actually lives called?

a. Life span

b. Life expectancy

c. Adulthood

d. Childhood

15. The science that defines how individuals are genetically programmed to respond to drugs is

    a. Pharmacology

    b. Genetics

    c. Pharmacogenomics

    d. Genometrics

16. The science of determining how genes cause the expression of certain traits in individuals is

    a. Advanced genetics

    b. Pharmacology

    c. Pharmacogenomics

    d. Genometrics

17. What is the process called that involves correcting defective genes responsible for disease?

    a. Genetics

    b. Genomics

    c. Pharmacology

    d. Gene therapy

LO 13.4

18. Which of the following is *not* recommended as a future focus for health care?

    a. Policy

    b. Common interests

    c. Markets

    d. Physician training

19. Which of the following is likely for the future of health care?

    a. A focus on health of the entire population

    b. Free health care for everyone

    c. A refusal to treat anyone without insurance

    d. None of these

20. Areas within health care likely to change in the future include

    a. Personal involvement in all aspects of care

    b. The ended licensure of some practitioners

    c. Less demanding courses of study for practitioners

    d. Data and connectivity

LO 13.1 to LO 13.4

An article by Robert J. Samuelson in the December 10, 2007, issue of *Newsweek* stated, "The politics of health care rests on a mass illusion: Most Americans think that someone else pays for their care."

21. As an employee working in a job with health care benefits, who pays for your care?

_____

_____

22. Who pays for the health care of the uninsured?

_____

_____

23. As the number of people 65 and older increases, who will pay for higher Medicare spending?

_____

_____

24. In your opinion, what are the implications for future health care practitioners in the United States if health care costs continue to rise?

_____

_____

25. How can the major stakeholders in the American health care system work to improve the system?

_____

_____

26. How do increasing numbers of uninsured Americans add to health care costs?

_____

_____

Case Studies

Use your critical thinking skills to answer the questions that follow each case study.

LO 13.3

Medical tourism is a recent trend in health care. Patients go to a different country for either urgent or elective medical procedures. The procedures are the same procedures being done in U.S. hospitals and outpatient surgery centers, often by American-trained physicians who have moved back home. Medical tourism is fast becoming a worldwide, multibillion-dollar industry. In fact, some insurance companies are paying for the cost of the procedures, as costs are far less than those charged in the United States. Sometimes the insurance company even pays for the plane fare and hotel costs—so a patient gets a vacation in addition to the needed surgical procedure. The reasons patients travel for treatment vary from the lower costs (for Americans) to shorter waiting times (for those in countries where there is national health insurance). There is no regulation by the U.S. government of medical tourism. Many patients come back enthusiastic about not only the success of their treatment, and the integrity and skill of all the providers, but also the high-class hotel-like accommodations while in the foreign hospital. India is one of the major countries advertising these services.

27. If other countries are able to do similar procedures as those done in the United States for lower fees, and with the same or better outcomes, why can't the United States offer the same services?

_____

_____

_____

28. If your insurance company wanted you to go to another country for a procedure because it was less expensive, would you do it? Explain your answer.

_____

_____

_____

In 2014, American patients with recurring head and neck cancers were traveling to China to receive gene therapy via a drug designed to activate the p53 gene, which is supposed to turn off cells that multiply abnormally, but often malfunctions, letting cancerous tumors grow. Since the drug was not FDA-approved in the United States, patients traveled to China to receive it, at a cost of $20,000 for the two-month treatment. No studies had yet been conducted to determine the efficacy of the treatment, but many patients believed their tumors were receding. A genetic research company in the United States was threatening to sue the Chinese company manufacturing the drug, alleging patent infringement.

29. In your opinion, should American patients be prohibited from traveling to foreign countries to receive unproven and possibly dangerous medical treatment? Explain your answer.

_____

_____

_____

Internet Activities LO 13.2 and LO 13.3

Complete the activities and answer the questions that follow.

30. Visit **http://nhqrnet.ahrq.gov/inhqrdr/state/select** to see how well your state is doing in health care quality, as measured by the National Healthcare Quality Report. In which area does your state excel? Where does your state still lag behind?

_____

_____

31. Visit the Quantified Self at **http://quantifiedself.com/about/**. How does this site fit one of the visions for the future of health care mentioned in the text?

_____

_____

32. Visit Patients Like Me at **www.patientslikeme.com/**. What service does the site offer, and how, in your opinion, is it useful?

_____

_____

Resources

Aetna—The Facts about Rising Health Care Costs: **www.aetna.com/health-reform-connection/aetnas-vision/facts-about-costs.html**.

Agency for Healthcare Research and Quality: **www.ahrq.gov/**.

Agency for Healthcare Research and Quality data sources: **www.ahrq.gov/data/dataresources.htm**.

Agency for Healthcare Research and Quality Report for Access and Quality: **http://www.ahrq.gov/research/findings/nhqrdr/nhqr12/2012nhqr.pdf**.

American Nurses Association: **http://nursingworld.org/MainMenuCategories/WorkplaceSafety/Healthy-Work-Environment/DPR/TheLawEthicsofDisasterResponse/AdaptingStandardsofCare.pdf**.

Commonwealth Fund study 2013: **www.commonwealthfund.org/Publications/In-the-Literature/2013/Nov/Access-Affordability-and-Insurance.aspx**.

Government spending charts: **www.usgovernmentspending.com/.**

Health Care Cost Institute: **www.healthcostinstitute.org/.**

Health care spending as a percentage of GDP: **http://data.worldbank.org/indicator/SH.XPD.TOTL.ZS/.**

Institute of Medicine reports: **www.iom.edu/Reports.aspx.**

Kaiser Permanente, "Our Vision for the Future of Health Care": **http://xnet.kp.org/future.**

National Center for Health Statistics: **www.cdc.gov/nchs/.**

National Center for Policy Analysis, health care information: **www.ncpa.org/healthcare.**

National Strategy for Quality Improvement in Health Care: **www.ahrq.gov/workingforquality/nqs/nqs2013annlrpt.htm.**

Tissue engineering: **www.wakehealth.edu/Research/.**

Total spent for health care: **www.kaiseredu.org/Issue-Modules/US-Health-Care-Costs/Background-Brief.aspx.**

Glossary

A

access The availability of health care and the means to purchase health care services.

Accountable Care Organization (ACO) A health care payment and delivery model that could reward doctors and hospitals for controlling costs and improving patient outcomes by allowing them to keep a portion of what they save if standards of quality are met.

accreditation Official authorization or approval for conforming to a specified standard.

active euthanasia A conscious medical act that results in death.

administer To instill a drug into the body of a patient.

administrative law Enabling statutes enacted to define powers and procedures when an agency is created.

affirmative action Programs that use goals and quotas to provide preferential treatment for minority persons determined to have been underutilized in the past.

affirmative defenses Defenses used by defendants in medical professional liability suits that allow the accused to present factual evidence that the patient's condition was caused by some factor other than the defendant's negligence.

Agency for Healthcare Research and Quality (AHRQ) The lead federal agency responsible for tracking and improving the quality, safety, efficiency, and effectiveness of health care for Americans.

allopathic Literally, "different suffering"; referring to the medical philosophy that dictates training physicians to intervene in the disease process, through the use of drugs and surgery.

alternative dispute resolution (ADR) Settlement of civil disputes between parties using neutral mediators or arbitrators without going to court.

Amendments to the Older Americans Act A 1987 federal act that defines elder abuse, neglect, and exploitation, but does not deal with enforcement.

American Medical Association Principles A code of ethics for members of the American Medical Association written in 1847.

American Recovery and Reinvestment Act (ARRA); Also called the Recovery Act. A 2009 act that made substantive change to HIPAA's privacy and security regulations.

amniocentesis A test whereby the physician withdraws a sample of amniotic fluid (the fluid surrounding the developing fetus inside the mother's womb) from the uterus of a pregnant woman. The fluid is then tested for genetic or other conditions that may lead to abnormal development of the fetus.

artificial insemination The mechanical injection of viable semen into the vagina.

associate practice A medical management system in which two or more physicians share office space and employees but practice individually.

assumption of risk A legal defense that holds the defendant is not guilty of a negligent act, since the plaintiff knew of and accepted beforehand any risks involved.

autonomy (or self-determination) The word *autonomy* comes from the Greek words *auto* (self) and *nomos* (governance). It is generally understood as the capacity to be one's own person, to make decisions based on one's own reasons and motives, not manipulated or dictated to by external forces.

autopsy A postmortem examination to determine the cause of death or to obtain physiological evidence, as in the case of a suspicious death.

B

beneficence Refers to the acts health care practitioners perform to help people stay healthy or recover from an illness.

bioethicists Specialists who consult with physicians, researchers, and others to help them make difficult ethical decisions regarding patient care.

bioethics A DIscipline dealing with the ethical implications of biological research methods and results, especially in medicine.

brain death Final cessation of bodily activity, used to determine when death actually occurs; circulatory and respiratory functions have irreversibly ceased, and the entire brain (including the brain stem) has irreversibly ceased to function.

breach Any unauthorized acquisition, access, use, or disclosure of personal health information which compromises the security or privacy of such information.

breach of contract Failure of either party to comply with the terms of a legally valid contract.

C

case law Law established through common law and legal precedent.

categorical imperative This principle means that there are no exceptions (categorical) from the rule (imperative). The right action is one based on a determined principle, regardless of outcome.

certification A voluntary credentialing process whereby applicants who meet specific requirements may receive a certificate.

Chemical Hygiene Plan The Standard for Occupational Exposures to Hazardous Chemicals in Laboratories, which clarifies the handling of hazardous chemicals in medical laboratories.

Child Abuse Prevention and Treatment Act A federal law passed in 1974 requiring physicians to report cases of child abuse and to try to prevent future cases.

chromosome A microscopic structure found within the nucleus of a plant or animal cell that carries genes responsible for the organism's characteristics.

civil law Law that involves wrongful acts against persons.

claims-made insurance A type of liability insurance that covers the insured only for those claims made (not for any injury occurring) while the policy is in force.

Clinical Laboratory Improvement Act (CLIA) Also called Clinical Laboratory Improvement Amendments. Federal statutes passed in 1988 that established minimum quality standards for all laboratory testing.

clone An organism begun asexually, usually from a single cell of the parent.

cloning The process by which organisms are created asexually, usually from a single cell of the parent organism.

code of ethics A system of principles intended to govern behavior—here, the behavior of those entrusted with providing care to the sick.

coma A condition of deep stupor from which the patient cannot be roused by external stimuli.

common law The body of unwritten law developed in England, primarily from judicial decisions based on custom and tradition.

common sense Sound practical judgment.

comparative negligence An affirmative defense claimed by the defendant, alleging that the plaintiff contributed to the injury by a certain degree.

compassion The identification with and understanding of another's situation, feelings, and motives.

confidentiality The act of holding information in confidence, not to be released to unauthorized individuals.

Confidentiality of Alcohol and Drug Abuse, Patient Records A federal statute that protects patients with histories of substance abuse regarding the release of information about treatment.

consent Permission from a patient, either expressed or implied, for something to be done by another. For example, consent is required for a physician to examine a patient, to perform tests that aid in diagnosis, and/or to treat for a medical condition.

consequence-oriented (or teleological) theories Consequence-oriented or teleological theories judge the rightness of a decision based on the outcome or predicted outcome of the decision.

constitutional law Law that derives from federal and state constitutions.

contract A voluntary agreement between two parties in which specific promises are made for a consideration.

contributory negligence An affirmative defense that alleges that the plaintiff, through a lack of care, caused or contributed to his or her own injury.

Controlled Substances Act The federal law giving authority to the Drug Enforcement Administration to regulate the sale and use of drugs.

coroner A public official who investigates and holds inquests over those who die from unknown or violent causes; he or she may or may not be a physician, depending on state law.

corporation A body formed and authorized by law to act as a single person.

cost In this context, the amount individuals, employers, state and federal governments, HMOs, and insurers spend on health care in the United States.

courtesy The practice of good manners.

covered entity Health care providers and clearinghouses that transmit HIPAA transactions electronically, and must comply with HIPAA standards and rules.

Criminal Health Care Fraud Statute A section of the united states code that prohibits fraud against any health care benefit program.

criminal law Law that involves crimes against the state.

critical thinking The ability to think analytically, using fewer emotions and more rationality.

curative care Treatment directed toward curing a patient's disease.

D

damages Monetary awards sought by plaintiffs in lawsuits.

defendant The person or party against whom criminal or civil charges are brought in a lawsuit.

de-identify To remove all information that identifies patients from health care transactions.

denial A defense that claims innocence of the charges or that one or more of the four Ds of negligence are lacking.

deontological (or duty-oriented) theory Focuses on the essential rightness or wrongness of an act, not the consequences of the act.

deposition Sworn testimony given and recorded outside the courtroom during the pretrial phase of a case.

discrimination Prejudiced or prejudicial outlook, action, or treatment.

dispense To deliver controlled substances in some type of bottle, box, or other container to a patient.

DNA (deoxyribonucleic acid) The combination of proteins, called nucleotides, that is arranged to make up an organism's chromosomes.

doctrine of informed consent The legal basis for informed consent, usually outlined in a state's medical practice acts.

doctrine of professional discretion A principle under which a physician can exercise judgment as to whether to show patients who are being treated for mental or emotional conditions their records. Disclosure depends on whether, in the physician's judgment, such patients would be harmed by viewing the records.

do-not-resuscitate (DNR) orders Orders written at the request of patients or their authorized representatives that cardiopulmonary resuscitation not be used to sustain life in a medical crisis.

Drug Enforcement Administration (DEA) A branch of the U.S. Department of Justice that regulates the sale and use of drugs.

durable power of attorney An advance directive that confers on a designee the authority to make a variety of legal decisions on behalf of the grantor, usually including health care decisions.

duty of care The obligation of health care professionals to patients and, in some cases, nonpatients.

duty-oriented (or deontological) theory See *deontological (or duty-oriented) theory*.

E

electronic health record (EHR) Contains the same information as any medical record, but in electronic form and is a collection of all the medical records for a single patient.

Electronic medical record (EMR) Contains all patient medical records for one practice or one organization.

emancipated minors Individuals in their mid- to late teens who legally live outside their parents' or guardians' control.

emergency A type of affirmative defense in which the person who comes to the aid of a victim in an emergency is not held liable under certain circumstances.

employment-at-will A concept of employment whereby either the employer or the employee can end the employment at any time, for any reason.

encryption The scrambling or encoding of information before sending it electronically.

endorsement The process by which a license may be awarded based on individual credentials judged to meet licensing requirements in a new state.

epigenetics The study of changes in gene activity that do not involve alterations to the genetic code, but are still passed down to at least one successive generation.

ethics Standards of behavior, developed as a result of one's concept of right and wrong.

ethics committee Committee made up of individuals who are involved in a patient's care, including health care practitioners, family members, clergy, and others, with the purpose of reviewing ethical issues in difficult cases.

ethics guidelines Publications that detail a wide variety of ethical situations that professionals (in this case, health care practitioners) might face in their work and offer principles for dealing with the situations in an ethical manner.

etiquette Standards of behavior considered to be good manners among members of a profession as they function as individuals in society.

executive order A rule or regulation issued by the president of the United States that becomes law without the prior approval of Congress.

expressed contract A written or oral agreement in which all terms are explicitly stated.

F

Fair Debt Collection Practices Act (FDCPA) A federal statute prohibiting certain unfair and illegal practices by debt collectors and creditors. It prohibits certain methods of debt collection, including harassment, misrepresentation, threats, dissemination of false information about the debtor, and engagement in unfair or illegal practices in attempting to collect a debt.

Federal Anti-Kickback Law Prohibits knowingly and willfully receiving or paying anything of value to influence the referral of federal health care program business.

Federal False Claims Act A law that allows for individuals to bring civil actions on behalf of the U.S. government for false claims made to the federal government, under a provision of the law called *qui tam* (from Latin meaning "to bring an action for the king and for oneself").

federal preemption A doctrine that can bar injured consumers from suing in state court when the products that hurt them had met federal standards.

federalism The sharing of power among national, state, and local governments.

felony An offense punishable by death or by imprisonment in a state or federal prison for more than one year.

fiduciary duty A physician's obligation to his or her patient, based on trust and confidence.

firewall Hardware, software, or both designed to prevent unauthorized persons from accessing electronic information.

Food and Drug Administration (FDA) A federal agency within the Department of Health and Human Services that oversees drug quality and standardization and must approve drugs before they are released for public use.

forensics A division of medicine that incorporates law and medicine and involves medical issues or medical proof at trials having to do with malpractice, crimes, and accidents.

fraud Dishonest or deceitful practices in depriving, or attempting to deprive, another of his or her rights.

G

gene A tiny segment of DNA found on a chromosome in a cell. Each gene holds the formula for making a specific enzyme or protein.

gene therapy The insertion of a normally functioning gene into cells in which an abnormal or absent element of the gene has caused disease.

General Duty Clause A section of the Hazard Communication Standard that states that any equipment that may pose a health risk must be specified as a hazard.

genetic counselor An expert in human genetics who is qualified to counsel individuals who may have inherited genes for certain diseases or conditions.

genetic discrimination Differential treatment of individuals based on their actual or presumed genetic differences.

genetic engineering Manipulation of DNA within the cells of plants and animals, through synthesis, alteration, or repair, to ensure that certain harmful traits will be eliminated in offspring and that desirable traits will appear and be passed on.

genetics The science that accounts for natural differences and resemblances among organisms related by descent.

genome All the DNA in an organism, including its genes.

genometrics The science of determining how genes cause the expression of certain traits in individuals.

Good Samaritan acts State laws protecting physicians and sometimes other health care practitioners and laypersons from charges of negligence or abandonment if they stop to help the victim of an accident or other emergency.

gross domestic product (GDP) America's total value for all goods and services produced.

group practice A medical management system in which a group of three or more licensed physicians share their collective income, expenses, facilities, equipment, records, and personnel.

H

Hazard Communication Standard (HCS) An OSHA standard intended to increase health care practitioners' awareness of risks, to improve work practices and appropriate use of personal protective equipment, and to reduce injuries and illnesses in the workplace.

Health Care and Education Reconciliation Act (HCERA) Enacted in 2010, a federal law that added to regulations imposed on the insurance industry by the Patient Protection and Affordable Care Act.

health care practitioners Those who are trained to administer medical or health care to patients.

health care proxy A durable power of attorney issued for purposes of health care decisions only.

Health Care Quality Improvement Act (HCQIA) of 1986 A federal statute passed to improve the quality of medical care nationwide. One provision established the National Practitioner Data Bank.

health information technology (HIT) The application of information processing, involving both computer hardware and software, that deals with the storage, retrieval, sharing, and use of health care information, data, and knowledge for communication and decision making.

Health Information Technology for Economic and Clinical Health Act (HITECH) A section of the American Recovery and Reinvestment Act (ARRA) that strengthened certain HIPAA privacy and security provisions.

Health Insurance Portability and Accountability Act (HIPAA) of 1996 A federal law passed in 1996 to protect privacy and other health care rights for patients. The act helps workers keep continuous health insurance coverage for themselves and their dependents when they change jobs, and protects confidential medical information from unauthorized disclosure and/or use. It was also intended to help curb the rising cost of health care fraud and abuse.

health maintenance organization (HMO) A health plan that combines coverage of health care costs and delivery of health care for a prepaid premium.

heredity The process by which organisms pass on genetic traits to their offspring.

heterologous artificial insemination The process in which donor sperm is mechanically injected into a woman's vagina to fertilize her eggs.

Hippocratic oath A pledge for physicians, developed by the Greek physician Hippocrates circa 400 B.C.E.

homologous artificial insemination The process in which a husband's sperm is mechanically injected into his wife's vagina to fertilize her eggs.

hospice A facility or program (often carried out in a patient's home) in which teams of health care practitioners and volunteers provide a continuing environment that focuses on the emotional and psychological needs of the dying patient.

Human Genome Project A scientific project funded by the U.S. government, begun in 1990 and successfully completed in 2000, for the purpose of mapping all of a human's genes. This Web site is an excellent resource: **www.ornl.gov/sci/techresources/Human_Genome/home.shtml.**

I

implied contract An unwritten and unspoken agreement whose terms result from the actions of the parties involved.

implied limited contract A contract created when a physician or other health care worker treats a patient in an emergency situation. The agreement does not extend to the relationship after the emergency ends.

individual (or independent) practice association (IPA) A type of HMO that contracts with groups of physicians who practice in their own offices and receive a per-member payment (capitation) from participating HMOs to provide a full range of health services for HMO members.

infertility The failure to conceive for a period of 12 months or longer due to a deviation from or interruption of the normal structure or function of any reproductive part, organ, or system.

intentional tort See *tort.*

interrogatory A written set of questions requiring written answers from a plaintiff or defendant under oath.

in vitro fertilization (IVF) Fertilization that takes place outside a woman's body, literally, "in glass," as in a test tube.

involuntary euthanasia The act of ending a terminal patient's life by medical means without his or her permission.

J

jurisdiction The power and authority given to a court to hear a case and to make a judgment.

just cause An employer's legal reason for firing an employee.

justice What is due an individual.

L

law Rule of conduct or action prescribed or formally recognized as binding or enforced by a controlling authority.

law of agency The law that governs the relationship between a principal and his or her agent.

legal precedents Decisions made by judges in the various courts that become rule of law and apply to future cases, even though they were not enacted by legislation.

liability insurance Contract coverage for potential damages incurred as a result of a negligent act.

liable Legally responsible or obligated.

libel Expressing through publication in print, writing, pictures, or signed statements that injure the reputation of another.

licensure A mandatory credentialing process established by law, usually at the state level, that grants the right to practice certain skills and endeavors.

life expectancy The number of years an individual can expect to live, calculated from his or her birth.

life span The number of years an individual actually lives.

limited data set Protected health information from which certain specified, direct identifiers of individuals have been removed.

litigious Prone to engage in lawsuits.

living will An advance directive that specifies an individual's end-of-life wishes.

M

malfeasance The performance of a totally wrongful and unlawful act.

managed care A system in which financing, administration, and delivery of health care are combined to provide medical services to subscribers for a prepaid fee.

mature minors Individual in their mid- to late teens, who, for health care purposes, are considered mature enough to comprehend a physician's recommendations and give informed consent.

medical boards Bodies established by the authority of each state's medical practice acts for the purpose of protecting the health, safety, and welfare of health care consumers through proper licensing and regulation of physicians and other health care practitioners.

medical ethicists Specialists who consult with physicians, researchers, and others to help them make difficult ethical decisions regarding patient care.

medical examiner A physician who investigates suspicious or unexplained deaths.

medical practice acts State laws written for the express purpose of governing the practice of medicine.

medical record A collection of data recorded when a patient seeks medical treatment.

Medical Waste Tracking Act The federal law that authorizes OSHA to inspect hazardous medical wastes and to cite offices for unsafe or unhealthy practices regarding these wastes.

mentally incompetent Unable to fully understand all the terms and conditions of a transaction, and therefore unable to enter into a legal contract.

minor Anyone under the age of majority: 18 years in most states, 21 years in some jurisdictions.

misdemeanor A crime punishable by fine or by imprisonment in a facility other than a prison for less than one year.

misfeasance The performance of a lawful act in an illegal or improper manner.

moral values One's personal concept of right and wrong, formed through the influence of the family, culture, and society.

multipotent stem cells Stem cells that can become a limited number of types of tissues and cells in the body.

mutation A permanent change in DNA.

mutual assent An understanding and consent to the terms of an agreement by both parties for the contract to be legally valid.

N

National Childhood Vaccine Injury Act A federal law passed in 1986 that created a no-fault compensation program for citizens injured or killed by vaccines, as an alternative to suing vaccine manufacturers and providers.

National Organ Transplant Act Passed in 1984, a statute that provides grants to qualified organ procurement organizations and established an Organ Procurement and Transplantation Network (OPTN).

National Practitioner Data Bank (NPDB) A repository of information about health care practitioners, established by the Health Care Quality Improvement Act of 1986.

National Vaccine Injury Compensation Program (VICP) A no-fault federal system of compensation for individuals or families of individuals injured by childhood vaccinations.

needs-based motivation Human behavior is based on specific human needs that must often be met in a specific order. Abraham Maslow is the best-known psychologist for this theory.

negligence An unintentional tort alleged when one may have performed or failed to perform an act that a reasonable person would not or would have done in similar circumstances.

nonfeasance The failure to act when one should.

nonmaleficence As paraphrased from the Hippocratic oath, means the duty to "do no harm."

O

Occupational Exposure to Bloodborne Pathogen Standard An OSHA regulation designed to protect health care workers from the risk of exposure to bloodborne pathogens.

Occupational Safety and Health Administration (OSHA) Established by the Occupational Safety and Health Act, the organization that is charged with writing and enforcing compulsory standards for health and safety in the workplace.

occurrence insurance A type of liability insurance that covers the insured for any claims arising from an incident that occurred, or is alleged to have occurred, during the time the policy is in force, regardless of when the claim is made.

open access plan A managed care feature whereby subscribers may see any in-network health care provider without a referral.

P

palliative care Treatment of a terminally ill patient's symptoms to make dying more comfortable; also called comfort care.

parens patriae A legal doctrine that gives the state the authority to act in a child's best interest.

partnership A form of medical practice management system whereby two or more parties practice together under a written agreement specifying the rights, obligations, and responsibilities of each partner.

passive euthanasia The act of allowing a patient to die naturally, without medical interference.

patient portal A secure online Web site that gives patients 24-hour availability to health care providers.

Patient Protection and Affordable Care Act (PPACA) A federal law enacted in 2010, to expand health insurance coverage and otherwise regulate the health insurance industry. Many provisions of the law were scheduled to take effect in 2014 and 2015.

Patient Self-Determination Act A federal law passed in 1990 that requires hospitals and other health care providers to provide written information to patients regarding their rights under state law to make medical decisions and execute advance directives.

permissions Reasons under HIPAA for disclosing patient information.

persistent vegetative state (PVS) Severe mental impairment characterized by irreversible cessation of the higher functions of the brain, most often caused by damage to the cerebral cortex.

personalized medicine The products and services that leverage the science of genomics and proteomics and capitalize on the trends toward wellness and consumerism to enable tailored approaches to prevention and care.

pharmacogenomics The science that defines how individuals are genetically programmed to respond to drugs.

physician-hospital organization (PHO) A health care plan in which physicians join with hospitals to provide a medical care delivery system and then contract for insurance with a commercial carrier or an HMO.

plaintiff The person bringing charges in a lawsuit.

pluripotent stem cells Stem cells that can become almost all types of tissues and cells in the body.

point-of-service (POS) plan A health care plan that allows members to seek health care from nonnetwork physicians but pays the highest benefits for care when it is given by the primary care physician (PCP) or via a referral from the PCP.

precedent Decisions made by judges in the various courts that become rule of law and apply to future cases, even though they were not enacted by a legislature; also known as case law.

preferred provider organization (PPO) A network of independent physicians, hospitals, and other health care providers who contract with an insurance carrier to provide medical care at a discount rate to patients who are part of the insurer's plan. Also called preferred provider association (PPA).

prescribe To issue a medical prescription for a patient.

primary care physician (PCP) The physician responsible for directing all of a patient's medical care and determining whether the patient should be referred for specialty care.

principle of utility Requires that the rule used to make a decision bring about positive results when generalized to a wide variety of situations.

prior acts insurance coverage A supplement to a claims-made policy that can be purchased when health care practitioners change insurance carriers.

privacy Freedom from unauthorized intrusion.

privileged communication Information held confidential within a protected relationship.

procedural law Law that defines the rules used to enforce substantive law.

prosecution The government as plaintiff in a criminal case.

protected health information (PHI) Information that contains one or more patient identifiers.

proteomics The study of the proteins that genes create or "express."

protocol A code prescribing correct behavior in a specific situation, such as a situation arising in a medical office.

public policy The common law concept of wrongful discharge when an employee has acted for the "common good."

Q

quality The degree of excellence of health care services offered.

quality assurance See *quality improvement (QI).*

quality improvement (QI) A program of measures taken by health care providers and practitioners to uphold the quality of patient care. Also called quality assurance.

R

reasonable person standard That standard of behavior that judges a person's actions in a situation according to what a reasonable person would or would not do under similar circumstances.

reciprocity The process by which a professional license obtained in one state may be accepted as valid in other states by prior agreement without reexamination.

registration A credentialing procedure whereby one's name is listed on a register as having paid a fee and/or met certain criteria within a profession.

release of tortfeasor A technical defense to a lawsuit that prohibits a lawsuit against the person who caused an injury (the tortfeasor) if he or she was expressly released from further liability in the settlement of a suit.

res ipsa loquitur Literally, "the thing speaks for itself"; a situation that is so obviously negligent that no expert witnesses need be called. Also known as the doctrine of common knowledge.

res judicata Literally, "the thing has been decided"; legal principle that a claim cannot be retried between the same parties if it has already been legally resolved.

respondeat superior Literally, "let the master answer." A doctrine under which an employer is legally liable for the acts of his or her employees, if such acts were performed within the scope of the employees' duties.

revocation The cancellation of a professional license.

right-to-know laws State laws that allow employees access to information about toxic or hazardous substances, employer duties, employee rights, and other workplace health and safety issues.

risk management The taking of steps to minimize danger, hazard, and liability.

role fidelity All health care practitioners have a specific scope of practice, for which they are licensed, certified, or registered, and from which the law says they may not deviate.

rule A document that includes the HIPAA standards or requirements.

S

safe haven laws State laws that allow mothers to abandon newborns to designated safe facilities without penalty.

security The use of policies and procedures to protect electronic information from unauthorized access.

self-determination (or autonomy) See *autonomy.*

self-insurance coverage An insurance coverage option whereby insured subscribers contribute to a trust fund to be used in paying potential damage awards.

Smallpox Emergency Personnel Protection Act (SEPPA) A no-fault program to provide benefits and/or compensation to certain individuals, including health care workers and emergency responders, who are injured as the result of the administration of smallpox countermeasures, including the smallpox vaccine.

sole proprietorship A form of medical practice management in which a physician practices alone, assuming all benefits and liabilities for the business.

stakeholders Those who have a vested interest in the health care industry in the United States, and in any efforts to reform the industry.

standard A general requirement under HIPAA.

standard of care The level of performance expected of a health care worker in carrying out his or her professional duties.

Stark Law Prohibits physicians or their family members who own health care facilities from referring patients to those entities if the federal government, under Medicare or Medicaid, will pay for treatment.

state preemption If a state's privacy laws are stricter than HIPAA privacy standards, state laws take precedence.

statute of frauds State legislation governing written contracts.

statute of limitations That period of time established by state law during which a lawsuit may be filed.

statutory law Law passed by the U.S. Congress or state legislatures.

stem cells Cells that have the potential to become any type of body cell.

subpoena A legal document requiring the recipient to appear as a witness in court or to give a deposition.

subpoena duces tecum A legal document requiring the recipient to bring certain written records to court to be used as evidence in a lawsuit.

substantive law The statutory or written law that defines and regulates legal rights and obligations.

summary judgment A decision made by a court in a lawsuit in response to a motion that pleads there is no basis for a trial.

summons A written notification issued by the clerk of the court and delivered with a copy of the complaint to the defendant in a lawsuit, directing him or her to respond to the charges brought in a court of law.

surety bond A type of insurance that allows employers, if covered, to collect up to the specified amount of the bond if an employee embezzles or otherwise absconds with business funds.

surrogate mother A woman who becomes pregnant, usually by artificial insemination or surgical implantation of a fertilized egg, and bears a child for another woman.

T

tail coverage An insurance coverage option available for health care practitioners: When a claims-made policy is discontinued, it extends coverage for malpractice claims alleged to have occurred during those dates that claims-made coverage was in effect.

technical defenses Defenses used in a lawsuit that are based on legal technicalities.

telemedicine Remote consultation by patients with physicians or other health professionals via telephone, closed-circuit television, or the Internet.

teleological (or consequence-oriented) theories See *consequence-oriented (or teleological) theories.*

terminally ill Referring to patients who are expected to die within six months.

tertiary care settings Those care settings providing highly specialized services.

testimony Statements sworn to under oath by witnesses testifying in court and giving depositions.

thanatology The study of death and of the psychological methods of coping with it.

third-party payer contract A written agreement signed by a party other than the patient who promises to pay the patient's bill.

tort A civil wrong committed against a person or property, excluding breach of contract.

tortfeasor The person guilty of committing a tort.

U

Unborn Victims of Violence Act Also called Laci and Conner's Act, a federal law passed in 2004 that provides for the prosecution of anyone who causes injury to or the death of a fetus in utero.

Uniform Anatomical Gift Act A national statute allowing individuals to donate their bodies or body parts, after death, for use in transplant surgery, tissue banks, or medical research or education.

Uniform Determination of Death Act A proposal that established uniform guidelines for determining when death has occurred.

Uniform Rights of the Terminally Ill Act A 1989 recommendation of the National Conference of Commissioners on Uniform State Laws that all states construct laws to address advance directives.

United Nations Globally Harmonized System of Classification and Labeling of Chemicals Led to a 2012 revision of the Hazard Communication Standard, in order to transform "right to know" to "right to understand," in line with GHS.

utilitarianism A person makes value decisions based on results or a rule that will produce the greatest balance of good over evil, everyone considered.

V

veracity Truth telling.

virtue ethics Focuses on the traits, characteristics, and virtues that a moral person should have.

vital statistics Numbers collected for the population of live births, deaths, fetal deaths, marriages, divorces, induced terminations of pregnancy, and any change in civil status that occurs during an individual's lifetime.

void Without legal force or effect.

voidable Able to be set aside or to be revalidated at a later date.

voluntary euthanasia The act of ending a patient's life by medical means with his or her permission.

W

workers' compensation A form of insurance established by federal and state statutes that provides reimbursement for workers who are injured on the job.

wrongful death statutes State statutes that allow a person's beneficiaries to collect for loss to the estate of the deceased for future earnings when a death is judged to have been due to negligence.

wrongful discharge A concept established by precedent that says an employer risks litigation if he or she does not have just cause for firing an employee.

Photo Credits

Chapter 1

Opener: © Stockbyte/Getty RF.

Chapter 2

Opener: © Tim Robberts/Getty Images. **2.1a** (*bottom left*): © BananaStock/age fotostock RF. **2.1b** (*bottom right*): © Plush Studios/BrandX/JupiterImages RF. **2.1c** (*top right*): © Stockbyte/Getty RF. **2.1d** (*top left*): © Mark Scott/Getty RF.

Chapter 3

Opener: © Blend Images/ArielSkelley/Getty Images.

Chapter 4

Opener: © Ryan McGinnis/Getty RF. **4.2:** © Royalty-Free/Corbis. **4.3:** © Michael Grimm/Getty Images.

Chapter 5

Opener: © Fuse/Getty RF.

Chapter 6

Opener: © Martin Poole/Getty.

Chapter 7

Opener: © Chris Ryan/OJO Images/Getty RF.

Chapter 8

Opener: © Image Source/JupiterImages RF.

Chapter 9

Opener: © Janis Christie/Getty RF.

Chapter 10

Opener: © Stephen Marks/Getty Images.

Chapter 11

Opener: © Stephen Marks/Getty Images.

Chapter 12

Opener: © David Sacks/Getty.

Chapter 13

Opener: © Javier Pierini/Getty RF. **13.3:** © Glow Images/Getty RF. **13.6:** © Royalty-Free/Corbis.

Index

Note: Page numbers followed by f indicate figures; those followed by t indicate tables.

Motivation, needs-based, 33
Motivation and Personality
(Maslow), 32
Mucopolysaccharidosis (MPS), 297t
Multipotent stem cells, 304
Munoz v. Clark, 129
Mutations, 297–298
National Board of Medical Examiners
(NBME), 55
National Board of Osteopathic Medical Examiners, 56
National Childhood Vaccine Injury
Act of 1986, 243–246, 244f,
245t, 247
National Committee for Quality
Assurance (NCQA), 54–55, 66
National Coordinator for Health
Information Technology, 190
National Family Caregiver Support
Program, 249
National Organ Transplant Act, 337
National Practitioner Data Bank
(NPDB), 70
National Vaccine Injury Compensation program (VICP), 244, 245t
Native Americans, adoption and, 308
NBME Diplomates, 55
Needlestick Safety and Prevention
Act, 274
Needs, Maslow's hierarchy of, 32f,
32–33
Needs-based motivation, 33
Negligence, 92, 94, 127–135
Chafee v. Seslar (physician sued for
negligence), 93
comparative, 159
contributory. *See* Contributory
negligence
damage awards and medical
malpractice insurance and,
133–134, 134t
Dempsey v. Pease, Mercy Health Services, St. Joseph Mercy Hospital
(breach of contract also charged
in medical negligence suit), 97
"four Ds" of, 130
The Joint Commission and, 130–131
Longnecker v. Loyola University Medical Center (Chicago hospital's
negligence clarified by Illinois
Appellate Court), 93
Munoz v. Clark (physician tried for
negligence), 129
911 operators sued (*Estate of
Turner v. Nichols*), 6
Pearson and Fahy v. Kancilla (chiropractor's outrageous conduct
results in trial), 93
res ipsa loquitur and, 131–133
Webb v. Smith (no expert testimony
needed), 133
wrongful death statutes and,
134–135
Networking bandwidths, advances
in, 373

Neurofibromatosis, 297t
New York Medical College, 329
Newborn, rights of, 309
Newborn screening tests, 296
Diagnostic genetic testing, 296
Ninth Amendment, 206
No expert testimony needed (*Webb v.
Smith*), 133
Nominal damages, 134t
Non-English speakers, inability to
give informed consent and, 186
Nonfeasance, 129–130
Nonmalficence, 40
"Nose" coverage, 166
Not guilty of breach of confidentiality
(*Cruz v. Angelides*), 182
Nuisance, 92t
Numbness, grieving and, 342
Nurse sues employer after fall at work
(*Mosseau v. Davita, Inc.*), 122
Obama, Barack, 190, 271, 303
Obesity, 372f, 372–373
Occupational Exposure to Bloodborne
Pathogen Standard, 274–275
Occupational Safety and Health Act
of 1970, 271, 272
Occupational Safety and Health
Administration (OSHA),
272–274
Occurrence insurance, 165
Office of Civil Rights (OCR), 216
Office of Inspector General (OIG),
fraud and abuse and, 218, 218t
Officers of the court, 94–95
Online education, 71
Open access plans, 65
Opening statements, 137
*OPIS Management Resources LLC v.
Secretary Florida Agency for
Health Care Administration,* 208
Organ Donation and Recovery
Improvement Act, 338
Organ donor directives, 338
Organ Procurement and Transplantation Network (OPTN), 337
Organ procurement organizations
(OPOs), 337
Organ transplantation, 337–340
frequently asked questions about,
339–340
National Organ Transplant Act
and, 337
organ donor directives and,
338, 338f
Uniform Anatomical Gift Act and,
338–339
Osteopaths, 56
O'Sullivan v. Mallon, 267
Pachowitz v. Ledoux, 212
Palliative care, 326–327
Parens patriae, 308–309
Parkinson's disease, stem cell research
and, 303
Partnership, 62
Passive euthanasia, 332

Paternalism, 39, 43
Patient(s). *See* Health care
consumers
Patient can contribute to negligence
(*Margaret Lyons as the administratrix of the estate of Kenneth
Cook, deceased v. Walker Regional
Medical Center, Inc. and Laurie
Hunter*), 160
"Patient Care Partnership: Understanding Expectations, Rights and
Responsibilities" (AHA), 104
Patient education, informed consent
and, 186
Patient portals, 71
Patient Protection and Affordable
Care Act (PPACA) of 2010,
67t–68t, 67–69
cost containment and, 208t,
360–361
on genetic discrimination, 299
patient rights under, 222–223
Patient Safety and Quality Improvement Act (PSQIA), 208t
Patient Self-Determination Act, 334
Patient sues over drug labeling issue
(*Wyeth v. Levine*), 8
Patient-Centered Medical Home
(PCMH), 66
Patients' Bill of Rights (AHA), 104,
222t, 222–224, 223t
Pearson and Fahy v. Kancilla, 93
People skills, 17
People v. Dr. Kevorkian, 39
People v. Lage, 251
Percival, Thomas, 12
Percival's Medical Ethics (Percival), 12
Permissions, disclosure of protected
health information and, 210
Persistent vegetative state (PVS), 325
Personalized medicine, 371–372,
377–378
Peterson, Conner, 249
Peterson, Laci, 249
Pharmaceutical companies, as health
care system stakeholders, 358
Pharmacogenomics, 369
Phenylketonuria (PKU), 297t
Photocopiers, confidentiality and, 193
Photographs, of patients, 178
Physician(s)
education of, 55–56, 71
guidelines for preventing liability
suits and, 151, 153–154
liability of, 121–122, 123–125
licensing of, 57f, 57–58
online education for, 71
primary care (gatekeeper), 65
rights and responsibilities of,
102–104
transfer between, release of information for, 182
Physician charged in assisted suicide
case (*People v. Dr. Kevorkian*),
court cases, 39